Therapeutic Measurement and Testing

THE BASICS OF ROM, MMT, POSTURE, AND GAIT ANALYSIS

Lisa Jennings Weaver and Amanda L. Ferg

Therapeutic Measurement and Testing

THE BASICS OF ROM, MMT, POSTURE, AND GAIT ANALYSIS

Lisa Jennings Weaver, PTA, CMT Northeast Wisconsin Technical College
Amanda L. Ferg, PTA

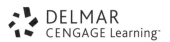

DELMAR
CENGAGE Learning

Australia • Brazil • Japan • Korea • Mexico • Singapore • Spain • United Kingdom • United States

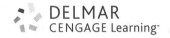

**Therapeutic Measurement and Testing:
The Basics of ROM, MMT, Posture, and
Gait Analysis**

Vice President, Career and Professional
  Editorial: Dave Garza

Director of Learning Solutions:
  Matthew Kane

Senior Acquisitions Editor: Sherry Dickinson

Managing Editor: Marah Bellgarde

Product Manager: Laura J. Wood

Editorial Assistant: Anthony R. Souza

Vice President, Career and Professional
  Marketing: Jennifer McAvey

Executive Marketing Manager:
  Wendy E. Mapstone

Senior Marketing Manager: Nancy Bradshaw

Marketing Coordinator: Scott A. Chrysler

Production Director: Carolyn Miller

Production Manager: Andrew Crouth

Senior Content Project Manager:
  Stacey Lamodi

Senior Art Director: David Arsenault

Technology Project Manager: Christopher
  Catalina

For product information and technology assistance, contact us at
Cengage Learning Customer & Sales Support, 1-800-354-9706

For permission to use material from this text or product,
submit all requests online at **www.cengage.com/permissions**.
Further permissions questions can be e-mailed to
permissionrequest@cengage.com

Library of Congress Control Number: 2008937969

ISBN-13: 978-1-4180-8080-8
ISBN-10: 1-4180-8080-2

Delmar
5 Maxwell Drive
Clifton Park, NY 12065-2919
USA

Cengage Learning is a leading provider of customized learning solutions
with office locations around the globe, including Singapore, the United
Kingdom, Australia, Mexico, Brazil and Japan. Locate your local office at:
international.cengage.com/region

Cengage Learning products are represented in Canada by Nelson
Education, Ltd.

To learn more about Delmar, visit **www.cengage.com/delmar**
Purchase any of our products at your local college store or at our
preferred online store **www.ichapters.com**

Notice to the Reader

Publisher does not warrant or guarantee any of the products described herein or perform any independent analysis in connection with
any of the product information contained herein. Publisher does not assume, and expressly disclaims, any obligation to obtain and
include information other than that provided to it by the manufacturer. The reader is expressly warned to consider and adopt all safety
precautions that might be indicated by the activities described herein and to avoid all potential hazards. By following the instructions
contained herein, the reader willingly assumes all risks in connection with such instructions. The publisher makes no representations
or warranties of any kind, including but not limited to, the warranties of fitness for particular purpose or merchantability, nor are any
such representations implied with respect to the material set forth herein, and the publisher takes no responsibility with respect to such
material. The publisher shall not be liable for any special, consequential, or exemplary damages resulting, in whole or part, from the
readers' use of, or reliance upon, this material.

Printed in the United States of America
2 3 4 5 6 7   17 16 15 14

CONTENTS

CHAPTER **3**   THE KNEE 69

CHAPTER **4** THE ANKLE AND FOOT 91

CHAPTER **7** THE ELBOW AND FOREARM 203

CHAPTER 11   POSTURE............................375

CHAPTER 12   GAIT 391

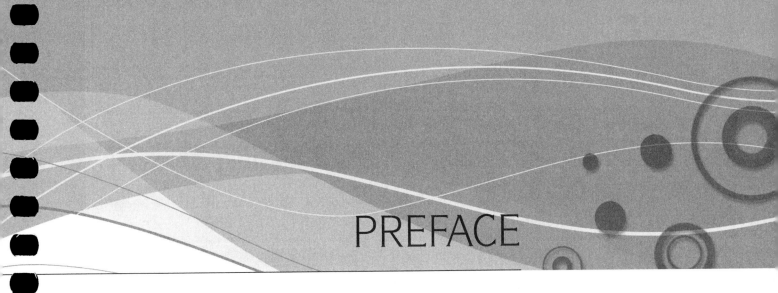

PREFACE

Therapeutic Measurement and Testing is a worktext designed to accompany assessment and kinesiology coursework in PTA and OTA programs. It provides an excellent foundation for beginning students to learn and master proper positioning, assessment, and measurement techniques and grading outcomes of the variety of patient situations encountered in the PTA and OTA settings. It is suggested that students keep this worktext after their coursework is complete for use as a clinical reference.

Conceptual Approach: What Is a Worktext?

Organized by body part, joint, and muscle, this worktext provides all assessment and measurement tools in an easy-to-use and consistent manner. A worktext is designed to provide an interactive learning experience for the student. Not only can *Therapeutic Measurement and Testing* be used in your introductory classroom discussions to provide an overview of measurement and testing techniques, it is ideal to use as a reference in the laboratory setting due to its step-by-step discussions of proper patient and therapist positioning, grading measurements, and proper instrument positioning.

Organization

Therapeutic Measurement and Testing is organized into 12 chapters and contains two appendices and a glossary for quick reference. An introductory chapter provides general information related to terminology, planes of motion, goniometry, and principles of muscle testing and ROM, among other topics. This introduction is followed by nine chapters that each focus on a specific body area, including the hip, knee, ankle and foot, shoulder, hand, and trunk. These chapters include tables that detail the primary and accessory muscle groups involved in movement of the particular body part being discussed. Therapist and patient positions, spoken directions for patients, and the grading parameters of muscle testing are provided in an easy-to-follow format. Range of motion is discussed in a separate section that provides proper positioning for the therapist, patient, and assessment tools.

Chapter 11 presents an in-depth discussion of posture, including abnormal and normal positions. Chapter 12 rounds out the discussion with a thorough examination of gait, including swing and stance phases. Appendix A provides a quick reference guide to kinesiology that discusses each body region in a concise and detailed listing that includes the action, innervations, origin, and insertion point for associated muscle groups. Appendix B offers a comprehensive table on joint movements. A glossary provides definitions to all key terms that are highlighted in boldface throughout the worktext.

Features

- A *Color Plate* includes approximately 45 full-color, detailed anatomy and physiology illustrations to help visualize and master the content discussed.

- Helpful, practical *Tips of the Trade* for working with patients are denoted throughout each chapter in order to provide clinically based applications of material.

- More than *150 photographs* clearly demonstrate the proper positioning for assessment and measurement techniques. Arrows are used on some photographs to emphasize the specific movement of the patient (black arrows) and/or the therapist (white arrows).

- *Key terms* are bolded throughout the worktext and defined in a *Glossary* for quick reference.

- *Tables* organize and present data in a clear and consistent manner for learning retention.

- *Learner Challenge* activities offer additional practice exercises to conduct in individual classroom and group laboratory settings.

- Potential *Substitutions* are provided for all manual muscle testing sections throughout the worktext.

For the Student

A CD-ROM in the back of the book contains an *Image Library,* which includes full-color versions of all images in the worktext, plus additional photographs and images that depict proper patient positioning and anatomical reference points.

For the Instructor

An Instructor Resources CD-ROM provides you with tools to aid you in facilitating students' learning. An *Instructor's Manual* provides case scenarios, suggested activities, and test questions written according to the format for the National Physical Therapy Examination. Also included is an *Image Library* that contains full-color versions of all images in the worktext. Use as handouts, on overheads, or incorporated into slide shows for in-class lectures.

About the Authors

Lisa Jennings Weaver graduated from Vincennes University in 1977 and spent 16 years practicing as a PTA in a wide variety of treatment settings. In 1993 she began teaching in the PTA program at Northeast Wisconsin Technical College. Lisa has taught extensively in the program, including courses in orthopedics, therapeutic exercise, and therapeutic measurement and testing as well as developing curriculum and teaching kinesiology. As a PTA, as well as an instructor, she is in a unique position of being able to understand both the role and function of a PTA in the clinical assessment/treatment process and the teaching methods best suited to meeting the needs of students.

Amanda L. Ferg (Mandy) is a PTA who graduated from Northeast Wisconsin Technical College in Green Bay, Wisconsin, in 2005. She also has a Bachelor of Science degree in Health Promotion and Wellness from the University of Wisconsin–Stevens Point and completed her internship at the Duke Center for Living in Durham, North Carolina. Mandy has worked in the therapy field for three years and is currently employed at Greentree Health and Rehabilitation, a skilled nursing facility in Clintonville, Wisconsin.

Reviewers

We would like to thank the reviewers whose constructive suggestions helped shape and develop this worktext:

Dolores Bertoti, MS, PT
Associate Professor and Chair AT/OT/SW
Alvernia College
Reading, PA

Ronald De Vera Barredo, PT, DPT, Ed.D., GCS
Assistant Dean and Associate Professor
Tennessee State University, College of Health Sciences
Nashville, TN

Toby Long, Ph.D., PT
Center for Child and Human Development
Georgetown University
Washington, DC

William M. Marcil, Ph.D., OTR, FAOTA
Director, Occupational Therapy Assistant Program
Tidewater Community College
Virginia Beach, VA

Michelle Parolise, MBA, OTR/L
Coordinator, Occupational Therapy Assistant Program
Santa Ana College
Santa Ana, CA

Becky Robler, Med, OTR
Instructor, OTA Program
Pueblo Community College
Pueblo, CO

Kevin Tenpenny, PTA
Associate Professor
Kaskaskia College PTA Program
Centralia, IL

Maggie Thomas, PT, MA
Physical Therapist Assistant Program Director
Kirkwood Community College
Cedar Rapids, IA

Marla Wonser, MSOT, OTR/L
Director, Occupational Therapy Assistant Program
Casper College
Casper, WY

Student Models

We would also like to extend our gratitude to the wonderful staff and students of the Physical Therapy program at the Sage Graduate College in Troy, New York. Without their time and enthusiasm for this project, the photographs displayed throughout this worktext would not be nearly as accurate, authentic, and impressive. A special thanks to Dr. Marjane Selleck, PT, DPT, MS, PCS, Chair and Director of the DPT Program, and Dr. James R. Brennan, PT, Ph.D., who helped to coordinate the use of the facility and student participation.

The students who you see in the photographs throughout this worktext are first-year students in the doctoral program in physical therapy at Sage. Their enthusiasm and dedication to the field was evident throughout the photo shoot and shines through in these beautiful photographs. The student models include: Alexandra Adams, Vernon A. Alexander, Jr., Kathryn Baird, Bridges B. Darko, Tara Dutcher, Lex Harding, Shane Henderson, Courtney Hines, Caritia Orozco, Dereck Silverman, and Cynthia Toth. Special thanks is extended to our outstanding photographer, Tom Stock, and his gracious assistant, Cassandra Swoto, as well as Delmar's own Stacey Lamodi and Jim Zayicek, who generously offered to assist as models.

Author Acknowledgements

This project has truly been a labor of love. It would not have been possible without the encouragement and challenges provided by both past and present PTA program students at Northeast Wisconsin Technical College in Green Bay, Wisconsin. You know who you are and you know why you matter so much to me.

Many thanks to Lisa Kihl, a former PTA program student who contributed material she painstakingly compiled to enhance her own learning experience. That material is found in Appendix A.

The Health Science Department Administration as well as the PTA program faculty at Northeast Wisconsin Technical College provided much support as this work progressed.

Many thanks to the patient and efficient staff at Delmar.

Co-author Mandy Ferg was indispensible as we divided work and collaborated on every aspect of this process. This wouldn't have been possible without her.

My family's support and encouragement has enabled me to achieve far more in my life than I ever would have dreamed possible. Thanks to my mother, Jeanne Riggs Jennings, and children Benjamin, Chelsea, and Nicholas.

I may be contacted via e-mail at lisa.weaver@nwtc.edu.

—Lisa Jennings Weaver, PTA, CMT

I would like to express my sincere thanks to all of the people who contributed to this book, especially the people at Delmar/Cengage Learning who gave us the opportunity to make Lisa's vision a reality. My deepest gratitude to my husband and family for always believing in me and providing constant support and encouragement in this project and in life in general. I would not be where I am today without them. I would also like to thank my daughter Zoey, who provided inspiration even from the womb. Awaiting her birth during the development of this book further motivated me to stay focused and do my best. Finally, a special thank you to Lisa, my teacher, mentor, and friend, for the amazing opportunity to participate in this learning experience and allowing me to challenge myself and grow both personally and professionally. It was truly a joy working together. I am very proud of what we accomplished.

—Amanda (Mandy) L. Ferg, PTA

INTRODUCTION

1

OBJECTIVES

Upon completion of this chapter the reader will be able to:

- Define positional terminology.

- Identify planes and axes of joint movement.

- Discuss goniometric terms and concepts.

- List basic requirements of assessment for documentation.

- Explain the types of ROM.

- Define both normal and abnormal end-feels.

- Define capsular patterns.

- Explain both numeric and named grading scales for manual muscle testing.

- Discuss terms and concepts of manual muscle testing.

INTRODUCTION TO BASIC TESTING

Because the human body is in almost constant motion, specific universal terminology must be used to describe body positions accurately. This is especially useful when discussing hand placement for muscle testing and goniometric placement for ROM. As the body changes position, so does the relationship of body parts to each other. These distinctions are crucial when collecting objective data during range of motion (ROM) and manual muscle testing (MMT) assessment.

Positional Terminology

Most communication regarding our methods of testing begins with the body at a starting point known as anatomical position. **Anatomical position** (see Figure 1-1) is with the body in an upright and forward-facing position. The arms are at the side with the palms facing forward. As you first practice this position, it seems a bit unnatural, but it is the standard placement for testing purposes, as you will see in future chapters. A more normal and comfortable position is called **fundamental position** (see Figure 1-2). This is essentially the same position, but the palms face the side of the body.

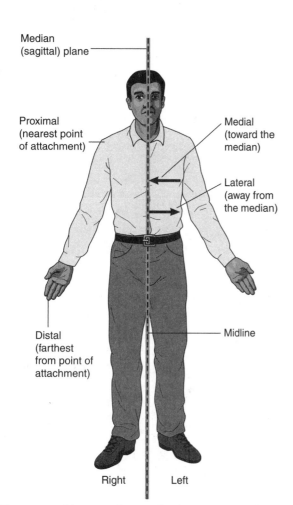

Figure 1-1 Directional terms, body in anatomical position (*See color plate*).

Source: Delmar/Cengage Learning

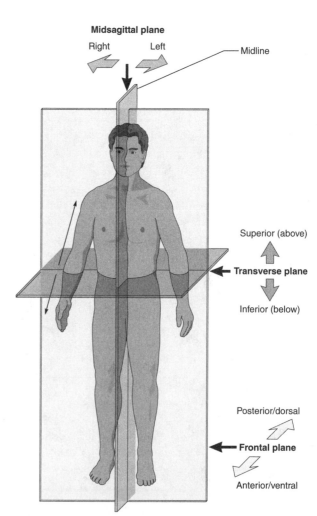

Figure 1-2 Planes of movement, body in fundamental position (*See color plate*).

Source: Delmar/Cengage Learning

As a review from anatomy and physiology, we must cover some terms that describe location of body parts in relation to other structures. The front surface of the body is referred to as the **anterior** or **ventral** portion. These terms can also be used to describe a position closer to the front than another position. **Posterior** is the term used for the back side of the body or positions closer to the back than another position. A synonym is **dorsal.** When speaking with other health professionals, use the terms *ventral* and *dorsal.* When speaking with patients, you may use the lay terms *front* and *back* to communicate clearly. Always remember to adjust your language to the audience to whom you are speaking.

> **TIPS** *of the* **Trade**
>
> If the terms *ventral* and *dorsal* are new for you, you can keep them straight by remembering the movie *Jaws.* A shark's dorsal fin is on its back.

The terms **medial** and **lateral** are used when describing locations in reference to the midline of the body. Locations closer to the midline are referred to as *medial* and those farther away as *lateral.* For example, the tibia is medial to the fibula.

Distal and **proximal** are terms referring to positions on the extremities. Locations farther away from the trunk are more distal. Locations closer to the trunk are more proximal.

> **TIPS** *of the* **Trade**
>
> Remember these terms are always used in reference to two points and their relative location to the trunk. Example: The knee is distal to the hip, but proximal to the ankle.

The terms used to depict structures being above or below another structure are **superior** and **inferior.** They can be used to depict positions of whole structures as they relate to another, as in "The fourth rib is inferior to the second," or they can be used to describe portions of individual structures, as in "the superior lobe of the right lung." Two other terms commonly used to depict this up and down position are **cephalad** and **caudal.** *Cephalad* refers to the head and *caudal* (which means "tail") refers to the foot.

Two final positional terms are **superficial** and **deep.** These are relatively self-explanatory in that they refer to a structure's position from the skin to the core of the body. For example, the trapezieus musculature is superficial to the rhomboids. If you were to dissect the area, the first muscles you would reach would be the trapezieus muscles. You would need to dissect deeper to reach the rhomboids.

Planes of Motion

Now that we have the positional terms down, we need to look at how the body is divided. These are called **planes of motion** (see Figure 1-3).

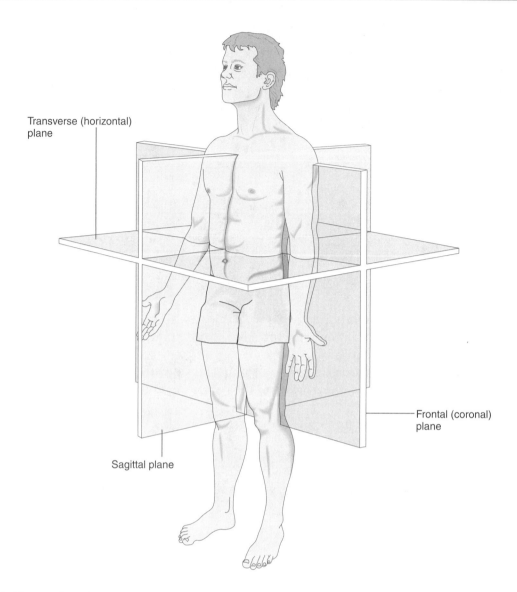

Transverse (horizontal) plane

Frontal (coronal) plane

Sagittal plane

Figure 1-3 Planes of motion. Source: Delmar/Cengage Learning

The **frontal plane** divides the body in half from front to back. The **sagittal plane** divides the body from side to side. The **transverse plane** divides the body in half from top to bottom. These planes help define the movement of a body part. For example, if a joint flexes or extends starting from anatomical position, it is moving along the lines of the sagittal plane. If a joint abducts or adducts, it is moving along the frontal plane. Finally, all rotational movements occur in the transverse planes.

We also need terms to define the direction of activity at the joint involved. For this we use the term **axis of motion** (see Figure 1-4), meaning the point around which movement occurs. The three axes are the **sagittal axis, frontal axis,** and **vertical axis.** Motion occurs around the axis in a rotational manner perpendicular to the movement of the body part. For example, the motions of flexion and extension occur in the sagittal plane, but move around the frontal axis because that axis is perpendicular to the sagittal plane. Likewise, abduction and adduction occur in the frontal plane around the sagittal axis, and rotational motions occur in the transverse plane about the vertical axis. Some clinicians refer to these axes as the *antero-posterior*, *medio-lateral*, and *vertical*, respectively.

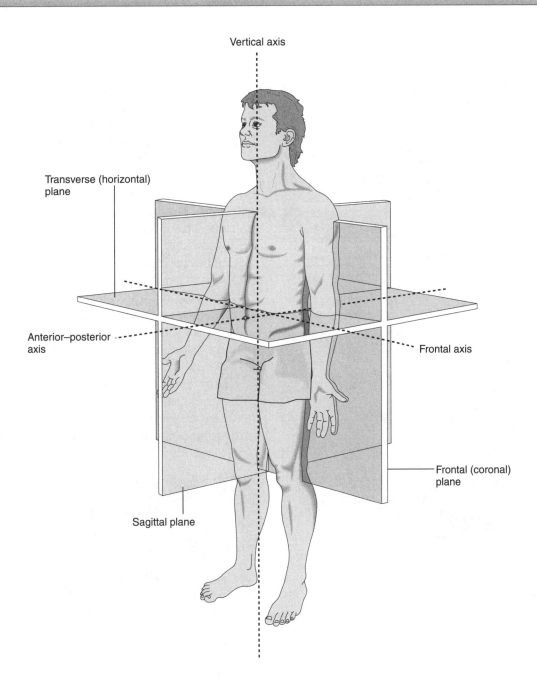

Figure 1-4 Planes with axes of the body. Source: Delmar/Cengage Learning

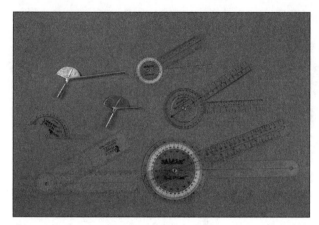

Figure 1-5 Goniometer examples. Source: Delmar/Cengage Learning

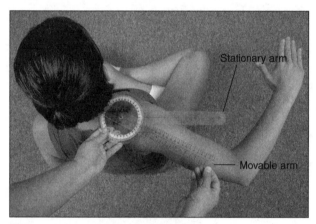

Figure 1-6 Goniometer with labels. Source: Delmar/Cengage Learning

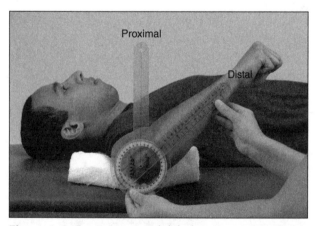

Figure 1-7 Goniometer with labels. Source: Delmar/Cengage Learning

Goniometry: Terms and Concepts

Goniometry is a medical term that refers to measuring joint movements. It comes from the Greek words *gonia*, meaning angle, and *metron*, meaning measure. These measurements are taken using a device called a **goniometer** (see Figure 1-5).

The goniometer has three parts. The body of the goniometer is typically a round or half-circle portion where the scale of degrees is located. The center is considered the axis or fulcrum. This center is aligned with the axis of motion on the joint being measured. The goniometer has two arms. One arm is an extension of the body called the *stationary arm*. The other is a freely moving separate piece affixed to the body through its attachment at the fulcrum. The second arm is called the *movable arm*, appropriately named because it moves with the body part being measured (see Figure 1-6).

During the measurement of a joint, these arms may be called by their reference points—or the *proximal arm* and the *distal arm* as they relate to the joint being measured (see Figure 1-7).

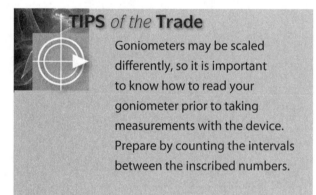

TIPS *of the* **Trade**

Goniometers may be scaled differently, so it is important to know how to read your goniometer prior to taking measurements with the device. Prepare by counting the intervals between the inscribed numbers.

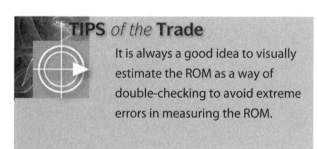

TIPS *of the* **Trade**

It is always a good idea to visually estimate the ROM as a way of double-checking to avoid extreme errors in measuring the ROM.

Accurate goniometric measurements are only as good as the documentation of the data collected. It is important to gather all pertinent information during the session, so you can record information that can be accurately assessed. You should include the following information at a minimum:

- Patient information such as name, ID number, age, gender, and diagnosis
- Specific body part and its position during the test
- Full ROM (include starting motion measurement as well as ending measurement)
- Type of motion (active or passive)
- Patient's response to testing (c/o pain, tenderness, tightness)
- Pertinent objective information gathered during testing (end-feels, joint sounds such as cracking or popping)
- Your signature, credentials, and the date

Many facilities document ROM information on flow charts, in which case your information would simply be entered in the appropriate boxes. In other cases, you will need to be prepared to document the information in a SOAP note or narrative fashion.

TIPS *of the* **Trade**

Some situations may call for goniometric measurements of PROM, AROM, or both. It is critical that your documentation reflects exactly what type of measurement you assessed.

Regardless of the type of measurement assessed, all information should be documented fully.

Principles of ROM

The principles of AROM vs. PROM, end-feels, and capsular vs. noncapsular patterns are crucial considerations.

Types of ROM

It is important to know the differences between **active range of motion (AROM)** and **passive range of motion (PROM)** when assessing ROM. AROM is the unassisted and voluntary motion of a joint. It demonstrates the patient's willingness/ability to move a particular joint. AROM, or lack thereof, can also provide information about the structures involved. Pain with active movement can be the result of stretching or contraction of contractile and/or noncontractile tissues. **Contractile tissue** refers to muscles and their tendonous attachments to the bone, while **noncontractile tissue** refers to ligaments, joint capsules, bursae, and facsia. If a patient can complete full range of motion without pain, it is a good indicator that further testing of motion of that joint is not needed.

PROM, as the name suggests, is movement without assistance from the patient. It is performed solely by the therapist and provides information about the integrity of articular surfaces and noncontractile tissues around a joint. If pain is experienced during PROM, it usually signals a problem with a joint's noncontractile tissue. However, pain at the end of PROM can also be from stretching the contractile tissues. Keep in mind that each joint has a small amount of motion available at end range that is not under voluntary control. This extra range absorbs outside forces, which helps to protect the joint. That is why PROM is usually slightly greater than AROM. Finally, PROM should always be assessed before MMT because the grading of MMT is based on the completion of a motion through full range.

End-feels

End-feels are assessed to determine the nature of resistance at the end of PROM of a joint. An **end-feel** is defined as the characteristic feeling of resistance to motion experienced by therapists as they passively take a joint to its end range. Distinguishing between the different end-feels is important in identifying structural limitations. To determine end-feels, movement must be carried out carefully and slowly to detect end range and distinguish between normal and abnormal end-feels. There are three normal end-feels (see Table 1-1) and five abnormal end-feels (see Table 1-2). Remember, it takes practice to become good at detecting these different feelings.

TABLE 1-1   NORMAL END-FEELS

END-FEEL	STRUCTURE	EXAMPLE
Soft	The range is limited by soft tissue compression.	Elbow flexion (the forearm pressing against the bulk of the bicep)
Firm	Firm or slightly springy feel at end of range as if it has some "give" to it.	Hip flexion with knee straight (passive elastic tension of hamstring muscles)
Hard	Bone contacting bone resulting in a hard yet painless end-feel.	Elbow extension (contact between olecranon process of ulna and olecranon fossa of humerus)

TABLE 1-2   ABNORMAL (PATHOLOGICAL) END-FEELS

END-FEEL	EXPLANATION	EXAMPLES
Soft	Occurs sooner in the ROM than is typical, or in a joint that normally has a firm or hard end-feel. Feels boggy.	Soft tissue edema Synovitis
Firm	Occurs sooner in the ROM than is typical, or in a joint that normally has a soft or hard end-feel.	Increased muscular tone Capsular or soft tissue shortening
Hard	Occurs sooner in the ROM than is typical or in a joint that normally has a soft or firm end-feel. A bony grating or bony block is felt.	Chondromalacia Osteoarthritis Loose bodies in joint
Empty	No end-feel is reached because pain or other symptoms limit the ROM before resistance is felt.	Acute joint inflammation Bursitis Psychogenic disorders

Capsular Patterns

When limitation in joint motion is noted, the therapist's natural inclination is to determine the cause of the restriction. Many conditions involving structures other than the joint capsule may cause limitation in ROM, such as muscle strains or internal joint derangement. This is referred to as a **noncapsular pattern** of restriction. Cyriax and Coldham (1984) were the first to propose that when a pathological condition involves the entire joint capsule, that joint will exhibit a certain predictable pattern of restriction. This specific pattern of restriction is called a **capsular pattern.** These patterns of restriction usually occur as a result of widespread effusion or inflammation in the joint or as a result of considerable joint fibrosis. These patterns are not the same for all joints. For example, not all joints show the most restriction in external rotation. However, the capsular pattern of a given joint is the same from patient to patient.

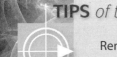

TIPS *of the* **Trade**

Remember that with a capsular pattern of restriction, the specific ROM will not be the same from patient to patient, but the pattern of most to least restriction will.

Although there are some differences of opinion regarding capsular patterns in some joints, most therapists embrace the work started by Cyriax and Coldham (1984) and carried on and refined by other therapists. The following lists the capsular patterns by joint, from most to least restriction:

- Shoulder: External rotation, abduction, flexion, internal rotation (Saunders, 1994)
- Elbow: Flexion, extension, pronation, and supination-full range (Saunders, 1994)
- Forearm (proximal and distal radio-ulnar joints): Pronation, supination (Cyriax & Coldham, 1984)
- Wrist (radio-carpal and midcarpal joints): Equal loss of flexion and extension
- Thumb carpometacarpal: Abduction, extension
- Metacarpophalangeal: Flexion, extension
- Interphalangeal: Flexion, extension
- Hip: Internal rotation, abduction, flexion, extension, adduction, external rotation
- Knee: Flexion (great), extension (slight)
- Ankle: Plantar flexion, dorsiflexion
- Metatarsophalangeal: Extension, flexion
- Interphalangeal: Extension, flexion (Saunders, 1994)

Principles of Muscle Testing

Muscle testing is used to gather objective information related to the strength of a muscle or group of muscles during a particular motion. There are two common grading scales, one numerical and the other qualitative in nature (see Table 1-3).

TABLE 1-3		MUSCLE TESTING GRADING SCALES
GRADE NAME	**GRADE NUMBER**	**DEFINITION**
Normal	5	Moves against gravity, through full ROM and holds against maximal resistance
Good	4	Moves against gravity, through full ROM and holds against moderate but not full resistance
Fair	3	Moves against gravity, through full ROM but cannot hold against resistance
Poor	2	Moves through full ROM in gravity decreased position but tolerates no resistance
Trace	1	Unable to move through ROM but contraction can be noted visually or palpably
Zero	0	No contraction noted

TIPS *of the* Trade

In many clinics a plus/minus system is incorporated to allow for more variances in the grading. For example, a therapist might decide on a 4+ grade for someone who seems a bit stronger than a grade 4 but cannot tolerate full applied pressure. Take extreme care with these additions, which allow for more variances between therapists and can result in less objectivity in the grading system.

In applying full resistance, you must first place the body so that the activity is done against gravity. This means that the body part must be able to overcome gravity to lift itself through the full ROM. Remember if that is possible, the test already moves to at least a grade 3. Commonly used terms that apply here are **against-gravity** or **gravity resisted.** Both terms signify lifting the body part using gravity as part of the resistance. If the body part is unable to lift against gravity, you must reposition the patient or body part to allow for the motion to be done with as little gravitational interference as possible. The terms commonly used to identify this position are **gravity minimal** and **gravity decreased.** Both terms mean positioning so that gravity plays less of a role in the added resistance.

TIPS *of the* Trade

To achieve a gravity decreased or gravity minimal position, place the body so that the part moves in a direction parallel to the floor rather than perpendicular to the floor.

After positioning the body appropriately, you must determine when and where to apply manual resistance. As a general rule of thumb, if you are testing a **one-joint muscle,** the resistance should be given close to the end of the range to ensure accurate **repeatability.** If you are testing a **two-joint muscle,** you should choose a midrange point to reduce the chances of **active insufficiency** decreasing the available strength.

Where to test is a bit more involved. You should always test at the longest lever arm possible. Attempt to apply resistance at the distal end of the bony segment where the muscle attaches. For example, if you are grading hip flexion with the patient's leg out straight, you should place your hands to apply resistance at the ankle. If the knee is not a stable joint, you should resist at the lower end of the femur, just above the knee—which automatically reduces the testing grade to 4. The reasoning is that using a short lever arm reduces the amount of strength required to hold against your resistance. Any time you use a short lever arm, you must adjust your grading accordingly.

After you have positioned your patient and determined hand placement, you must apply resistance. The procedure currently used in muscle testing is called the **break test.** With the break test, the therapist applies pressure in the opposite direction of the body part's movement, thereby trying to force the body part back in the direction it came. Common instructions to the patient include "Hold this position and do not let me pull you out of it" or "Try to resist me and don't let me move your leg/arm." If you succeed in causing the body part to "break" its position, the muscle test would be rated no higher than grade 4. Remember when applying pressure, it is important to gradually apply it until full resistance is achieved to allow maximum tolerable intensity. It is helpful to count to 5 and increase intensity as you go. This also helps decrease the chance of the body part being injured.

If patients are unable to lift the body part against gravity (grade 3), they must be placed in a gravity minimal/gravity decreased position and asked to perform the same task. If they are unable to move the part, your kinesiology knowledge becomes even more valuable. You will need to place your hands over the muscles responsible for the action to palpate for any muscle activity that might not be visible. Either seeing or palpating a twitch in the muscle constitutes a grade 1 or Trace value.

As with all activities performed on a patient, documentation is essential. When recording information on MMT, you should include the following information at a minimum:

- Patient information such as name, ID number, age, gender, and diagnosis
- Specific body part and its position during the test
- Grade of MMT earned by patient
- Patient's response to testing (c/o pain, tenderness, tightness)
- Pertinent objective information gathered during testing (end-feels, cracking, or popping)
- Your signature, credentials, and the date

PRACTICAL APPLICATION

Beginning with Chapter 2, we will move through the body to address individual joints and the muscles surrounding them. We will discuss the most commonly used manual muscle testing techniques and goniometric techniques to be used with each. The final two chapters pull these individual structures together as a whole to explore posture and gait analysis. Throughout this worktext, it will be important to keep a few overriding principles in mind.

- Be knowledgeable of the direction of the muscle fibers being tested and their line of pull.
- Be able to identify patterns of substitution to increase testing accuracy.
- Know the muscle location as well as its points of origin and insertion.
- Detect contractile activity visually and through palpation when testing minimally active muscles.
- Be aware of laxity or deformity of a joint as well as its available ROM. If a condition such as contracture limits ROM, the available ROM becomes the full ROM.
- Stabilize the proximal segment of the joint being tested.

- Be aware of ways to modify test procedures when necessary without compromising the test results.
- Keep in mind that muscles, especially if already compromised, can fatigue easily during long testing sessions.
- Resist the temptation to take shortcuts with muscle testing. It is imperative to master the basic procedures first.
- It is not necessary or efficient to test every muscle in the body. General observations of the patient doing functional tasks like walking into the room or taking off a jacket can help you target the problem areas.
- Be a good listener and stay attentive to patient reactions during the tests. They can offer important clues.
- As with all patient interactions, make sure the patient is positioned as comfortably as possible and appropriately draped.

Periodically review this list to make these practices part of your standard procedures as you begin your journey toward mastery of the key assessment techniques of MMT, ROM, posture, and gait analysis.

THE HIP

CHAPTER 2

OBJECTIVES

Upon completion of this chapter, the reader will be able to:

- Describe the hip joint.
- Identify the bones and bony landmarks significant to the hip.
- Name the major ligaments of the hip and their purpose.
- Identify any supporting structures important to the hip.
- Describe the major motions of the hip and name the muscles that perform them.
- Identify the origins, insertions, and innervations of the muscles of the hip.
- Perform proper manual muscle testing on the major muscles of the hip grades 5–0.
- Be aware of possible substitutions during manual muscle testing on the hip.
- Accurately perform range of motion testing using the goniometer on the hip joint.

MUSCULOSKELETAL OVERVIEW

The lower extremities are made up of the pelvis, thigh, leg, and foot. Because they support the entire weight of the erect human body, the bones making up these structures must be strong and thick. Unlike the upper extremities, the bones of the lower extremities are specialized for stability and weight bearing to allow them to handle the exceptional forces created during weight-bearing activities like running, walking, and jumping. The pelvis contains the two hip bones, the sacrum and the coccyx, and plays a key role in weight bearing. In addition to receiving the forces from the vertebral column and distributing them to the sturdy hip bones, the pelvis receives the forces generated from the foot contacting the ground and distributes them up toward the vertebral column. The hip's responsibility for handling such large forces from repetitive loads makes it susceptible to various injuries.

Joints

The hip joint itself is very strong and stable and is comprised of the pelvis and the femur. The head of the femur articulates with the acetabulum of the hip bone. The hip is the most proximal joint of the lower extremity and attaches the inferior **appendicular skeleton** to the **axial skeleton.** The various muscles and ligaments around the hip provide strength and support, allowing the extremities to complete complex movements through a full range of motion.

The hip is categorized as a **synovial,** triaxial ball-and-socket joint, meaning it has motion in all three planes of movement. Like the shoulder, the hip can perform **flexion, extension,** hyperextension, **abduction, adduction, internal rotation,** and **external rotation.** However, it has less range of motion than the shoulder joint due to the increased stability from its ligaments and deeper socket. The capsular pattern for the hip is limitation of internal rotation and abduction more than flexion and extension.

Bones

The main bones making up the hip joint are the hip bones, also known as *coxal bones,* and the femur. The hip bone is irregularly shaped and consists of the ilium, ischium, and pubis. By adulthood, these three bones are fused to form the pelvic or hip bone. The ilium is a large fan-shaped bone that forms the superior portions of the hip bone. The ischium is arc shaped and forms the posterior inferior part of the hip bone. Its thicker superior body joins the ilium, while the thinner inferior portion connects to the pubis bone. The pubis bone is essentially V-shaped and forms the anterior inferior portion of the hip bone. It can be divided into the inferior ramus, the body, and the superior ramus. The acetabulum is formed at the point where the ilium, ischium, and pubis are fused. This deep hemispherical socket on the lateral surface of the pelvis articulates with the smooth head of the femur. The femur is the longest and strongest bone in the body and the only bone in the thigh. It helps to distribute and absorb the vigorous forces that are placed on it during weight-bearing activities.

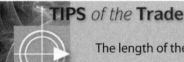

TIPS *of the* **Trade**

The length of the femur is one-fourth of a person's height.

The following are the bony landmarks significant to the hip joint.

Hip bones

- **Os coxae or hip bone:** Made up of an ilium, ischium, and pubis bone and forming the pelvic girdle by uniting with its partner anteriorly and the sacrum posteriorly (see Figure 2-1)

Ilium

- **Iliac fossa:** Large smooth **concave** area that deepens the anterior surface of the ilium (see Figure 2-2)

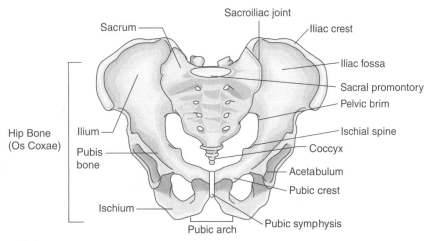

Figure 2-1 Pelvic girdle bones. Source: Delmar/Cengage Learning

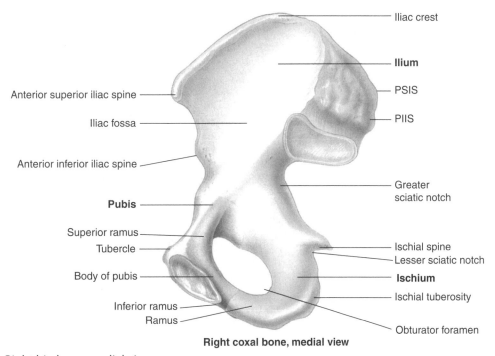

Right coxal bone, medial view

Figure 2-2 Right hip bone medial view. Source: Delmar/Cengage Learning

- **Iliac crest:** The large rounded bony superior border of the ilium lying between the anterior superior iliac spine and the posterior superior iliac spine

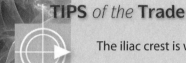

TIPS *of the* Trade

The iliac crest is where you place your hands when resting on your hips.

- **Anterior superior iliac spine (ASIS):** Bony protrusion on the anterior portion of the iliac crest
- **Anterior inferior iliac spine (AIIS):** Bony protrusion just inferior to ASIS
- **Posterior superior iliac spine (PSIS):** Bony protrusion posteriorly on the iliac crest
- **Posterior inferior iliac spine (PIIS):** Found below the PSIS

Ischium

- **Body:** Thicker superior portion of the ischium connecting to the ilium and making up two-fifths of the acetabulum (see Figure 2-3)
- **Ramus:** Thinner portion of the ischium extends medially from the body to join the inferior ramus of the pubis
- **Spine:** Projects medially into the pelvic cavity and is found posteriorly on the ischial body and inferiorly to the border of the greater sciatic notch
- **Ischial tuberosity:** Thick and rough projection of the inferior surface of the ischial body

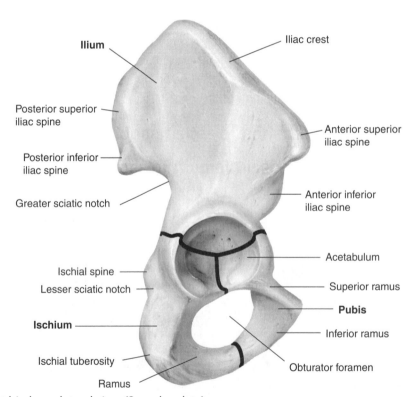

Figure 2-3 Right hip bone lateral view *(See color plate).* Source: Delmar/Cengage Learning

TIPS *of the* **Trade**

The ischial tuberosity is the part of the body that bears weight when sitting.

- **Lesser sciatic notch:** Inferior to the ischial spine where numerous nerves and blood vessels pass through

Pubis

- **Body:** Flat medial portion of the pubis between the inferior ramus and the superior ramus making up one-fifth of the acetabulum
- **Superior ramus:** Located superior to the pubis body and the acetabulum
- **Inferior ramus:** Located posterior, lateral, and inferior to the body of the pubis
- **Symphysis pubis:** Connects the two bodies of the pubic bones by a fibrocartilage disc at the anterior midline
- **Pubic tubercle:** Bony notch by the symphysis pubis that projects anteriorly on the superior ramus

Other Landmarks

The following landmarks are important to the hip but do not belong to one bone in particular:

- **Acetabulum:** A deep socket that articulates with the head of the femur and is made up of almost equal portions of the ilium, ischium, and pubis bone
- **Obturator foramen:** A large opening created by the bodies and rami of the ischium and pubis
- **Greater sciatic notch:** Large notch inferior to the PIIS formed by the indentation and deepening of the ilium

Femur

- **Head:** Ball-like portion covered with articulation cartilage and articulates with the acetabulum
- **Neck:** Narrow portion between the trochanters that carries the head and angles laterally to join the shaft

TIPS *of the* **Trade**

The neck is the weakest part of the femur, resulting in common fractures called hip fractures.

- **Greater trochanter:** Large lateral projection where neck and shaft meet
- **Lesser trochanter:** Small medial projection posterior and distal to the greater trochanter

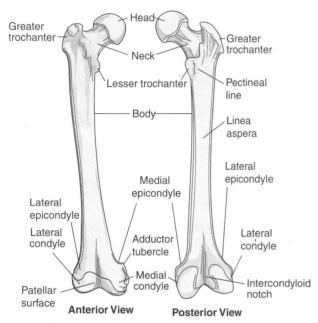

Figure 2-4 Femur *(See color plate).* Source: Delmar/Cengage Learning

- **Body or shaft:** Located between the bone ends, long and cylindrical in shape bowing slightly anteriorly (see Figure 2-4)
- **Medial condyle:** Distal medial end of femur
- **Lateral condyle:** Distal lateral end of femur
- **Medial epicondyle:** Protuberance proximal to the medial condyle of the femur
- **Lateral epicondyle:** Protuberance proximal to the lateral condyle of the femur
- **Intercondylar fossa:** Deep U-shaped space located posteriorly on the femur between the medial and lateral condyles
- **Adductor tubercle:** Small bump proximal to medial epicondyle
- **Linea aspera:** Vertical prominent ridge running posterior length of the femur

- **Pectineal line:** Found on the posterior femur and runs diagonally from below the lesser tubercle to the linea aspera
- **Patellar surface:** The area of the femur that articulates with the posterior surface of the patella located anteriorly between the medial and lateral condyle

Ligaments

As previously mentioned, the hip is a synovial ball-and-socket joint that plays a key role in stability. Like all synovial joints, the hip has a thick fibrous articular surface that spans the joint and completely encloses it. The capsule extends from the rim of the acetabulum distally to the neck of the femur in a type of cylindrical sleeve. The joint capsule is reinforced by strong ligaments that help provide stability. The iliofemoral, pubofemoral, and ischiofemoral ligaments are the three main reinforcing structures spirally wrapping around the hip joint as they attach to the femur (see Figure 2-5). They create a strong band of fibers, with each ligament responsible for stabilizing the joint surfaces from external force and limiting range of motion of certain movements.

The most important of the three ligaments is the iliofemoral. It spans the anterior surface of the hip joint and attaches proximally to the AIIS, reinforcing the joint capsule anteriorly. Then it splits distally and forms an inverted Y shape by attaching to the proximal medial region of the femur, medial to the greater trochanter. Because of this shape, it is also known as the Y ligament. The main function of the iliofemoral ligament is to limit hyperextension of the hip joint. Inferior to the iliofemoral ligament is the pubofemoral ligament. It spans the hip joint medially and inferiorly. This ligament runs from the medial part of the acetabular rim and superior ramus of the pubis down and back to the neck of the femur. It limits the hyperextension of the hip joint as well as extreme abduction. The final of the three main ligaments is the ischiofemoral ligament, which spans the joint capsule posteriorly. It attaches from the posterior or ischial portion of the acetabulum to the femoral neck. This ligament runs across the joint in a lateral and superior direction, and its fibers limit hyperextension and medial rotation of the hip. These three ligaments together limit motion in one direction while allowing full motion in the opposite direction. This means they are taut in hyperextension and become slack in hip flexion.

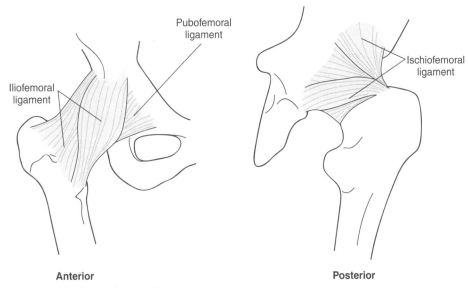

Iliofemoral
ligament

Pubofemoral
ligament

Ischiofemoral
ligament

Anterior

Posterior

Figure 2-5 Ligamentous reinforcement of hip joint. Source: Delmar/Cengage Learning

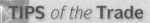

TIPS *of the* **Trade**

By thrusting the hips in front of the knees and shoulders, a person can stand in an upright posture resting on the iliofemoral ligament without using any muscles at all. This is how an individual with spinal cord paralysis can stand upright.

Two other ligaments in the hip should be mentioned: the ligamentum teres and the inguinal ligament. The ligamentum teres is a small, flat, intracapsular ligament that attaches from the distal femoral head to the lower lip of the acetabulum. Its importance is debatable (see Figure 2-6). Because it is slack during most hip movements, it does not play a role in stabilizing the hip joint surface, but it does contain an artery that supplies blood to the head of the femur. Although damage to this artery can lead to arthritis of the hip joint, it does not keep the head of the femur viable by itself.

The inguinal ligament attaches on the ASIS to the pubic tubercle (see Figure 2-7). It has no function at the hip joint, but it is the landmark that separates the anterior abdominal wall from the thigh.

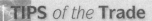

TIPS *of the* **Trade**

The external iliac artery and vein become the femoral artery and vein when they pass under the inguinal ligament.

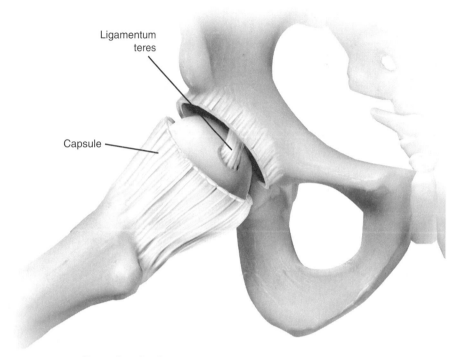

Figure 2-6 Ligamentum teres *(See color plate).* Source: Delmar/Cengage Learning

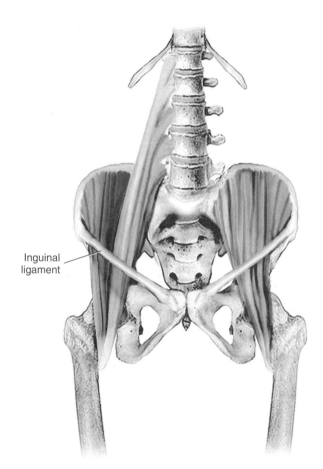

Figure 2-7 Inguinal ligament *(See color plate).*

Source: Delmar/Cengage Learning

Supporting Structures

Two other important structures worth mentioning are the acetabular labrum and the iliotibial band or tract. The acetabular labrum is a circular rim of fibrocartilage that enhances the depth of the acetabulum. The diameter of the labrum is less than that of the head of the femur, providing a snug fit for the femur in the acetabulum. This helps keep the femoral head in the acetabulum, making hip dislocation rare.

The iliotibial tract is found on the anterior portion of the iliac crest and runs superficially down the lateral side of the thigh attaching to the tibia. Although it does not play a role in supporting the hip joint, its long tendinous portion of the tensor fascia latae muscles provides an attachment place for muscles of the lower extremity.

MUSCLE TESTING OF THE HIP

As previously mentioned, the motions at the hip are flexion, extension, hyperextension, abduction, adduction, internal rotation, and external rotation. The following section reviews manual muscle testing for each of these motions.

Hip Flexion

It is important to have a good knowledge of the range of motion of the hip before completing manual muscle tests for hip strength. Poor working knowledge of hip range of motion can result in contaminated results. Because it is important to review the muscles associated with the movement, each section starts with a table of the muscles responsible for the movement being tested, followed by a drawing of the primary muscles. Table 2-1 details the primary and accessory muscles responsible for hip flexion. The iliopsoas and rectus femoris muscles are the primary movers for hip flexion (see Figures 2-8 and 2-9).

TABLE 2-1 MUSCLES RESPONSIBLE FOR HIP FLEXION

PRIMARY MUSCLES	ORIGIN	INSERTION	INNERVATIONS
Iliopsoas	Iliac fossa, anterior and lateral surfaces of T12-L5	Lesser trochanter of the femur	Iliacus: femoral nerve (L2, L3) Psoas major: (L2, L3)
Rectus femoris	Anterior inferior iliac spine (AIIS)	Tibial tuberosity via patellar tendon	Femoral (L2–L4)

ACCESSORY MUSCLES	ORIGIN	INSERTION	INNERVATIONS
Sartorious	Anterior superior iliac spine (ASIS)	Proximal medial aspect of tibia	Femoral (L2, L3)
Tensor fascia latae	ASIS	Lateral condyle of tibia	Superior gluteal (L4, L5)
Pectineus	Superior ramus of pubis	Pectineal line of femur	Femoral (L2, L3, L4)
Adductor magnus	Ischium and pubis	Linea aspera and adductor tubercle	Obturator and sciatic (L3, L4)
Adductor Longus	Pubis	Middle third of linea aspera	Obturator (L3, L4)
Adductor Brevis	Pubis	Pectineal line and proximal linea aspera	Obturator (L3, L4)
Gluteus medius	Outer surface ilium	Lateral surface greater trochanter	Superior gluteal (L4, L5, S1)

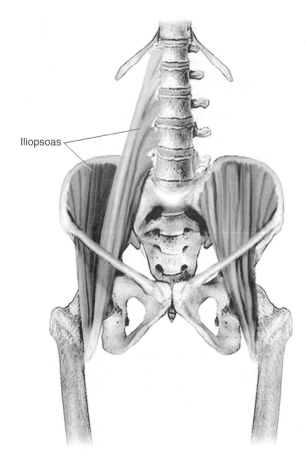

Iliopsoas

Figure 2-8 Iliopsoas *(See color plate).*

Source: Delmar/Cengage Learning

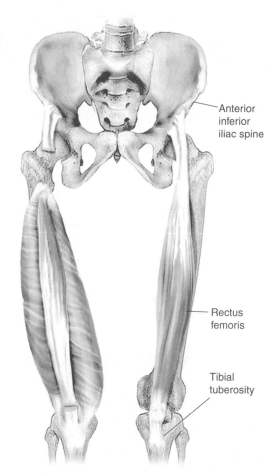

Anterior inferior iliac spine

Rectus femoris

Tibial tuberosity

Figure 2-9 Rectus femoris muscle anterior view *(See color plate).* Source: Delmar/Cengage Learning

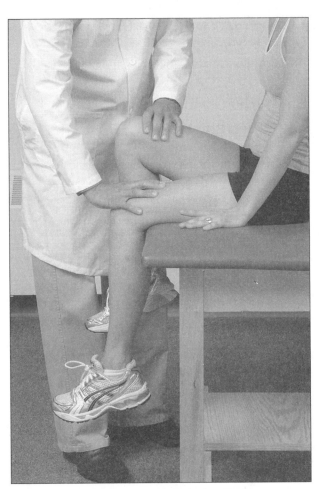

Figure 2-10 Proper positioning for hip flexion grades 5–3. Source: Delmar/Cengage Learning

Testing for Hip Flexion Grades 5, 4, 3 (Normal, Good, Fair) Gravity Resisted

POSITION OF PATIENT: Short sitting with arms at sides to provide trunk stability and thighs fully supported on table.

POSITION OF THERAPIST: Standing next to test limb or kneeling if patient is standing. Testing hand is contoured over thigh above the knee (see Figure 2-10). This hand provides resistance in a downward motion toward the floor.

TEST: Patient flexes hip until leg clears the table while maintaining neutral rotation.

DIRECTIONS: Say to the patient, "Lift your leg off the table and don't let me push it down."

GRADING:

- **Grade 5 (Normal):** Patient flexes the hip and clears the table while holding against therapist's maximum resistance without breaking.
- **Grade 4 (Good):** Patient flexes the hip and holds against therapist's strong to moderate resistance and then breaks.
- **Grade 3 (Fair):** Patient flexes the hip through full range and holds at end range, but no resistance is tolerated.

TIPS *of the* **Trade**

If the trunk is weak, perform the test from a supine position to make the test more accurate.

TIPS *of the* **Trade**

Because hip flexion is not a strong movement, experience will teach you what constitutes a normal level of resistance.

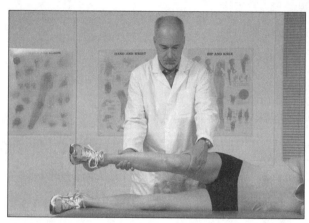

Figure 2-11 Proper positioning for hip flexion grade 2.

Source: Delmar/Cengage Learning

Testing for Hip Flexion Grade 2 (Poor) Gravity Minimal

POSITION OF PATIENT: Side-lying with bottom leg flexed for stability and top leg (test limb) supported by the therapist.

POSITION OF THERAPIST: Behind patient cradling test limb with one arm with hand supporting under knee. Other hand helps maintain trunk alignment at hip (see Figure 2-11). No resistance is applied.

TEST: Patient is to flex the hip through available ROM. Knee is allowed to flex to decrease tension on the hamstrings.

DIRECTIONS: Say to patient, "Bend your hip up toward your chest."

GRADING:

- **Grade 2 (Poor):** Able to complete hip flexion through full ROM with gravity minimized.

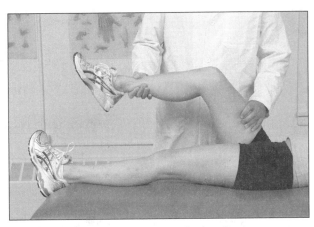

Figure 2-12 Proper positioning for hip flexion grades 1–0. Source: Delmar/Cengage Learning

Testing for Hip Flexion Grades 1, 0 (Trace, None) Gravity Minimal

POSITION OF PATIENT: Supine with test limb knee bent and being supported by therapist.

POSITION OF THERAPIST: Next to test limb with one hand supporting under calf with hand behind the knee. Other hand palpates just distal to the inguinal ligament on medial side of sartorius (see Figure 2-12).

TEST: Patient tries to flex the hip.

DIRECTIONS: Say to patient, "Try to bend your hip."

GRADING:

- **Grade 1 (Trace):** Tendon movement is palpable but there is no visible movement.
- **Grade 0 (None):** Unable to palpate any contraction of the muscles or tendons.

Hip Extension

Table 2-2 details the primary and accessory muscles responsible for hip extension. The gluteus maximus, semitendinosus, semimembranosus, and biceps femoris (see Figure 2-13) are the primary movers for hip extension.

TABLE 2-2	MUSCLES RESPONSIBLE FOR HIP EXTENSION		
PRIMARY MUSCLES	**ORIGIN**	**INSERTION**	**INNERVATIONS**
Gluteus maximus (see Figure 2-14)	Posterior sacrum and ilium	Posterior femur distal to greater trochanter and iliotibial band	Inferior gluteal (L5, S1, S2)
Semitendinosus	Ischial tuberosity	Anteromedial surface of proximal tibia	Sciatic (L5, S1, S2)
Semimembranosus	Ischial tuberosity	Posterior surface of medial condyle of tibia	Sciatic (L5, S1, S2)
Biceps femoris	Long head: ischial tuberosity Short head: lateral lip of linea aspera	Fibular head Fibular head	Sciatic (S1, S2, S3) Common peroneal (L5, S1, S2)
ACCESSORY MUSCLES	**ORIGIN**	**INSERTION**	**INNERVATIONS**
Adductor magnus (inferior)	Ischium and pubis	Entire linea aspera and adductor tubercle	Obturator and sciatic (L3, L4)
Gluteus medius (posterior)	Outer surface ilium	Lateral surface greater trochanter	Superior gluteal (L4, L5, S1)

For any patient, the therapist should perform a general test that evaluates the strength of the hip extensor muscles together. If any asymmetry is noted, the therapist can isolate the gluteus maximus to find the exact weakness.

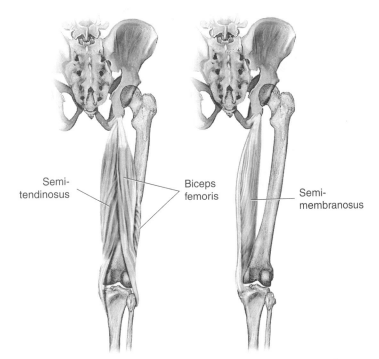

Figure 2-13 Hamstring muscles: semitendinosus, biceps femoris, and semimembranosus *(See color plate)*.

Source: Delmar/Cengage Learning

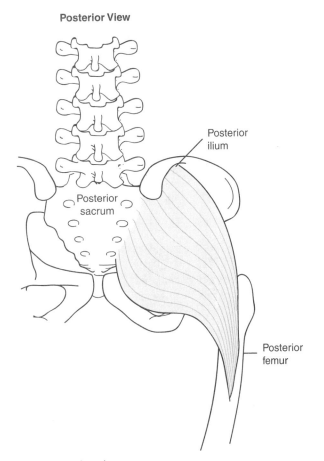

Posterior View

Figure 2-14 Gluteus maximus posterior view. Source: Delmar/Cengage Learning

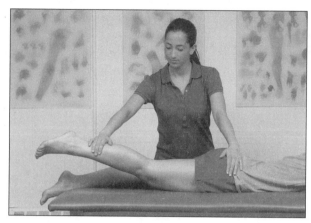

Figure 2-15 Proper positioning for hip extension grades 5–3. Source: Delmar/Cengage Learning

Testing for Hip Extension Grades 5, 4, 3 (Normal, Good, Fair) Gravity Resisted

POSITION OF PATIENT: Prone with arms at sides or overhead for stability.

POSITION OF THERAPIST: Standing at test side at level of the pelvis. Testing hand is placed on posterior of leg above the ankle and applies resistance down toward the floor (see Figure 2-15). The stabilizing hand is placed on the posterior superior spine of the ilium to maintain pelvis alignment.

> **TIPS** *of the* **Trade**
>
> Because the lever arm here is the longest, this test is the most demanding. A less demanding alternative is to place the testing hand on the posterior thigh just above the knee (Hislop & Montgomery, 2002).

TEST: Patient extends hip through available ROM.

DIRECTIONS: Say to patient, "Lift your leg off the table as high as you can, and keep your knee straight."

GRADING:

- **Grade 5 (Normal):** Patient extends the hip through full ROM and holds against therapist's maximum resistance without breaking.
- **Grade 4 (Good):** Patient extends the hip through full ROM and holds against therapist's strong to moderate resistance and then breaks.
- **Grade 3 (Fair):** Patient extends the hip through full ROM and holds at end range but no resistance is tolerated.

> **TIPS** *of the* **Trade**
>
> Be aware that the hip extensors are among the most powerful muscles in the body, making them difficult for most therapists to break in a grade 5 hip extension muscle test. Be careful not to overgrade a grade 4 muscle.

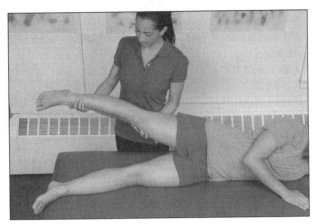

Figure 2-16 Proper positioning for hip extension grade 2. Source: Delmar/Cengage Learning

Testing for Hip Extension Grade 2 (Poor) Gravity Minimal

POSITION OF PATIENT: Side-lying with bottom leg flexed for stability and top leg (test limb) straight and supported by the therapist.

POSITION OF THERAPIST: Behind patient with one arm cradling the test limb with the hand just below the knee. The other hand is placed over the pelvic crest to help maintain hip and pelvic alignment (see Figure 2-16). No resistance is applied.

TEST: Patient is to extend the hip through full ROM without any resistance or assistance from the therapist.

DIRECTIONS: Say to the patient, "Try to bring your leg back toward me, while keeping your knee straight."

GRADING:

- **Grade 2 (Poor):** Able to complete hip extension through full ROM with gravity minimized.

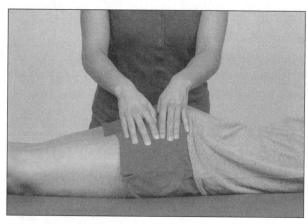

Figure 2-17 Proper positioning for hip extension grades 1–0. Source: Delmar/Cengage Learning

Testing for Hip Extension Grades 1, 0 (Trace, None) Gravity Minimal

POSITION OF PATIENT: Prone

POSITION OF THERAPIST: Standing next to test limb with one hand palpating deep into the tissue for the hamstrings at the ischial tuberosity and the other hand palpating the gluteus maximus over the center of the buttocks (see Figure 2-17).

TEST: Patient attempts to extend hip or squeeze buttocks together.

DIRECTIONS: Say to the patient, "Try to lift your leg from the table or squeeze your butt together."

GRADING:

- **Grade 1 (Trace):** Tendon movement is palpable but there is no visible movement.
- **Grade 0 (None):** Unable to palpate any contraction of the muscles or tendons.

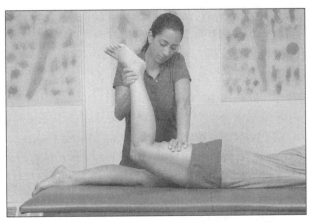

Figure 2-18 Proper positioning for hip extension isolate gluteus maximus grades 5–3. Source: Delmar/Cengage Learning

Testing for Isolation of Gluteus Maximus for Hip Extension Grades 5, 4, 3 Gravity Resisted

The strength testing for the isolation of the gluteus maximus is similar to the general testing of the hip extensors with a few minor differences.

POSITION OF PATIENT: Prone with knee flexed to 90°. An alternative position will be discussed for patients with hip flexion **contractures.**

POSITION OF THERAPIST: Standing by the test limb at the level of the pelvis. Testing hand is contoured over the posterior thigh above the knee and applies resistance in a downward motion. The stabilizing hand helps maintain alignment of the pelvis (see Figure 2-18).

TEST: Patient extends hip through available ROM with knee flexed.

DIRECTIONS: Say to patient, "Lift your foot to the ceiling, and don't let me push it down."

GRADING:

- **Grade 5 (Normal):** Patient extends the hip through full ROM and holds against therapist's maximum resistance without breaking.
- **Grade 4 (Good):** Patient extends the hip through full ROM and holds against therapist's strong to moderate resistance and then breaks.
- **Grade 3 (Fair):** Patient extends the hip through full ROM and holds at end range but no resistance is tolerated.

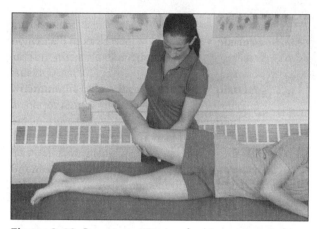

Figure 2-19 Proper positioning for hip extension isolate gluteus maximus grade 2. Source: Delmar/Cengage Learning

Testing for Isolation of Gluteus Maximus for Hip Extension Grade 2 (Poor) Gravity Minimal

POSITION OF PATIENT: Side-lying with bottom leg straight for stability and top leg (test limb) flexed at the knee and supported by the therapist.

POSITION OF THERAPIST: Behind patient with one arm cradling the test limb with the hand just below the knee. The other hand is placed over the pelvic crest to help maintain hip and pelvic alignment (see Figure 2-19). No resistance is applied.

TEST: Patient is to extend the hip with flexed knee supported.

DIRECTIONS: Say to patient, "Try and bring your leg back toward me."

GRADING:

• **Grade 2 (Poor):** Able to complete hip extension through available ROM with gravity minimized.

Testing for Isolation of Gluteus Maximus for Hip Extension Grades 1, 0 (Trace, None) Gravity Minimal

The testing for these two grades is identical to the ones for the aggregate hip extension testing (refer to Figure 2-17).

TIPS *of the* **Trade**

Tension in the rectus femoris muscle when the knee is flexed results in a decrease in hip extension ROM. Therefore, it is common to see a diminished ROM when isolating the gluteus maximus muscle during muscle testing.

GRADING

• **Grade 1 (Trace):** Tendon movement is palpable but there is no visible movement.

• **Grade 0 (None):** Unable to palpate any contraction of the muscles or tendons.

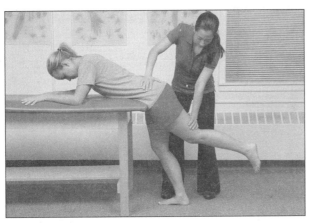

Figure 2-20 Proper positioning for modified hip extension grades 5–3. Source: Delmar/Cengage Learning

Modified Hip Extension Tests

When testing the hip extensor muscles with a patient with a hip flexion contracture, a modified position must be used for the testing of grades 5, 4, and 3. In this situation, the patient needs to stand and lean over the edge of the table to allow the patient to move against gravity through the available ROM by decreasing the influence of the hip flexion contracture.

POSITION OF PATIENT: Standing with torso prone on the table and the hips flexed. The nontest knee should be flexed to allow the test limb to begin resting on the floor, and the arms can hug the table for stability.

POSITION OF THERAPIST: Standing at the side of the test limb with the testing hand over the posterior thigh above the knee to provide resistance in a downward and forward motion. The stabilizing hand is placed over the pelvis laterally to maintain hip and pelvis posture (see Figure 2-20).

TEST: Patient extends hip through available ROM. Have the patient keep the testing limb straight to test all hip extensor muscles or have the knee bent to isolate the gluteus maximus muscle.

DIRECTIONS: Say to patient, "Lift your foot off the floor as high as you can, and don't let me push it down."

GRADING:

- **Grade 5 (Normal):** Patient extends the hip through available ROM and holds against therapist's maximum resistance without breaking.
- **Grade 4 (Good):** Patient extends the hip through available ROM and holds against therapist's strong to moderate resistance and then breaks.
- **Grade 3 (Fair):** Patient extends the hip through available ROM and holds at end range but no resistance is tolerated.

Modified Hip Extension Grades 2, 1, 0 (Poor, Trace, None)

Testing for patients with hip flexion contractures and weak extensors (less than grade 3) should not be done in the standing position. These tests should be done as described in the aggregate extensor muscle testing section for grades 2–0 or the isolated gluteus maximus testing.

Hip Abduction

Table 2-3 shows the primary and accessory muscles responsible for hip abduction. The gluteus medius (see Figure 2-21) and gluteus minimus (see Figure 2-22) are the primary movers for hip abduction.

TABLE 2-3	MUSCLES RESPONSIBLE FOR HIP ABDUCTION		
PRIMARY MUSCLES	**ORIGIN**	**INSERTION**	**INNERVATIONS**
Gluteus medius	Outer surface ilium	Lateral surface greater trochanter	Superior gluteal (L4, L5, S1)
Gluteus minimus	Lateral ilium	Anterior surface greater trochanter	Superior gluteal (L4, L5, S1)
ACCESSORY MUSCLES	**ORIGIN**	**INSERTION**	**INNERVATIONS**
Gluteus maximus	Posterior sacrum and ilium	Posterior femur distal to greater trochanter and iliotibial band	Inferior gluteal (L5, S1, S2)
Tensor fascia latae	ASIS	Lateral condyle tibia	Superior gluteal (L4, L5)
Obturator internus	Rami of pubis and ischium	Greater trochanter	Nerve to obturator internus
Gemellus superior	Ischium	Greater trochanter	Nerve to obturator internus
Gemellus inferior	Ischial tuberosity	Greater trochanter	Nerve to quadratus femoris
Sartorius	ASIS	Proximal medial aspect of tibia	Femoral (L2, L3)

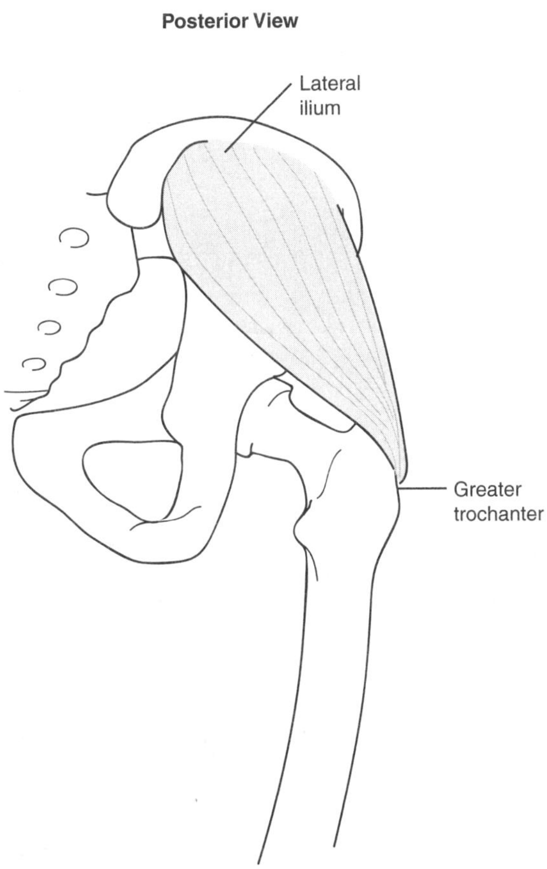

Posterior View

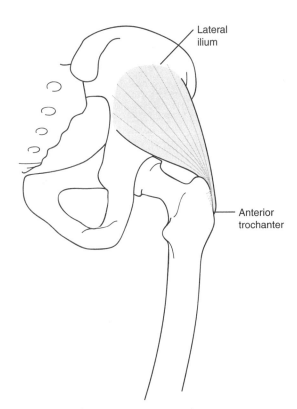

Lateral
ilium

Greater
trochanter

Figure 2-21 Gluteus medius muscle.

Source: Delmar/Cengage Learning

Posterior View

Lateral
ilium

Anterior
trochanter

Figure 2-22 Gluteus minimus muscle.

Source: Delmar/Cengage Learning

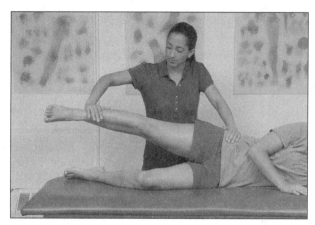

Figure 2-23 Proper positioning for hip abduction grades 5–3. Source: Delmar/Cengage Learning

Testing for Hip Abduction Grades 5, 4, 3 (Normal, Good, Fair) Gravity Resisted

POSITION OF PATIENT: Side-lying with bottom leg bent for stability. Top limb (test limb) straight and extended slightly beyond the midline with pelvis rotated slightly forward.

POSITION OF THERAPIST: Standing behind the patient with the test hand placed across the lateral surface of the knee applying resistance in a straight downward motion. The stabilizing hand is placed proximal to the greater trochanter of the femur to palpate the gluteus medius muscle (see Figure 2-23).

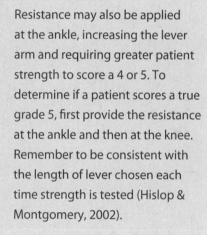

TIPS *of the* **Trade**

Resistance may also be applied at the ankle, increasing the lever arm and requiring greater patient strength to score a 4 or 5. To determine if a patient scores a true grade 5, first provide the resistance at the ankle and then at the knee. Remember to be consistent with the length of lever chosen each time strength is tested (Hislop & Montgomery, 2002).

TEST: Patient completes abduction through full available ROM. No hip flexion or rotation is visible.

DIRECTIONS: Say to patient, "Lift your leg up in the air and hold it. Do not let me push it down."

GRADING:

- **Grade 5 (Normal):** Patient abducts hip through available ROM and holds against therapist's maximum resistance without breaking.

- **Grade 4 (Good):** Patient abducts hip through available ROM and holds against therapist's strong to moderate resistance and then breaks.

- **Grade 3 (Fair):** Patient abducts hip through available ROM and holds at end range but no resistance is tolerated.

TIPS *of the* **Trade**

The hip has tremendous strength in its intrinsic muscles, often masking significant weakness in grade 4 with the abductor muscles. A good way to overcome this problem is to provide resistance at the ankle instead of the knee.

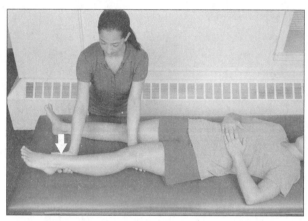

Figure 2-24 Proper positioning for hip abduction grade 2. Source: Delmar/Cengage Learning

Testing for Hip Abduction Grade 2 (Poor) Gravity Minimal

POSITION OF PATIENT: Supine.

POSITION OF THERAPIST: Standing next to the test limb with one hand under the ankle to slightly lift and support the test limb off the table. This hand should not provide assistance or resistance. It is used to decrease the friction from the table. This may not be necessary when using smooth surfaces. The other hand is placed just proximal to the greater trochanter of the femur to palpate the gluteus medius (see Figure 2-24).

TEST: Patient is to abduct the hip through full available ROM.

DIRECTIONS: Say to patient, "Bring your leg out to the side, while keeping the knee cap pointing toward the ceiling."

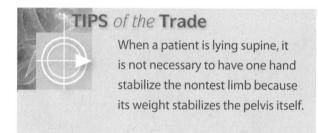

TIPS *of the* **Trade**

When a patient is lying supine, it is not necessary to have one hand stabilize the nontest limb because its weight stabilizes the pelvis itself.

GRADING:

- **Grade 2 (Poor):** Able to complete hip abduction through full ROM with gravity minimized.

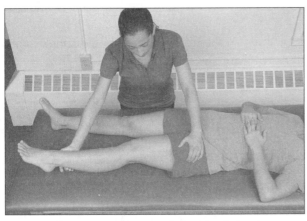

Figure 2-25 Proper positioning for hip abduction grades 1–0. Source: Delmar/Cengage Learning

Testing for Hip Abduction Grades 1, 0 (Trace, None) Gravity Minimal

POSITION OF PATIENT: Supine.

POSITION OF THERAPIST: Standing next to the test limb with one hand under the ankle for stability. The other hand is placed on the lateral aspect of the hip just proximal to the greater trochanter of the femur to palpate the gluteus medius (see Figure 2-25).

TEST: Patient tries to abduct the hip.

DIRECTIONS: Say to patient, "Try to bring your leg out to the side."

GRADING:

- **Grade 1 (Trace):** Tendon movement of gluteus medius is palpable but there is no visible movement.
- **Grade 0 (None):** Unable to palpate any contraction of the muscles or tendons.

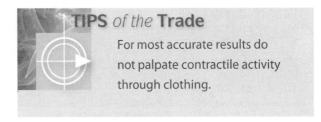

TIPS *of the* **Trade**

For most accurate results do not palpate contractile activity through clothing.

Hip Adduction

Table 2-4 lists the primary and accessory muscles responsible for hip adduction. The adductor magnus, adductor brevis, adductor longus, pectineus, and gracilis are the primary movers for hip adduction (see Figure 2-26).

TABLE 2-4	MUSCLES RESPONSIBLE FOR HIP ADDUCTION		
PRIMARY MUSCLES	**ORIGIN**	**INSERTION**	**INNERVATIONS**
Adductor magnus	Ischium and pubis	Entire linea aspera and adductor tubercle	Obturator and sciatic (L3, L4)
Adductor brevis	Pubis	Pectineal line and proximal linea aspera	Obturator (L3, L4)
Adductor longus	Pubis	Middle third of linea aspera	Obturator (L3, L4)
Pectineus	Superior ramus of pubis	Pectineal line of femur	Femoral (L2, L3, L4)
Gracilis	Pubis	Anterior middle surface of proximal end of tibia	Obturator (L2, L3)
ACCESSORY MUSCLES	**ORIGIN**	**INSERTION**	**INNERVATIONS**
Obturator externus	Rami of pubis and ischium	Trochanteric fossa	Obturator
Gluteus maximus	Posterior sacrum and ilium	Posterior femur distal to greater trochanter and iliotibial band	Inferior gluteal (L5, S1, S2)

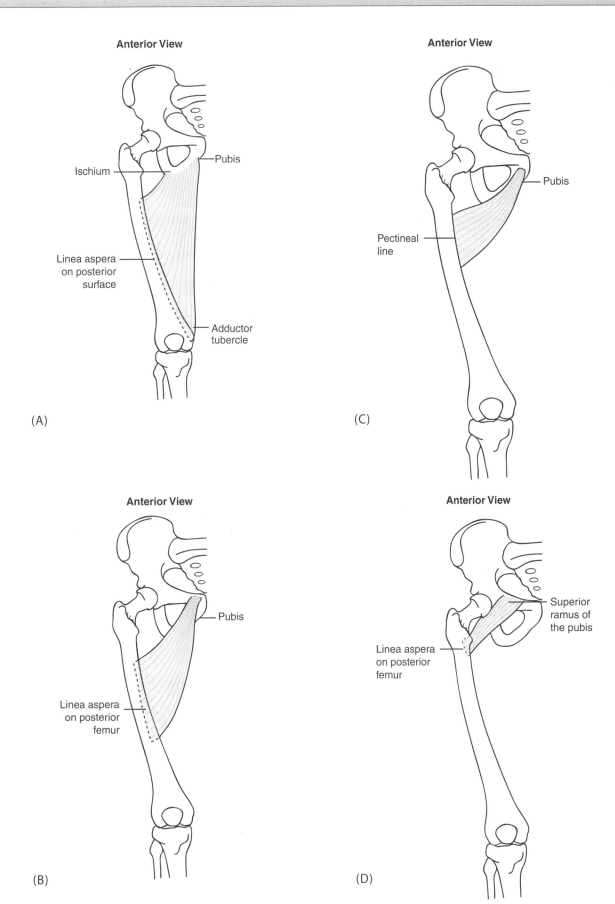

Anterior View

Ischium — — Pubis

Linea aspera on posterior surface

Adductor tubercle

(A)

Anterior View

— Pubis

Linea aspera on posterior femur

(B)

Anterior View

Pectineal line — — Pubis

(C)

Anterior View

Superior ramus of the pubis

Linea aspera on posterior femur

(D)

Figure 2-26 Adductor muscles: (A) Adductor magnus, (B) Adductor longus, (C) Adductor brevis, (D) Pectineus.

Source: Delmar/Cengage Learning

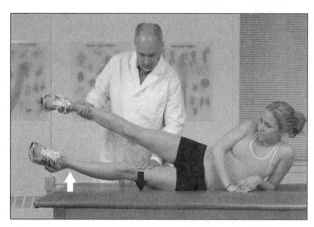

Figure 2-27 Proper positioning for hip adduction grades 5–3. Source: Delmar/Cengage Learning

Testing for Hip Adduction Grades 5, 4, 3 (Normal, Good, Fair) Gravity Resisted

POSITION OF PATIENT: Side-lying with top leg in 25° of abduction supported by the therapist and the test limb is resting on the table.

POSITION OF THERAPIST: Standing behind the patient cradling the top leg with the forearm and stabilizing hand supporting the medial surface of the knee. The testing hand is placed on the medial surface of the knee of bottom limb (test limb) and applies resistance straight down toward the table (see Figure 2-27).

TEST: Patient adducts hip bringing lower limb in contact with upper limb.

DIRECTIONS: Say to patient, "Lift your bottom leg up to the top one and hold it. Do not let me push it down."

GRADING:

- **Grade 5 (Normal):** Patient adducts the hip through available ROM and holds against therapist's maximum resistance without breaking.
- **Grade 4 (Good):** Patient adducts hip through available ROM and holds against therapist's strong to moderate resistance and then breaks.
- **Grade 3 (Fair):** Patient adducts hip through available ROM and holds at end range but no resistance is tolerated.

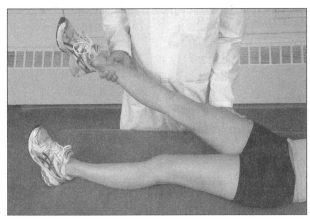

Figure 2-28 Proper positioning for hip adduction grade 2. Source: Delmar/Cengage Learning

Testing for Hip Adduction Grade 2 (Poor) Gravity Minimal

POSITION OF PATIENT: Supine with the nontest limb slightly abducted to decrease interference with the test limb when moving.

POSITION OF THERAPIST: Standing next to the test limb with one hand under the ankle to slightly lift and support the test limb off the table. This hand should not provide assistance or resistance. It is used to decrease the friction from the table. This may not be necessary when using smooth surfaces. The other hand is placed on the inside of the proximal thigh to palpate the adductor muscles (see Figure 2-28).

TEST: Patient is to adduct the hip through full available ROM without rotating the hip.

DIRECTIONS: Say to patient, "Bring your leg in toward the other one, while keeping the knee cap pointing up."

GRADING:

- **Grade 2 (Poor):** Able to complete hip adduction through full ROM with gravity minimized.

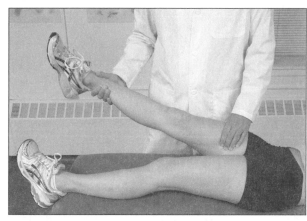

Figure 2-29 Proper positioning for hip adduction grades 1–0. Source: Delmar/Cengage Learning

Testing for Hip Adduction Grades 1, 0 (Trace, None) Gravity Minimal

POSITION OF PATIENT: Supine.

POSITION OF THERAPIST: Standing next to the test limb with one hand under the ankle for stability. The other hand is placed on the inside of the proximal thigh to palpate the adductor muscles (see Figure 2-29).

TEST: Patient tries to adduct the hip.

DIRECTIONS: Say to patient, "Try to bring your leg in."

GRADING:

• **Grade 1 (Trace):** Tendon movement of adductors is palpable but there is no visible movement.

• **Grade 0 (None):** Unable to palpate any contraction of the muscles or tendons.

Hip External Rotation

Table 2-5 highlights the primary and accessory muscles responsible for hip external rotation. The obturator externus, obturator internus, quadratus femoris, piriformis, gemellus superior, gemellus inferior, and gluteus maximus are the primary movers for hip external rotation (see Figure 2-30).

TABLE 2-5	MUSCLES RESPONSIBLE FOR HIP EXTERNAL ROTATION		
PRIMARY MUSCLES	**ORIGIN**	**INSERTION**	**INNERVATIONS**
Obturator externus	Rami of pubis and ischium	Trochanteric fossa	Obturator
Obturator internus	Rami of pubis and ischium	Greater trochanter	Nerve to obturator internus
Quadratus femoris	Ischial tuberosity	Intertrochanteric crest	Nerve to quadratus femoris
Piriformis	Sacrum	Greater trochanter	S1, S2
Gemellus superior	Ischium	Greater trochanter	Nerve to obturator internus
Gemellus inferior	Ischial tuberosity	Greater trochanter	Nerve to quadratus femoris
Gluteus maximus	Posterior sacrum and ilium	Posterior femur distal to greater trochanter and iliotibial band	Inferior gluteal (L5, S1, S2)
ACCESSORY MUSCLES	**ORIGIN**	**INSERTION**	**INNERVATIONS**
Sartorius	ASIS	Proximal medial aspect of tibia	Femoral (L2, L3)
Biceps femoris (long head)	Long head: ischial tuberosity	Fibular head	Sciatic (S1, S2, S3)
Gluteus medius (posterior)	Outer surface ilium	Lateral surface greater trochanter	Superior gluteal (L4, L5, S1)
Adductor magnus	Ischium and pubis	Linea aspera and adductor tubercle	Obturator and sciatic (L3, L4)
Adductor Longus	Pubis	Middle third of linea aspera	Obturator (L3, L4)
Popliteus (if the tibia is fixed)	Lateral condyle of femur	Posterior medial condyle of tibia	Tibial (L4-S1)

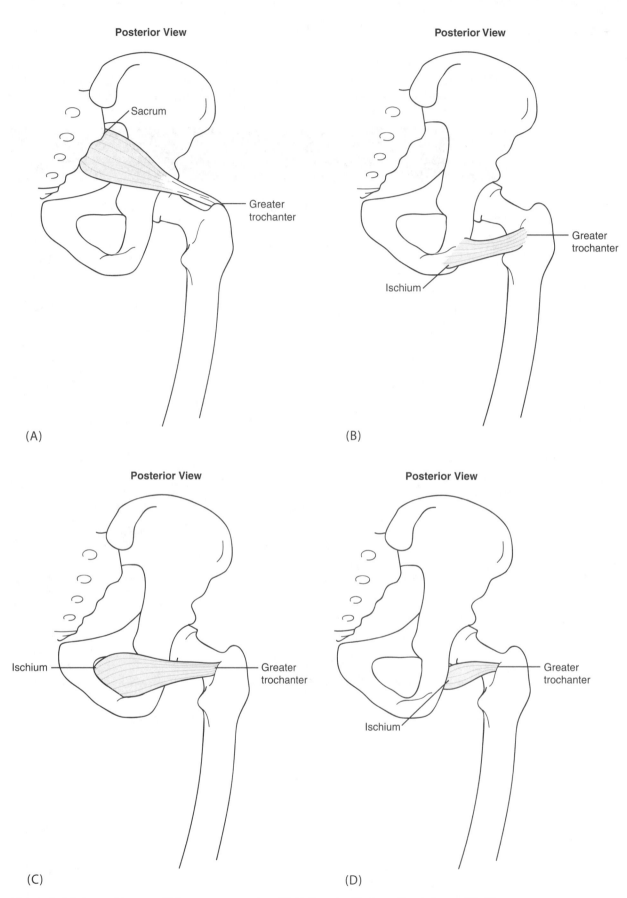

Figure 2-30 Lateral/external hip rotator muscles: (A) Piriformis, (B) Gemellus inferior, (C) Obturator internus, (D) Obturator externus, (E) Gemellus superior, (F) Quadratus femoris. Source: Delmar/Cengage Learning

Posterior View

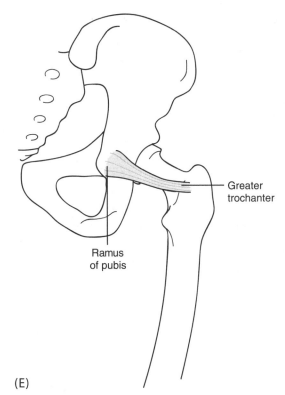

Greater
trochanter

Ramus
of pubis

(E)

Posterior View

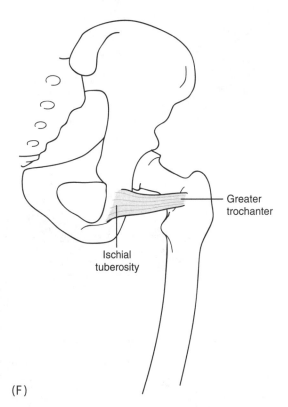

Greater
trochanter

Ischial
tuberosity

(F)

Figure 2-30 *(continued)*. Source: Delmar/Cengage Learning

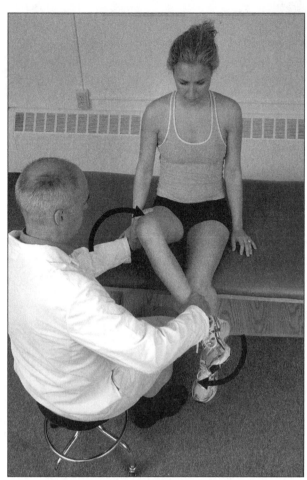

Figure 2-31 Proper positioning for hip external rotation grades 5–3. Source: Delmar/Cengage Learning

Testing for Hip External Rotation Grades 5, 4, 3 (Normal, Good, Fair) Gravity Resisted

POSITION OF PATIENT: Short sitting with hands at sides to support trunk.

TIPS *of the* **Trade**

To avoid adding visual distortion and contamination to the external rotation test results, do not allow a patient to abduct the test hip, increase flexion of the test knee, lift the opposite buttock off the table, or lean in any direction, thus lifting the pelvis off the table.

POSITION OF THERAPIST: Kneeling or on a low stool next to test limb. One hand placed around ankle just above the medial malleolus and applies resistance outward toward the ankle. The other hand is placed over the lateral thigh above the knee and offers counterpressure by providing resistance medially toward the knee. The two forces are applied together in counterdirections for this test (see Figure 2-31).

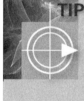

TIPS *of the* **Trade**

When testing a patient in short sitting, it is often helpful to place a towel roll under the knee to keep the knee in a horizontal plane.

TEST: Patient externally rotates the hip.

TIPS *of the* **Trade**

For this test, it may be easier for the therapist to place the limb in the end position instead of having the patient move it there.

DIRECTIONS: Say to patient, "Don't let me turn your leg out."

GRADING:

- **Grade 5 (Normal):** Patient holds at end range against therapist's maximum resistance without breaking.
- **Grade 4 (Good):** Patient holds at end range against therapist's strong to moderate resistance and then breaks.
- **Grade 3 (Fair):** Patient holds at end range but no resistance is tolerated.

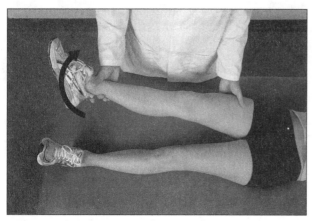

Figure 2-32 Proper positioning for hip external rotation grades 2–0. Source: Delmar/Cengage Learning

Testing for Hip External Rotation Grade 2 (Poor) Gravity Minimal

POSITION OF PATIENT: Supine with test limb in internal rotation.

POSITION OF THERAPIST: Standing next to the test limb with one hand at the lateral hip to maintain pelvic alignment (see Figure 2-32).

TEST: Patient is to externally rotate the hip through full available ROM.

DIRECTIONS: Say to patient, "Roll your leg out."

GRADING:

- **Grade 2 (Poor):** Able to complete external rotation of hip through full ROM. When rolling past midline, the therapist can provide a small amount of resistance to offset the help of gravity.

Testing for Hip External Rotation Grades 1, 0 (Trace, None) Gravity Minimal

POSITION OF PATIENT: Supine with test limb in internal rotation.

POSITION OF THERAPIST: Standing next to the test limb.

TEST: Patient tries to externally rotate the hip.

DIRECTIONS: Say to patient, "Try to roll your leg out."

GRADING:

- **Grades 1, 0 (Trace, None):** There is no way to palpate any of the external rotator muscles, except the gluteus maximus. Therefore, any visible contractile activity should be given a grade of 1. If unsure, a lesser grade should always be assigned. In this situation, a grade of 0 would be appropriate if no movement is discerned.

Hip Internal Rotation

Table 2-6 illustrates the primary and accessory muscles responsible for hip internal rotation. The gluteus minimus, tensor fascia latae, and gluteus medius are the primary movers for hip internal rotation (see Figures 2-21, 2-22, and 2-33).

TABLE 2-6	MUSCLES RESPONSIBLE FOR HIP INTERNAL ROTATION		
PRIMARY MUSCLES	**ORIGIN**	**INSERTION**	**INNERVATIONS**
Gluteus minimus (anterior fibers)	Lateral ilium	Anterior surface greater trochanter	Superior gluteal (L4, L5, S1)
Tensor fascia latae	ASIS	Lateral condyle tibia	Superior gluteal (L4, L5)
Gluteus medius (anterior fibers)	Outer surface ilium	Lateral surface greater trochanter	Superior gluteal (L4, L5, S1)
ACCESSORY MUSCLES	**ORIGIN**	**INSERTION**	**INNERVATIONS**
Semitendinosus	Ischial tuberosity	Anteromedial surface of proximal tibia	Sciatic (L5-S2)
Semimembranosus	Ischial tuberosity	Posterior surface of medial condyle of tibia	Sciatic (L5-S2)
Adductor magnus	Ischium and pubis	Entire linea aspera and adductor tubercle	Obturator and sciatic (L3, L4)
Adductor longus	Pubis	Middle third of linea aspera	Obturator (L3, L4)

Anterior View

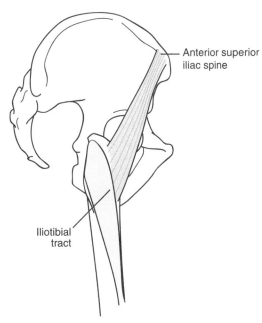

Anterior superior iliac spine

Iliotibial tract

Figure 2-33 Tensor fascia latae muscle. Source: Delmar/Cengage Learning

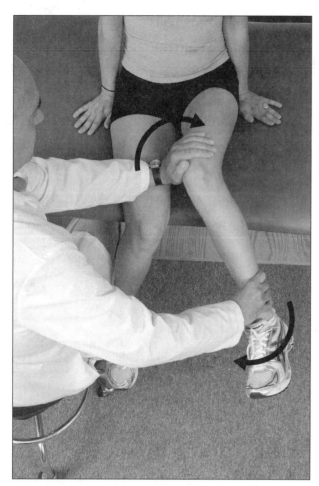

Figure 2-34 Proper positioning for hip internal rotation grades 5–3. Source: Delmar/Cengage Learning

Testing for Hip Internal Rotation Grades 5, 4, 3 (Normal, Good, Fair) Gravity Resisted

POSITION OF PATIENT: Short sitting with hands at sides to support trunk.

TIPS *of the* **Trade**

When testing a patient in short sitting position, it is often helpful to place a towel roll under the knee to keep the knee in a horizontal plane.

POSITION OF THERAPIST: Kneeling or sitting in front of patient. One hand placed around ankle just above the lateral malleolus and applies resistance inward toward the ankle. The other hand is placed over the medial thigh above the knee and offers counterpressure by providing resistance laterally toward the knee (see Figure 2-34). As with external rotation, the two forces are applied together in counterdirections.

TEST: For this test, best results are seen when the therapist places the limb in the end position instead of having the patient move it there. When short sitting, make sure the patient does not lift the pelvis off the mat on the test limb side. This can assist in internal rotation.

DIRECTIONS: Say to patient, "Don't let me move your leg in."

GRADING:

- **Grade 5 (Normal):** Patient holds at end range against therapist's maximum resistance without breaking.
- **Grade 4 (Good):** Patient holds at end range against therapist's strong to moderate resistance and then breaks.
- **Grade 3 (Fair):** Patient holds at end range but no resistance is tolerated.

TIPS *of the* **Trade**

To avoid contaminating the test results, make sure the patient avoids hip extension, hip adduction, or knee extension of the test limb.

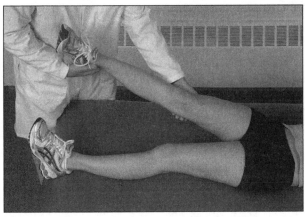

Figure 2-35 Proper positioning for hip internal rotation grades 2–0. Source: Delmar/Cengage Learning

Testing for Hip Internal Rotation Grade 2 (Poor) Gravity Minimal

POSITION OF PATIENT: Supine with test limb partially externally rotated.

POSITION OF THERAPIST: Standing next to the test limb with one hand over the anterolateral hip below the ASIS to palpate the tensor fascia latae. The other hand is placed proximal to the greater trochanter to palpate the gluteus medius (see Figure 2-35).

TEST: Patient is to internally rotate the hip through full available ROM.

DIRECTIONS: Say to patient, "Roll your leg in."

GRADING:

- **Grade 2 (Poor):** Able to complete internal rotation of hip through full ROM. When rolling past midline, the therapist can provide a small amount of resistance to offset the help of gravity.

Testing for Hip Internal Rotation Grades 1, 0 (Trace, None) Gravity Minimal

POSITION OF PATIENT: Supine with test limb in external rotation.

POSITION OF THERAPIST: Standing next to the test limb with one hand palpating the gluteus medius and the other the tensor fascia latae, as described previously.

TEST: Patient tries to internally rotate the hip.

DIRECTIONS: Say to patient, "Try to roll your leg in."

GRADING:

- **Grade 1 (Trace):** Able to palpate contractile activity in either or both muscles.
- **Grade 0 (None):** Unable to palpate any contraction of the muscles or tendons.

Combination Movement: Hip Flexion, Abduction, and External Rotation with Knee Flexion

The sartorius muscle is the primary mover for the combination movement of hip flexion, abduction, and external rotation with knee flexion (see Table 2-7 and Figure 2-36).

TABLE 2-7	MUSCLE RESPONSIBLE FOR COMBINATION MOVEMENT		
PRIMARY MUSCLE	**ORIGIN**	**INSERTION**	**INNERVATIONS**
Sartorius	ASIS	Tibia: proximal medial surface	Femoral (L2, L3)

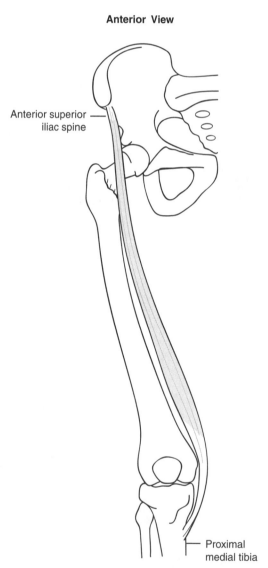

Anterior View

Anterior superior iliac spine

Proximal medial tibia

Figure 2-36 Sartorius muscle. Source: Delmar/Cengage Learning

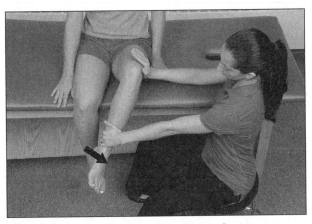

Figure 2-37 Proper positioning for hip flexion, abduction, and external rotation grades 5–3.

Source: Delmar/Cengage Learning

Testing for Combination Movement Grades 5, 4, 3 (Normal, Good, Fair) Gravity Resisted

POSITION OF PATIENT: Short sitting with hands at sides to support trunk and thighs supported by the table.

POSITION OF THERAPIST: Standing on the side of the test limb with one hand on the lateral knee providing resistance in a down and inward direction against flexion and abduction. The other hand is placed on the inside ankle around the medial malleolus and provides resistance in an up and outward motion against hip external rotation (see Figure 2-37).

TEST: With a flexed knee, patient brings hip into hip flexion while abducting and externally rotating hip.

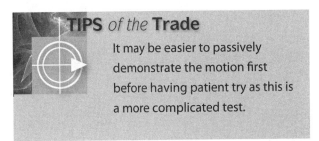

TIPS *of the* **Trade**

It may be easier to passively demonstrate the motion first before having patient try as this is a more complicated test.

DIRECTIONS: Say to patient, "Slide your heel up the shin of your other leg. Hold it and don't let me pull you out of this position."

GRADING:

- **Grade 5 (Normal):** Patient holds at end range against therapist's maximum resistance without breaking.
- **Grade 4 (Good):** Patient holds at end range against therapist's strong to moderate resistance and then breaks.
- **Grade 3 (Fair):** Patient holds at end range but no resistance is tolerated.

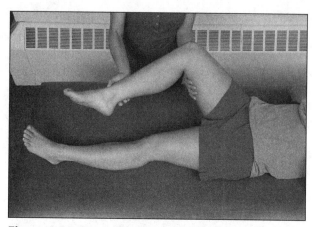

Figure 2-38 Proper positioning for hip flexion, abduction, and external rotation grade 2.

Source: Delmar/Cengage Learning

Testing for Combination Movement Grade 2 (Poor) Gravity Minimal

POSITION OF PATIENT: Supine with heel of test limb on contralateral shin.

POSITION OF THERAPIST: Standing next to the test limb supporting test limb to keep position as needed (see Figure 2-38).

TEST: Patient is to slide heel of test limb up contralateral shin to the knee.

DIRECTIONS: Say to patient, "Slide your heel up your shin to your knee."

GRADING:

- **Grade 2 (Poor):** Able to complete movement through full ROM.

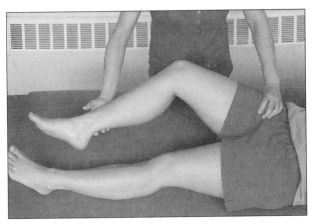

Figure 2-39 Proper positioning for hip flexion, abduction, and external rotation grades 1–0.

Source: Delmar/Cengage Learning

Testing for Combination Movement Grades 1, 0 (Trace, None) Gravity Minimal

POSITION OF PATIENT: Supine

POSITION OF THERAPIST: Standing next to the test limb with one hand cradling leg with hand under knee. Other hand palpates the sartorius muscle on the medial side of the thigh where it crosses the femur or near the muscle origin by the ASIS (see Figure 2-39).

TEST: Patient tries to slide heel up shin to knee.

DIRECTIONS: Say to patient, "Try to slide your heel up your shin."

GRADING:

- **Grade 1 (Trace):** Slight contraction of muscle is detected but no visible movement.
- **Grade 0 (None):** Unable to palpate any contraction of the muscles or tendons.

Substitutions

Important substitutions to watch for during manual muscle testing (MMT) of the hip are as follows:

- If hip external rotation and abduction are seen with hip flexion, the sartorius muscle is being used.

- If hip internal rotation and adduction are seen with hip flexion in the seated position, the tensor fascia latae muscle is being used. However, this is not the case when the patient is tested in supine due to gravity causing the limb to externally rotate.

- During abduction, a patient may try to externally rotate the hip during the movement to allow the oblique action of the hip flexors to substitute for the gluteus medius.

- The tensor fascia latae may be performing abduction if the patient is allowed to begin the test with active hip flexion or the hip partially flexed.

- By using a posterior pelvic tilt to internally rotate the hip, a patient may be substituting the hip flexors for weak adductors. The patient looks as if trying to move into a supine position from side-lying. This is why it is important to maintain a true side-lying position when testing adduction.

- By using an anterior pelvic tilt to externally rotate the hips, a patient may be substituting the hamstrings for weak adductors. This patient looks as if trying to move prone.

- When completing the combination of hip flexion, abduction, and external rotation, a substitution of the iliopsoas or rectus femoris muscle will result in pure hip flexion without the other movements.

RANGE OF MOTION

This section discusses the proper way to measure ROM for the six motions at the hip.

Hip Flexion

Hip flexion occurs in the sagittal plane around the medial-lateral axis. As previously mentioned, the primary muscles involved are the iliopsoas and rectus femoris. According to the American Academy of Orthopaedic Surgeons (1965), normal active range of motion (AROM) for hip flexion is 0°–120°. The end-feel for hip flexion should be soft due to the soft tissue contact between the anterior thigh and the lower abdominals. The proper positioning to measure hip flexion is described next.

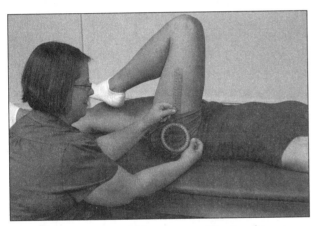

Figure 2-40 Proper goniometer positioning for hip flexion. Source: Delmar/Cengage Learning

POSITION OF PATIENT: Supine with legs extended straight and hip in neutral. As the patient brings the knee into the chest to measure, the knee is permitted to flex so the hamstring tension does not restrict the hip flexion motion.

POSITION OF THERAPIST: Sitting on a stool next to patient by test limb. One hand stabilizes the pelvis to prevent posterior tilting or rotation, and the other maintains hip flexion by pushing on the distal femur.

POSITION OF GONIOMETER:

- **Fulcrum:** Over the greater trochanter (see Figure 2-40)
- **Stationary arm:** Lateral midline of the pelvis up along the side of the trunk
- **Movable arm:** Lateral midline of the femur toward the lateral epicondyle

Hip Extension

Hip extension also occurs in the sagittal plane around the medial-lateral axis. As previously mentioned, the primary muscles involved are the semimembranosus, semitendinosus, biceps femoris, and gluteus maximus. According to the American Academy of Orthopaedic Surgeons (1965), normal AROM for hip extension is 0°–20°. A firm end-feel is expected due to the tension in the hip's anterior joint capsule and the surrounding ligaments.

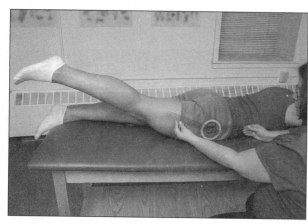

Figure 2-41 Proper goniometer positioning for hip extension. Source: Delmar/Cengage Learning

POSITION OF PATIENT: Prone with the hips in neutral position and flat against the mat. The knee is kept straight as the patient lifts the leg up toward the ceiling. This prevents tension from the rectus femoris muscle from restricting hip extension. It is best not to use a pillow under the patient's head.

POSITION OF THERAPIST: Sitting on a stool next to patient by test limb. One hand stabilizes the pelvis to prevent anterior tilting or rotation, and the other hand supports the distal femur.

POSITION OF GONIOMETER:

- **Fulcrum:** Over the greater trochanter (see Figure 2-41)

- **Stationary arm:** Lateral midline of the pelvis up along the side of the trunk

- **Movable arm:** Lateral midline of the femur toward the lateral epicondyle

Hip Abduction

Hip abduction occurs in the frontal plane around the anterior-posterior axis. As previously mentioned, the primary muscles involved are the gluteus minimus and medius. According to the American Academy of Orthopaedic Surgeons (1965), normal AROM for hip abduction is 0°–45°. A firm end-feel is expected due to the tension in the hip's medial joint capsule, the surrounding ligaments, and the tension in the muscles that perform adduction.

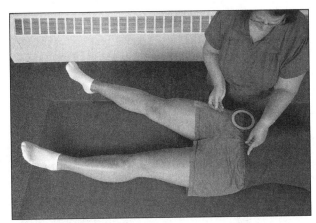

Figure 2-42 Proper goniometer positioning for hip abduction. Source: Delmar/Cengage Learning

POSITION OF PATIENT: Supine with the hip in neutral and the knee extended. The knee is kept straight as patient moves the leg out to the side.

POSITION OF THERAPIST: Sitting on a stool next to patient by test limb. One hand stabilizes the pelvis to prevent lateral tilting or rotation. The other hand cups the back of the ankle to guide the lower extremity into abduction while preventing lateral tilting of the pelvis.

POSITION OF GONIOMETER:

- **Fulcrum:** Over the ASIS of test limb (see Figure 2-42)
- **Stationary arm:** Pointing toward the ASIS of nontest limb
- **Movable arm:** Down the middle of the femur with the patella for a reference point

Hip Adduction

Hip adduction also occurs in the frontal plane around the anterior-posterior axis. As previously mentioned, the primary muscles involved are the adductor longus, brevis, and magnus as well as the pectineus and gracilis. According to the American Academy of Orthopaedic Surgeons (1965), normal AROM for hip adduction is 0°–30°. A firm end-feel is expected due to the tension in the hip's lateral joint capsule, the superior band of the iliofemoral ligament, and the tension in the muscles that perform abduction.

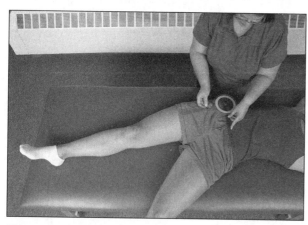

Figure 2-43 Proper goniometer positioning for hip adduction. Source: Delmar/Cengage Learning

POSITION OF PATIENT: Supine with the hip in neutral and the knee extended. The knee is kept straight as patient moves the leg out to the side. The **contralateral** hip is abducted to allow the test limb to complete full range of motion.

POSITION OF THERAPIST: Sitting on a stool next to patient by test limb. One hand stabilizes the pelvis to prevent lateral tilting or rotation. The other hand cups the back of the ankle to guide the lower extremity into adduction while preventing lateral tilting of the pelvis.

POSITION OF GONIOMETER:

- **Fulcrum:** Over the ASIS of test limb (see Figure 2-43)
- **Stationary arm:** Pointing toward the ASIS of nontest limb
- **Movable arm:** Down the middle of the femur with the patella for a reference point

Hip Medial/Internal Rotation

Hip internal rotation occurs in the transverse plane around a vertical axis. As previously mentioned, the primary muscles involved are the gluteus medius, gluteus minimus, and tensor fascia latae. According to the American Academy of Orthopaedic Surgeons (1965), normal AROM for hip internal rotation is 0°–45°. A firm end-feel is expected due to the tension in the hip's posterior joint capsule, the ischiofemoral ligament, and the tension in the muscles that perform lateral rotation.

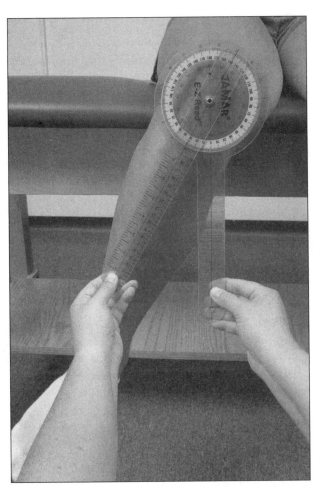

Figure 2-44 Proper goniometer positioning for hip internal rotation. Source: Delmar/Cengage Learning

POSITION OF PATIENT: Short sitting with hips and knees at 90° and hands at side for support. The hips are also in neutral alignment.

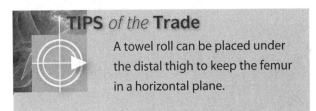

TIPS *of the* **Trade**

A towel roll can be placed under the distal thigh to keep the femur in a horizontal plane.

POSITION OF THERAPIST: Sitting on a stool next to patient by test limb. One hand stabilizes the distal end of the femur on the lateral side to prevent the hip from any adduction or flexion greater than 90°. The other hand is contoured behind the ankle to move it out to the side as the hip internally rotates.

POSITION OF GONIOMETER:

- **Fulcrum:** Middle of the patella (see Figure 2-44)
- **Stationary arm:** Perpendicular to the floor and hangs freely once test limb moves
- **Movable arm:** Crest of the tibia with a reference point between the two malleoli

Hip Lateral/External Rotation

Hip external rotation also occurs in the transverse plane around a vertical axis. As previously mentioned, the primary muscles involved are the deep rotators and the gluteus maximus. According to the American Academy of Orthopaedic Surgeons (1965), normal AROM for hip external rotation is 0°–45°. A firm end-feel is expected due to the tension in the hip's anterior joint capsule, the surrounding ligaments, and the tension in the muscles that perform adduction and internal rotation.

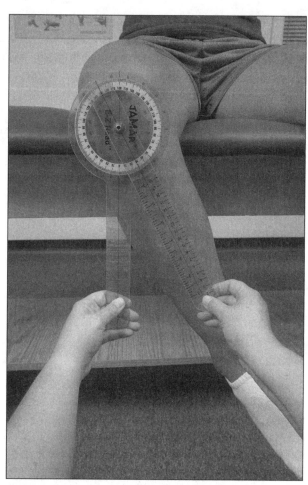

Figure 2-45 Proper goniometer positioning for hip external rotation. Source: Delmar/Cengage Learning

POSITION OF PATIENT: Short sitting with hips and knees at 90° and hands at side for support. The hips are also in neutral alignment. The contralateral knee should be flexed to provide enough room for the test limb to complete full ROM.

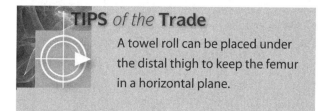

TIPS *of the* **Trade**

A towel roll can be placed under the distal thigh to keep the femur in a horizontal plane.

POSITION OF THERAPIST: Sitting on a stool next to patient by test limb. One hand stabilizes the distal end of the femur on the lateral side to prevent the hip from any abduction or flexion greater than 90°. The other hand is contoured behind the ankle to move it in as the hip externally rotates.

POSITION OF GONIOMETER:

- **Fulcrum:** Middle of the patella (see Figure 2-45)
- **Stationary arm:** Perpendicular to the floor and hangs freely once test limb moves
- **Movable arm:** Crest of the tibia with a reference point between the two malleoli

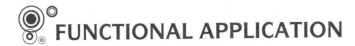

FUNCTIONAL APPLICATION

Normal strength and ROM of the hip joint are necessary for completing many of the functional tasks performed every day, such as walking, climbing stairs, and performing activities that require sitting and bending. Simply walking from one place to the other on level surfaces requires that the hip joint must have 30° of hip flexion, 10° of hip extension, and 5° of hip abduction, adduction, and internal and external rotation, according to the *Observational Gait Analysis Handbook* of the Professional Staff Association, Rancho Los Amigos Medical Center (1989). Livingston, Stevenson, and Olney (1991) studied stair ambulation and found that a person needs 1° of hip extension and 66° of hip flexion for ambulating up stairs and 1° of hip extension and 45° of hip flexion to ambulate down stairs. To sit comfortably, a person needs at least 90° of hip flexion. Simple tasks like getting up from a chair, putting on pants or socks, or tying shoes requires hip flexion greater than 90° (Norkin & White, 1995). These are only a few examples of the main functional tasks that require good hip strength and ROM. It is easy to see how limitations or deficits in either can result in the disruption of normal living.

LEARNER CHALLENGE

1. List all the hip motions and identify the plane and axis in which they occur.
2. Palpate the following hip landmarks: ASIS, PSIS, ischial tuberosity, greater trochanter, and sacrum.
3. To practice manual muscle testing (MMT), one lab partner acts as the therapist and performs MMT of hip flexion, hip adduction, and hip internal rotation grades 5–0. Then switch roles and the other lab partner performs MMT for hip extension, hip abduction, and hip external rotation grades 5–0.
4. Using a goniometer, measure ROM on your lab partner for hip flexion, hip abduction, and hip external rotation. Switch roles and have the other partner use the goniometer to measure hip extension, hip adduction, and hip internal rotation. Double-check for proper goniometer placement and compare your findings to normal ROM for each movement.
5. Fill in the following tables summarizing MMT and ROM measurements of the hip.

A) Manual Muscle Testing for Grades 5, 4, 3 Gravity Resisted			
MOTION	**TESTING POSITION**	**STABILIZING HAND**	**RESISTANCE HAND**
Hip Flexion			
Hip Extension General			
Isolation of Gluteus Maximus			

continues

A) Manual Muscle Testing for Grades 5, 4, 3 Gravity Resisted *(continued)*

MOTION	TESTING POSITION	STABILIZING HAND	RESISTANCE HAND
Modified Hip Extension			
Hip Abduction			
Hip Adduction			
Hip Internal Rotation			
Hip External Rotation			
Hip Combination Movement			

B) Manual Muscle Testing for Grades 2, 1, 0 Gravity Minimal

MOTION	TESTING POSITION	STABILIZING HAND	RESISTANCE HAND	PALPATION
Hip Flexion				
Hip Extension General				
Isolation of Gluteus Maximus				
Hip Abduction				
Hip Adduction				

continues

B) Manual Muscle Testing for Grades 2, 1, 0 Gravity Minimal *(continued)*

MOTION	TESTING POSITION	STABILIZING HAND	RESISTANCE HAND	PALPATION
Hip Internal Rotation				
Hip External Rotation				

C) Range of Motion

MOTION	MOVABLE ARM	STATIONARY ARM	FULCRUM	NORMAL ROM
Hip Flexion				
Hip Extension				
Hip Abduction				
Hip Adduction				
Hip Internal Rotation				
Hip External Rotation				

NOTES

THE KNEE

3

OBJECTIVES

Upon completion of this chapter, the reader will be able to:

- Describe the joints that make up the knee.

- Identify the bones and bony landmarks significant to the knee.

- Name the major ligaments of the knee and their purpose.

- Identify any supporting structures important to the knee.

- Describe the major motions of the knee and name the muscles that perform them.

- Become familiar with the origins, insertions, and innervations of the muscles of the knee.

- Perform proper manual muscle testing on the major muscles of the knee grades 5–0.

- Be aware of possible substitutions during manual muscle testing on the knee.

- Accurately perform range of motion testing using the goniometer on the knee joint.

MUSCULOSKELETAL OVERVIEW

The knee endures tremendous stress and strain. Whatever one's lifestyle or career, the knee undergoes constant stress. The more physical the lifestyle, the greater the stress. In addition, the knee is supported entirely by muscles and ligaments. There is no bony stability to support this joint. Given those factors, it is easy to see why the knee is the most commonly injured joint in the body.

Joints

The knee is comprised of two joints: the patellofemoral joint and the tibiofemoral joint. The patellofemoral joint consists of the articulation between the patella and the distal end of the femur. The smooth posterior of the patella glides over the patellar surface of the femur. The tibiofemoral joint includes the articulation between the lateral and medial condyles of the distal femur and the C-shaped menisci of the proximal tibia. The femoral condyles and the tibial plateaus are surrounded by the joint capsule, thus providing stability to the knee. The joint capsule also distributes synovial fluid to lubricate the articulating surfaces of the knee during movement.

The knee is categorized as a synovial **hinge joint,** making flexion and extension the main motions it performs. However, it is not a true hinge joint like the elbow because a small amount of rotation occurs when the knee is partially flexed. This rotation is possible because the femoral medial condyle's articular surface is longer than the lateral condyle's articular surface. When the knee is fully extended, rotation is limited by resistance from the ligaments and menisci in the knee. The capsular pattern of the knee is flexion limited more than extension.

Bones

The bones making up the knee joint are the distal end of the femur, the proximal end of the tibia, and the patella. The femur, or thigh bone, is the largest, longest, and strongest bone in the body. The tibia, the second strongest bone, receives the weight of the body from the femur and transmits it to the foot. The patella is found within the quadriceps tendon. It is categorized as a **sesamoid bone,** triangular in shape with the superior aspect broader than the pointier distal aspect. Its main functions are to guard the knee anteriorly and to act as a pulley, giving the quadriceps a mechanical advantage. The patella is susceptible to cumulative trauma secondary to the repetitive stresses placed on it daily, making it a common spot for pain and injury. The small sticklike bone lateral to the tibia is the fibula. It is not technically part of the knee joint because it does not articulate with the tibia. However, it serves as an attachment point for important muscles of the knee. The following sections detail bony landmarks significant to the knee on the femur (see Figure 3-1) and the tibia (see Figure 3-2).

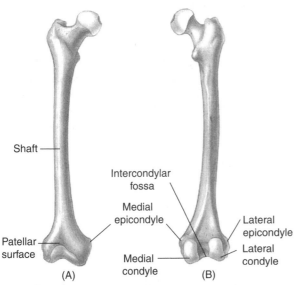

Shaft

Intercondylar
fossa

Medial
epicondyle

Lateral
epicondyle

Patellar
surface

Lateral
condyle

Medial
condyle

(A)   (B)

Figure 3-1 Femur: (A) Anterior view, (B) Posterior view.

Source: Delmar/Cengage Learning

Femur

- **Medial condyle:** Distal medial end of femur
- **Lateral condyle:** Distal lateral end of femur
- **Medial epicondyle:** Protuberance proximal to the medial condyle of the femur
- **Lateral epicondyle:** Protuberance proximal to the lateral condyle of the femur
- **Intercondylar fossa:** Deep U-shaped space located posteriorly on the femur between the medial and lateral condyles
- **Patellar surface:** The area of the femur that articulates with the posterior surface of the patella located anteriorly between the medial and lateral condyle

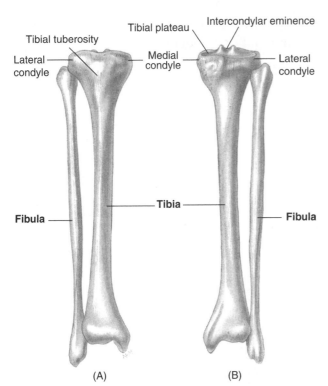

Tibial tuberosity

Tibial plateau

Intercondylar eminence

Lateral
condyle

Medial
condyle

Lateral
condyle

Tibia

Fibula   Fibula

(A)   (B)

Figure 3-2 Tibia: (A) Anterior view, (B) Posterior view.

Source: Delmar/Cengage Learning

Tibia

- **Medial condyle:** The proximal medial end of the tibia
- **Lateral condyle:** The proximal lateral end of the tibia
- **Tibial plateau:** The larger proximal end of the tibia, including the medial condyles, lateral condyles, and intercondylar eminence
- **Intercondylar eminence:** Double-pointed protrusion that extends into the intercondylar fossa of the femur and is found at the midpoint of the tibia on the proximal surface
- **Tibial tuberosity:** Enlarged protrusion on the anterior surface of the proximal end of the tibia midline

Ligaments

As previously mentioned, the stability of the knee is provided by the ligamentous structures of the knee, not by the bones. There are two sets of these ligaments: the cruciate ligaments and the collateral ligaments (see Figure 3-3). The cruciate ligaments consist of the anterior cruciate ligament (ACL) and the posterior cruciate ligament (PCL). Because these ligaments are located inside the joint capsule, they are categorized as intracapsular ligaments. The ACL extends from the anterior tibia to the posterior femur, and the PCL extends from the posterior tibia to anterior femur. The purpose of the cruciate ligaments is to stabilize the knee in the sagittal and rotational planes, preventing anterior-posterior and rotational movements. The ACL is the most commonly injured ligament, and its primary function is to prevent anterior translation of the tibia on the femur or posterior translation of the femur on the tibia when the knee is partially flexed. By tightening during extension, the ACL also helps prevent hyperextension of the knee joint. Of the two cruciate ligaments, the PCL is stronger and injured less often. Its primary purpose is to prevent posterior displacement of the tibia on the femur and to help prevent hyperextension. The ACL and PCL work together to resist rotational movements of the knee.

The collateral ligaments consist of the medial or tibial collateral and the lateral or fibular collateral ligaments. These ligaments are categorized as extracapsular because they are located outside the joint capsule. These ligaments are located on the sides of the knees and provide resistance against **varus** and **valgus** stresses in the frontal plane as well as rotation. The lateral collateral ligament (LCL) is strong and cordlike. It attaches at the lateral condyle of the femur and goes down to the head of the fibula. The LCL is more rigid during internal rotation and protects the knee from stresses to the medial aspect of the knee. If there is an excessive force to the medial knee, this ligament provides lateral stability. There is no attachment to the lateral meniscus, and it is not commonly injured.

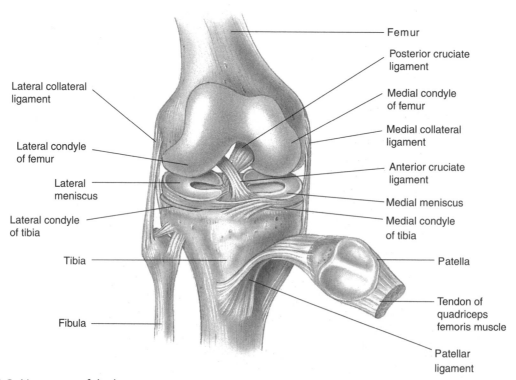

Figure 3-3 Ligaments of the knee. Source: Delmar/Cengage Learning

On the other hand, the MCL is weaker than the LCL and consists of a flat wide ligament that is attached to the medial condyles of the femur and tibia. A part of the MCL is connected to the medial meniscus, which means excessive stresses to the MCL often result in frequent tearing of the medial meniscus. The MCL is more rigid during internal rotation and protects the knee from excessive blows to the lateral side of the knee. MCL injuries are far more common than LCL injuries.

Supporting Structures

Besides ligaments and bones, other important structures contribute to the smooth functioning of the knee joint. These are the menisci and bursa. Each knee contains two half-moon, wedge-shaped fibrocartilage disks called *menisci*. They are found on the superior surface of the tibia and attach only to its outer margins. An important function of the meniscus is to deepen the fairly flat joint surfaces of the tibia. These disks also help to absorb shock and to prevent side-to-side rocking of the femur on the tibia (see Figure 3-4).

Bursae are sacs filled with synovial fluid that help reduce friction between the multiple tendons and bony areas of the knee. They blend with the joint capsule and are a common source of pain and inflammation.

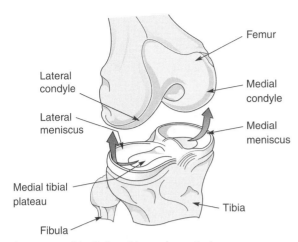

Figure 3-4 Medial and lateral menisci.

Source: Delmar/Cengage Learning

MUSCLE TESTING OF THE KNEE

As previously mentioned, the motions at the knee are flexion and extension. Although some rotation does occur, it is not under voluntary control so it is not significant enough to perform the MMT or break test. Because it is important to review the muscles associated with the movement, each section starts with a table of the muscles responsible for the movement being tested, followed by a drawing of the primary muscles.

Knee Flexion

Table 3-1 describes the primary and accessory muscles responsible for knee flexion. The biceps femoris, semitendinosus, and semimembranosus muscles are the primary movers for knee flexion (see Figure 3-5).

TABLE 3-1	MUSCLES RESPONSIBLE FOR KNEE FLEXION		
PRIMARY MUSCLES	**ORIGIN**	**INSERTION**	**INNERVATIONS**
Biceps femoris long head	Ischial tuberosity	Fibular head	Sciatic (L5-S2)
Biceps femoris short head	Lateral lip of linea aspera	Fibular head	Common peroneal (L5-S2)
Semitendinosus	Ischial tuberosity	Anteromedial surface of proximal tibia	Sciatic (L5-S2)
Semimembranosus	Ischial tuberosity	Posterior surface of medial condyle of tibia	Sciatic (L5-S2)
ACCESSORY MUSCLES	**ORIGIN**	**INSERTION**	**INNERVATIONS**
Gracilis	Pubis	Anterior medial surface of proximal tibia	Obturator and sciatic (L3, L4)
Tensor fascia latae (> 30° flex)	ASIS	Lateral condyle of tibia	Superior gluteal (L4, L5)
Sartorius	ASIS	Proximal medial aspect of tibia	Femoral (L2, L3)
Popliteus	Lateral condyle of femur	Posterior medial condyle of tibia	Tibial (L4-S1)
Gastrocnemius	Medial and lateral condyles of femur	Posterior of calcaneus	Tibial (S1, S2)
Plantaris	Posterior lateral condyle of femur	Posterior of calcaneus	Tibial (L4-S1)

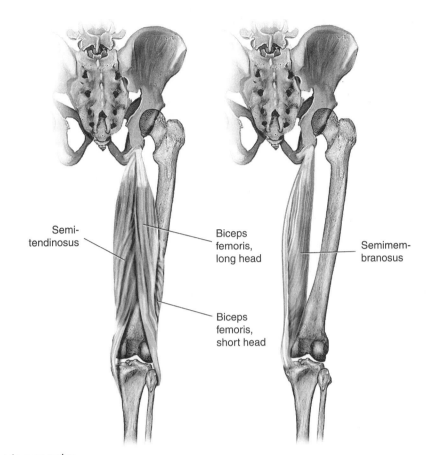

Figure 3-5 Hamstring muscles. Source: Delmar/Cengage Learning

Semi-
tendinosus

Biceps
femoris,
long head

Biceps
femoris,
short head

Semimem-
branosus

For any patient, the therapist should perform a general test evaluating the strength of the hamstring muscles together. If any asymmetry is noted, the therapist can isolate the hamstrings by testing the medial and lateral muscles separately to find the exact weakness. Asymmetry is present if lower extremity internal or external rotation is seen during knee flexion. If the leg externally rotates, the biceps femoris is stronger. Conversely, if the leg internally rotates, the medial muscles (semimembranosus and semitendinosus) are stronger. The strength testing of the medial and lateral hamstrings for grades 5–3 gravity resisted is similar to the general testing of the hamstrings with a few minor differences. The following information covers all three tests.

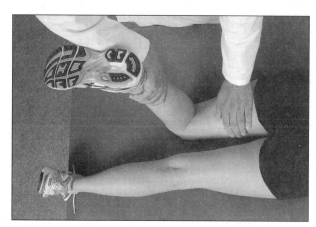

Figure 3-6 Proper positioning for knee flexion general hamstring muscle test grades 5–3. Source: Delmar/Cengage Learning

Testing for Knee Flexion General Hamstring Grades 5, 4, 3 (Normal, Good, Fair) Gravity Resisted

POSITION OF PATIENT: Prone with 45° knee flexion.

POSITION OF THERAPIST: Standing next to test limb. Testing hand is contoured around leg above the ankle (see Figure 3-6). This hand provides resistance in a downward motion in the direction of knee extension. The stabilizing hand is on the posterior thigh for support.

TEST: Patient is to flex the knee without allowing any rotation of the lower extremity.

DIRECTIONS: Say to the patient "Bend your knee and hold it there. Don't let me pull it straight."

GRADING:

- **Grade 3 (Fair):** Patient flexes the knee but no resistance is tolerated. It is important to watch for a tight rectus femoris because this can limit knee ROM. Hip flexion at the end of knee flexion is a good indication tightness is present.

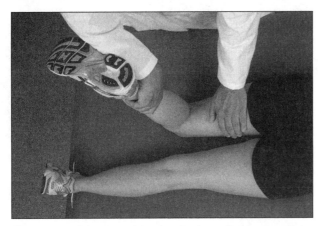

Figure 3-7 Proper positioning for knee flexion medial hamstring muscle test grades 5–3. Source: Delmar/Cengage Learning

Testing for Knee Flexion Medial Hamstring Grades 5, 4, 3 (Normal, Good, Fair) Gravity Resisted

POSITION OF PATIENT: Prone with knee flexed less than 90° with leg internally rotated. Patient's toes should be pointed inward.

POSITION OF THERAPIST: Testing hand placed around leg above ankle, providing resistance down and out to the side toward knee extension (see Figure 3-7). The stabilizing hand is placed on the midhamstrings to provide support.

TEST: Patient is to flex the knee while maintaining internal rotation (heel toward therapist).

DIRECTIONS: Say to patient, "Bend your knee, keeping the toes pointing in and hold it there. Do not let me straighten it."

GRADING:

- **Grade 3 (Fair):** Patient flexes the knee but no resistance is tolerated. It is important to watch for a tight rectus femoris because this can limit knee ROM. Hip flexion at the end of knee flexion is a good indication tightness is present.

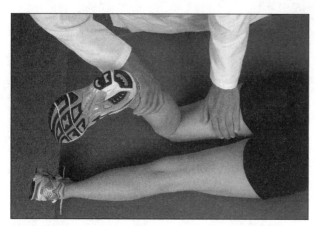

Figure 3-8 Proper positioning for knee flexion lateral hamstring muscle test grades 5–3. Source: Delmar/Cengage Learning

Testing for Knee Flexion Lateral Hamstring Grades 5, 4, 3 (Normal, Good, Fair) Gravity Resisted

POSITION OF PATIENT: Prone with knee flexed less than 90° with leg externally rotated. Patient's toes should be pointed out to side.

POSITION OF THERAPIST: Testing hand placed around leg above ankle providing resistance down and in toward knee extension (see Figure 3-8). The stabilizing hand is placed on the mid-hamstrings to provide support.

TEST: Patient flexes knee with toes pointing out while maintaining external rotation (heel away from therapist).

DIRECTIONS: Say to patient, "Bend your knee, keeping the toes pointing out and hold it there. Do not let me straighten it."

GRADING:

- **Grade 5 (Normal):** Patient flexes the knee and holds against therapist's maximum resistance without breaking (see Figure 3-8).

- **Grade 4 (Good):** Patient flexes the knee and holds against therapist's strong to moderate resistance and then breaks.

- **Grade 3 (Fair):** Patient flexes the knee but no resistance is tolerated.

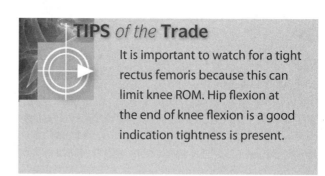

TIPS *of the* **Trade**

It is important to watch for a tight rectus femoris because this can limit knee ROM. Hip flexion at the end of knee flexion is a good indication tightness is present.

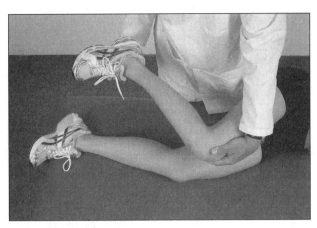

Figure 3-9 Proper positioning for knee flexion muscle test grade 2. Source: Delmar/Cengage Learning

Testing for Knee Flexion Grade 2 (Poor) Gravity Minimal

POSITION OF PATIENT: Side-lying with bottom leg flexed for stability and top leg (test limb) supported by the therapist.

POSITION OF THERAPIST: Behind patient with one arm around medial side of leg above the ankle, and the other arm cradles the thigh with hand supporting the medial side of the knee (see Figure 3-9). No resistance is applied.

TEST: Patient is to flex the knee through available ROM.

DIRECTIONS: Say to patient, "Bend your knee as far as possible."

GRADING:

- **Grade 2 (Poor):** Able to complete knee flexion through full ROM with gravity minimized.

TIPS *of the* Trade

Because the gastrocnemius assists in knee flexion, it is appropriate to begin the test with the knee at 10° of flexion for grades 2 and 3 when gastrocnemius weakness is present.

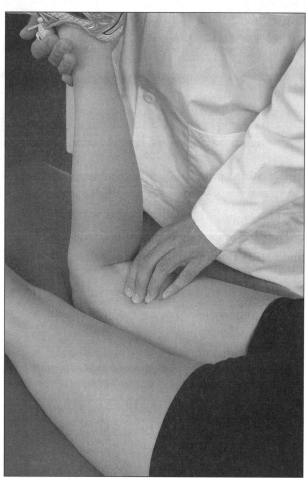

Figure 3-10 Proper positioning for knee flexion muscle test grades 1–0. Source: Delmar/Cengage Learning

Testing for Knee Flexion Grades 1, 0 (Trace, None) Gravity Minimal

POSITION OF PATIENT: Prone with legs straight and toes pointing down. Test limb is partially flexed and ankle supported by therapist.

POSITION OF THERAPIST: Next to test limb with one hand supporting the lower extremity at the ankle and the other palpating the medial and lateral hamstring tendons above the knee (see Figure 3-10).

TEST: Patient tries to flex the knee.

DIRECTIONS: Say to patient, "Try to bend your knee."

GRADING:

- **Grade 1 (Trace):** Tendon movement is palpable but there is no visible movement.
- **Grade 0 (None):** Unable to palpate any contraction of the muscles or tendons.

Knee Extension

The primary and accessory muscles responsible for knee extension are described in Table 3-2. The rectus femoris, vastus intermedius, vastus lateralis, and vastus medialis are the primary movers for knee extension (see Figure 3-11).

TABLE 3-2 MUSCLES RESPONSIBLE FOR KNEE EXTENSION

PRIMARY MUSCLES	ORIGIN	INSERTION	INNERVATIONS
Rectus femoris	Anterior inferior iliac spine (AIIS)	Tibial tuberosity via patellar tendon	Femoral (L2–L4)
Vastus intermedius	Anterior femur	Tibial tuberosity via patellar tendon	Femoral (L2–L4)
Vastus lateralis	Linea aspera	Tibial tuberosity via patellar tendon	Femoral (L2–L4)
Vastus medialis	Linea aspera	Tibial tuberosity via patellar tendon	Femoral (L2–L4)
ACCESSORY MUSCLE	**ORIGIN**	**INSERTION**	**INNERVATIONS**
Tensor fascia latae	ASIS	Lateral condyle of tibia	Superior gluteal (L4, L5)

Unlike the hamstrings, the heads of the quadriceps cannot be isolated for individual testing. Therefore, they are tested together as one functional unit.

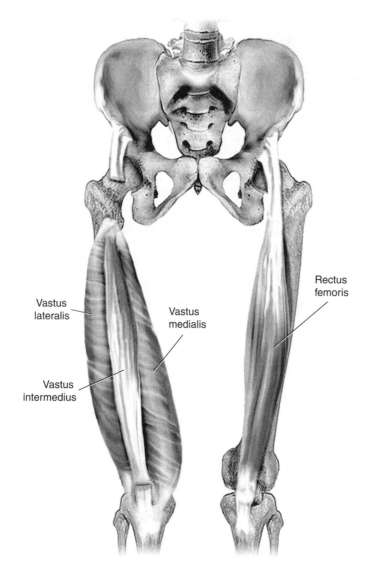

Vastus lateralis

Vastus medialis

Rectus femoris

Vastus intermedius

Figure 3-11 Quadriceps group (*See color plate*). Source: Delmar/Cengage Learning

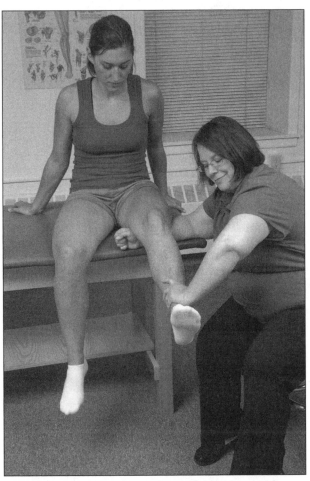

Figure 3-12 Proper positioning for knee extension muscle testing grades 5–3. Source: Delmar/Cengage Learning

Testing for Knee Extension Grades 5, 4, 3 (Normal, Good, Fair) Gravity Resisted

POSITION OF PATIENT: Short sitting with hands resting on table sides for stability. Leaning back is allowed to ease tension of tight hamstrings. Remind patient not to lock the knee into hyperextension.

POSITION OF THERAPIST: One hand is placed under the testing limb to keep the femur in alignment. The other hand is placed over the anterior portion of the lower extremity just above the ankle to provide resistance in a downward motion (see Figure 3-12).

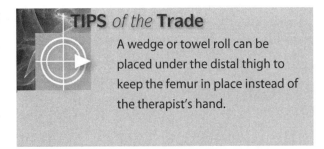
TIPS *of the* **Trade**
A wedge or towel roll can be placed under the distal thigh to keep the femur in place instead of the therapist's hand.

TEST: Patient moves the knee into extension, avoiding hyperextension.

DIRECTIONS: Say to patient, "Straighten your knee as much as possible but do not lock it. Hold it there and do not let me bend it."

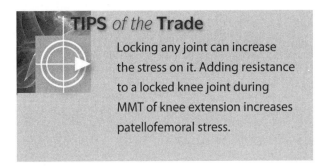
TIPS *of the* **Trade**
Locking any joint can increase the stress on it. Adding resistance to a locked knee joint during MMT of knee extension increases patellofemoral stress.

GRADING:

- **Grade 5 (Normal):** Patient extends the knee and holds against therapist's maximum resistance without breaking.
- **Grade 4 (Good):** Patient extends knee and holds against therapist's strong to moderate resistance and then breaks.
- **Grade 3 (Fair):** Patient extends knee but no resistance is tolerated.

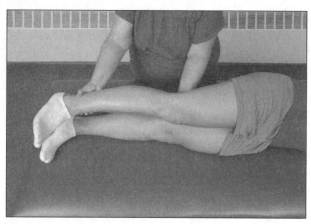

Figure 3-13 Proper positioning for knee extension muscle testing grade 2. Source: Delmar/Cengage Learning

Testing for Knee Extension Grade 2 (Poor) Gravity Minimal

POSITION OF PATIENT: Side-lying with bottom leg flexed for stability and top leg (test limb) supported by the therapist at 90° of knee flexion and hip in full extension.

POSITION OF THERAPIST: Behind patient with one arm cradling the thigh with the hand supporting the medial side of the knee. The other hand supports the leg under the medial malleolus. No resistance is applied (see Figure 3-13).

TEST: Patient is to extend the knee without any resistance or assistance from the therapist.

DIRECTIONS: Say to patient, "Extend your knee as far as possible."

GRADING:

- **Grade 2 (Poor):** Able to complete knee extension through full ROM with gravity minimized.

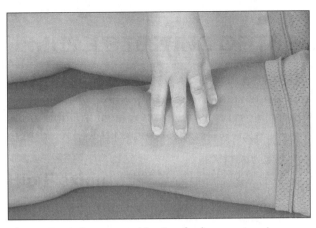

Figure 3-14 Proper positioning for knee extension muscle testing grades 1–0. Source: Delmar/Cengage Learning

Testing for Knee Extension Grades 1, 0 (Trace, None) Gravity Minimal

POSITION OF PATIENT: Supine.

POSITION OF THERAPIST: Next to test limb with one hand palpating the quadriceps tendon by gently holding it between the thumb and fingers. The other hand can palpate the patellar tendon below the knee (see Figure 3-14).

TEST: Patient tries to extend the knee.

DIRECTIONS: "Try to push the back of your knee into the table."

GRADING:

- **Grade 1 (Trace):** Tendon movement is palpable but there is no visible movement.
- **Grade 0 (None):** Unable to palpate any contraction of the muscles or tendons.

Substitutions

Important substitutions to watch for during MMT of the knee are as follows:

- While testing knee flexion with the patient prone, hip flexion substitution is present if the buttocks on the test side rise and the patient rolls slightly supine. This occurs as the hip flexes to help initiate knee flexion.
- A hip adduction movement during knee flexion indicates a gracilis muscle substitution.
- If the sartorius is contributing to knee flexion, knee flexion and hip external rotation will be seen together. This decreases the difficulty because the leg is not being raised vertically against gravity.
- A patient is to have the toes pointed down during knee flexion to avoid the substitution of the gastrocnemius muscle.
- When testing for knee extension in the side-lying position, be aware of hip internal rotator substitution. This will result in the knee falling into extension.

RANGE OF MOTION

The following section discusses measuring ROM for the two motions available at the knee joint.

Knee Flexion

Knee flexion occurs in the sagittal plane around the medial-lateral axis. The primary muscles involved are the hamstrings and gastrocnemius. According to the American Academy of Orthopaedic Surgeons (1965), normal active range of motion (AROM) for this motion is 0°–135° and passive range of motion (PROM) is between 0° and 140°–150°. The end-feel for knee flexion should be soft due to the soft tissue contact.

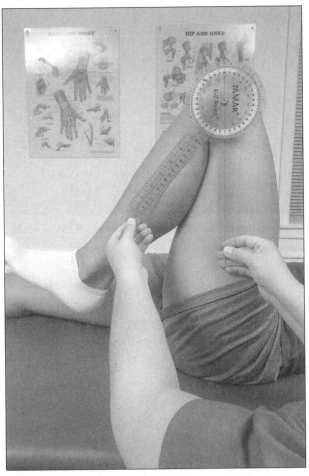

Figure 3-15 Proper goniometer positioning for knee flexion ROM. Source: Delmar/Cengage Learning

POSITION OF PATIENT: Supine with legs extended straight. Patient may also be prone with the hip in neutral and the foot over the edge of the table. This provides better stabilization. If there is limited ROM in the rectus femoris, this position is not appropriate.

POSITION OF THERAPIST: Sitting on a stool next to patient by test limb. One hand stabilizes the femur to prevent rotation, abduction, and adduction. This is done as the patient moves into flexion.

POSITION OF GONIOMETER:

- **Fulcrum:** Centered at the lateral joint line (see Figure 3-15)

TIPS *of the* Trade

Have patient flex knee. The joint line is the indentation felt below the lateral epicondyle of the femur.

- **Stationary arm:** Lateral midline of femur toward the greater trochanter
- **Movable arm:** Lateral midline of the fibula toward the lateral malleolus

Knee Extension

Knee extension also occurs in the sagittal plane around the medial-lateral axis. The primary muscles involved are the quadriceps. According to the American Academy of Orthopaedic Surgeons (1965), AROM for this motion is 0°–5°/10°. A firm end-feel is expected due to the tension in the knee's posterior joint capsule and the surrounding ligaments.

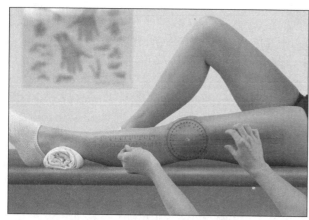

Figure 3-16 Proper goniometer positioning for knee extension ROM. Source: Delmar/Cengage Learning

POSITION OF PATIENT: Seated or supine with towel roll under test ankle to allow for full knee extension.

POSITION OF THERAPIST: Sitting on a stool next to patient by test limb. One hand stabilizes the femur to prevent rotation, abduction, and adduction.

POSITION OF GONIOMETER:

- **Fulcrum:** Centered at the lateral joint line (see Figure 3-16)

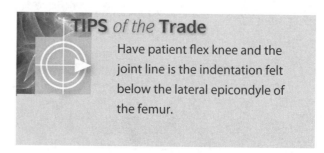

TIPS *of the* **Trade**

Have patient flex knee and the joint line is the indentation felt below the lateral epicondyle of the femur.

- **Stationary arm:** Lateral midline of femur toward the greater trochanter
- **Movable arm:** Lateral midline of the fibula toward the lateral malleolus

FUNCTIONAL APPLICATION

Like the hip, normal strength and ROM of the knee joint are necessary for meeting many of the mobility demands placed on the body when completing daily tasks. To walk on level surfaces, the knee joint needs 60° of flexion, according to the *Observational Gait Analysis Handbook* of the Professional Staff Association, Rancho Los Amigos Medical Center (1989). Livingston, Stevenson, and Olney (1991) studied stair ambulation and found that a person needs 105° of knee flexion for ambulating up stairs and 107° of knee flexion to ambulate down stairs. Jevsevar and colleagues (1993) found that 90.1° of knee flexion is required to get up from a chair and 106° is needed to tie shoes. Again, these are only a few examples of functional tasks that require good knee strength and ROM. Limitations or deficits in either can result in the compensation by other joints, often causing more problems down the road, as well as the disruption of normal living.

LEARNER CHALLENGE

1. List all the knee motions. Then identify the plane and axis in which they occur.
2. Palpate the following knee landmarks: medial and lateral condyles and epicondyles of the femur, the patella, medial and lateral condyles of the tibia, tibial plateau, and tibial tuberosity.
3. To practice manual muscle testing (MMT), one lab partner acts as the therapist and performs MMT of knee flexion grades 5–0. Then switch roles and the other lab partner performs MMT for knee extension.
4. Using a goniometer, measure ROM on your lab partner for knee flexion and extension. Switch roles and have the other partner use the goniometer to measure the same. Double-check for proper goniometer placement and compare your findings to normal ROM for each movement.
5. Fill in the following tables summarizing MMT and ROM measurements of the knee.

A)   Manual Muscle Testing for Grades 5, 4, 3 Gravity Resisted

MOTION	TESTING POSITION	STABILIZING HAND	RESISTANCE HAND
Knee Flexion General Hamstring Test			
Knee Flexion Medial Hamstring Test			
Knee Flexion Lateral Hamstring Test			
Knee Extension			

B)   Manual Muscle Testing for Grades 2, 1, 0 Gravity Minimal

MOTION	TESTING POSITION	STABILIZING HAND	RESISTANCE HAND	PALPATION
Knee Flexion General Hamstring Test				
Knee Extension				

C)   Range of Motion

MOTION	MOVABLE ARM	STATIONARY ARM	FULCRUM	NORMAL ROM
Knee Flexion				
Knee Extension				

THE ANKLE AND FOOT

CHAPTER **4**

OBJECTIVES

Upon completion of this chapter, the reader will be able to:

- Name the three functions of the ankle joint.

- Describe the three major joints that make up the ankle.

- Name the major joints of the foot.

- Identify the bones and bony landmarks significant to the ankle and foot.

- Name the major ligaments of the ankle.

- Identify any supporting structures important to the ankle and foot.

- Name the arches of the foot and their purpose.

- Describe the major motions of the ankle and foot and name the muscles that perform them.

- Become familiar with the origins, insertions, and innervations of the muscles of the ankle and foot.

- Perform proper manual muscle testing on the major muscles of the ankle grades 5–0.

- Perform proper manual muscle testing on the major muscles of the foot grades 5–0.

- Be aware of possible substitutions during manual muscle testing of the ankle and foot.

- Accurately perform range of motion testing using the goniometer on the ankle.

- Accurately perform range of motion testing using the goniometer on the foot.

MUSCULOSKELETAL OVERVIEW

Moving distally down the lower extremity from the knee are the ankle and foot. The ankle and foot are made up of a collection of complex structures with an elaborate arrangement of joints that act as support for the entire body and allow humans to move in an upright position. These two structures are made up of 28 bones and can be divided into four functional regions known as the ankle, rearfoot, midfoot, and forefoot. Together, they play a key role in balance and mobility required for gait.

The ankle and foot work as one unit to perform three major functions. The first is to act as a shock absorber by distributing the weight-bearing forces as the heel strikes the ground during the start of the stance phase of gait. The second function is to adapt to the various ground surface types during gait to help maintain balance. The segmentation of the foot makes it pliable and allows for this adaptation. Third, the ankle and foot provide a stable base of support and act as a lever to propel the body forward during ambulation. To provide both mobility and stability, the muscles and ligaments of these two structures must work together to find a proper balance for optimal function. Enough mobility is necessary to generate the forces needed for propulsion of the body, while stability is required to control these forces to prevent damaging the tissues and causing pain and dysfunction.

Joints

The ankle is comprised of three major joints, as well as many intertarsal joints that allow for gliding motions. The main ankle joint, talocrural or talotibial joint, consists of the articulations between the talus and the distal end and medial malleolus of the tibia and the distal end and lateral malleolus of the fibula. The talocrural joint is also described as a tenon-mortise or peg and socket joint.

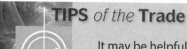

TIPS *of the* **Trade**

It may be helpful to think of the talocrural joint in carpentry terms. A mortise is an indentation cut into a piece of wood to make room for the projecting piece shaped to go into that notch. In the ankle joint, the talus bone is the peg or tenon that fits into the notch or mortise made by the lateral and medial malleoli.

The results of this arrangement are an increase in stability with a decrease in unwanted lateral and medial movements, thus decreasing the chance of injury. The talocrural joint is a synovial, uniaxial, hinge joint, making dorsiflexion and plantar flexion the main motions it performs. This joint is considered to be triplanar because the motions occurring here are around an oblique axis of rotation. In short, it passes through all three planes. There are no true plane movements. During dorsiflexion, the ankle dorsiflexes and inverts, bringing the foot up and slightly lateral. Conversely in plantarflexion, the ankle plantar flexes and everts, bringing the foot down and slightly medial (see Figure 4-1). When standing in anatomical position, the ankle is in neutral. The capsular pattern for the talocrural joint is plantarflexion limited greater than dorsiflexion.

The other two joints in the ankle are the subtalar or talocalcaneal joint and the transverse tarsal or midtarsal joint. For the subtalar joint, the inferior surface of the talus articulates with the superior surface of the calcaneus. The midtarsal or transverse joint is comprised of the anterior surface of the talus and calcaneus articulating with the posterior surface of the navicular and cuboid. Because functionally the subtalar and transverse tarsal joints cannot be separated, the motions they perform are inversion and eversion. As with the talocrural joint, these motions also occur around an oblique axis and are not true plane motions. Inversion is a composite of adduction, plantarflexion, and supination, while eversion consists of abduction, dorsiflexion, and pronation (see Figure 4-1). The capsular pattern is inversion limited more than eversion.

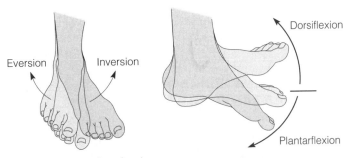

Figure 4-1 Ankle and foot motions *(See color plate).* Source: Delmar/Cengage Learning

Two other joints worth mentioning are the superior and inferior tibiofibular joints. While they are not actually part of the ankle joint, they do play a small role in its proper functioning. The superior tibiofibular joint is a uniaxial plane joint consisting of the articulation between the head of the fibula and the posterior aspect of the proximal tibia. The only motion present is a small amount of gliding. The inferior tibiofibular joint is a syndemosis joint between the distal tibia and distal fibula. The strong fibrous union holding this joint together provides much of the strength of the ankle joint.

The foot consists of the metatarsophalangeal, the proximal interphalangeal, distal interphalangeal, and the interphalangeal joints. Like the five metacarpophalangeal joints of the hand, the foot has five metatarsophalangeal (MTP) joints. They consist of the metatarsal heads articulating with the proximal phalanges (see Figure 4-2). The MTPs are synovial joints that allow for the motions of flexion, extension, hyperextension, abduction, and adduction (see Figure 4-3). Of the five MTP joints, the first one is much more mobile than the other four.

Also similar to the hand are the proximal interphalangeal (PIP) and distal interphalangeal (DIP) joints of toes two through five of the foot. Like the thumb, the great toe only has the one interphalangeal (IP) joint. The motions performed at these joints are flexion and extension. Due to the decreased need for dexterity in the foot versus the hand, the PIP and DIP joints in the foot are not as significant as they are in the hand (see Figure 4-2).

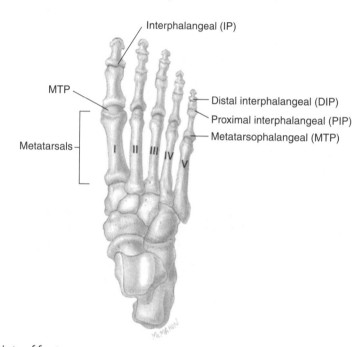

Figure 4-2 Phalange joints of foot. Source: Delmar/Cengage Learning

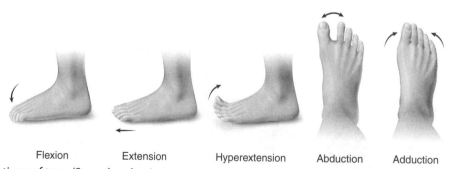

Flexion   Extension   Hyperextension   Abduction   Adduction

Figure 4-3 Motions of toes *(See color plate).* Source: Delmar/Cengage Learning

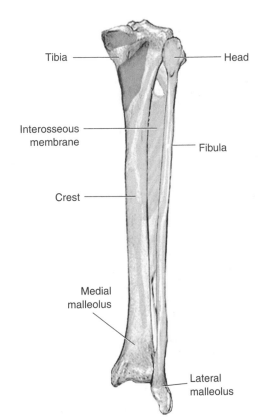

Figure 4-4 Tibia and fibula, anterior view *(See color plate)*. Source: Delmar/Cengage Learning

Bones

The tibia and fibula make up the part of the lower extremity going from the knee to the ankle that is known as the leg. These two bones along with the talus comprise the ankle joint. The tibia is triangular in shape and the larger of the two leg bones. As previously mentioned, it is the second strongest bone in the body and receives the weight of the body from the femur and transmits it to the foot. It is also the only true weight-bearing bone of the leg. The fibula is set back slightly posterior to the tibia and is long and thin (see Figure 4-4). The following section describes the bony landmarks of the leg significant to the ankle joint. Although the talus is part of the ankle, it will be discussed in the following section of the foot. Refer to Chapter 3 for a complete listing of landmarks for the tibia.

Tibia

- **Crest:** Anterior portion and the most prominent of the three borders
- **Medial malleolus:** Larger distal medial surface

Fibula

- **Head:** Larger proximal portion of bone
- **Lateral malleolus:** Larger distal end

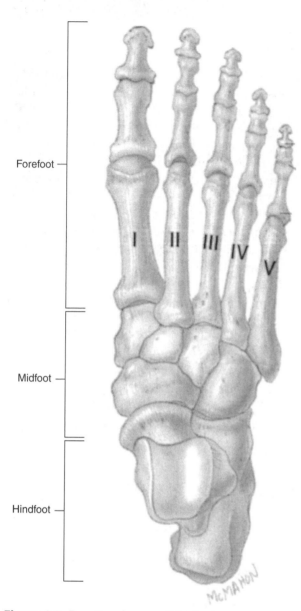

I II III IV V

Forefoot

Midfoot

Hindfoot

Figure 4-5 Functional areas of the foot.

Source: Delmar/Cengage Learning

The Foot

The bones of the foot consist of seven tarsals, five metatarsals, and fourteen phalanges. The foot consists of three functional areas known as the rearfoot, midfoot, and forefoot (see Figure 4-5). The tarsals make up the rear and midfoot, while the metatarsals and phalanges make up the forefoot.

The calcaneus and talus make up the rearfoot. The rearfoot is important because it is the first part of the foot to make contact with the ground during heel strike in the gait cycle. It also influences the function and movement of the other two portions of the foot. The navicular, cuboid, and three cuneiform bones form the midfoot. Its job is to provide mobility and stability to the foot as it transfers movement from rearfoot to forefoot during ambulation. The forefoot, consisting of the metatarsals and phalanges, is the last part of the foot to be in contact with the ground during the stance phase and is responsible for adapting to the various surface levels during ambulation. Of the five metatarsals, the first and fifth are weight-bearing bones. When standing, weight is borne from the base of the calcaneus up to the heads of the first and fifth metatarsals in a triangle shape. The phalanges or toes are important because they play a crucial role in ambulation. The following are the bony landmarks significant to the ankle and foot joints (see Figure 4-6).

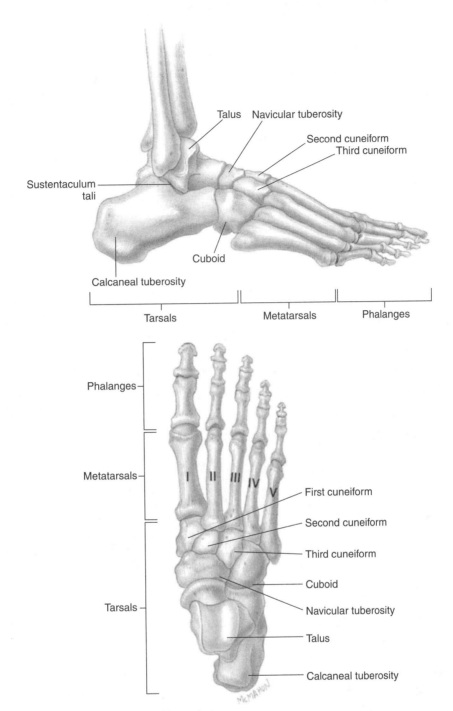

Figure 4-6 Bones of the foot: superior and lateral views. Source: Delmar/Cengage Learning

Tarsals

- **Calcaneus:** Largest posterior tarsal bone known as the heel
- **Calcaneal tuberosity:** Protrusion on the posterior inferior surface of calcaneus
- **Sustentaculum tali:** Medial superior protrusion supporting the medial side of the talus
- **Talus:** Second largest tarsal bone, wedge shaped and positioned on top of the calcaneus
- **Navicular:** Bone lying proximal to the cuneiforms and medially in front of the talus
- **Navicular tuberosity:** Protrusion on the navicular on the medial border of the foot
- **Cuboid:** Bone on the lateral foot distal to the calcaneus and proximal to the fourth and fifth metatarsals
- **Cuneiforms:** Three total with number one being the largest and located medially as they move laterally in line with the metatarsals

Metatarsals

- **Base:** Proximal end of each metatarsal
- **Head:** Distal end of each metatarsal
- **First:** Weight-bearing bone located on the medial side of the foot; the shortest and thickest of the five bones
- **Second:** The longest of the five bones; articulates with the second cuneiform
- **Third:** Articulates with the third cuneiform
- **Fourth:** Articulates with the cuboid
- **Fifth:** Articulates with the cuboid and has a prominent tuberosity on the lateral side of its base

Phalanges

- **First digit:** Known as the great toe; made up of a proximal and distal phalanx only
- **Second-fourth digits:** Known as lesser toes; made up of a proximal, middle, and distal phalanx

Ligaments

The ankle, like the other synovial joints in the body, is surrounded by a joint capsule and has a strong and intricate ligamentous support system that reinforces and strengthens the capsule to increase stability and help decrease the chance of injury. Because the ankle and foot consist of numerous bones, several ligaments provide support and stability between the bones they connect. For the purpose of this text, the focus will be on three main groups of ligaments known as the medial or deltoid ligaments, the lateral ligaments, and the tarsal ligaments.

The deltoid or medial ligaments consist of a triangular shaped group of four ligaments that begin along the tip of the medial malleolus of the tibia and fan out to attach to the talus, navicular, and calcaneus bones (see Figure 4-7). The anterior fibers of the deltoid ligament are known as the tibionavicular ligament, which runs from the tibia out to the navicular bone. The tibiocalcaneal ligament makes up the middle fibers and runs from the tibia to the sustentaculum tali of the calcaneus. The tibiotalar ligament runs from the tibia back to the talus and forms the posterior fibers of the deltoid ligament. The final ligament of this group is the anterior tibiotalar, which runs deep from the anterior tibia back to the talus. These ligaments work together to strengthen the medial side of the ankle, maintain the longitudinal arch, and hold the calcaneus and navicular against the talus.

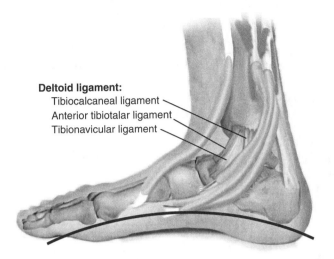

Figure 4-7 Deltoid ligament. Source: Delmar/Cengage Learning

Support to the lateral ankle is provided by a group of three ligaments known as the lateral ligaments. There are three parts to this ligament whose function is to connect the lateral malleolus to the talus and calcaneus, thus increasing ankle strength (see Figure 4-8). The anterior talofibular ligament runs from the lateral malleolus to the talus and is considered to be rather weak. The calcaneofibular ligament is the long, strong middle portion and runs laterally connecting the lateral malleolus to the talus. The talofibular ligament makes up the posterior portion of this group and is considered to be very strong. It runs horizontally connecting the lateral malleolus to the talus. In spite of all the ligamentous support, the ankle is still the most frequently injured joint in the body, with the lateral ligament being the one most commonly stretched or torn.

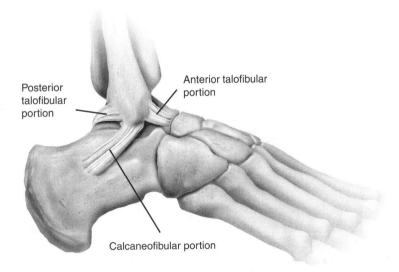

Figure 4-8 Lateral ligaments *(See color plate)*. Source: Delmar/Cengage Learning

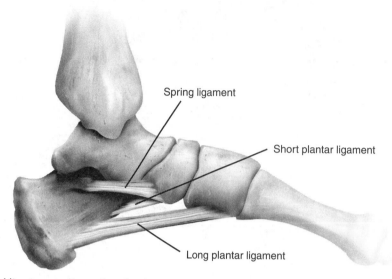

Figure 4-9 Tarsal ligaments *(See color plate).* Source: Delmar/Cengage Learning

The three tarsal ligaments are the spring or plantar calcaneonavicular ligament, the long plantar ligament, and the short plantar ligament (see Figure 4-9). The primary function of these ligaments is to help support the arches in the foot. The spring ligament is short and wide and runs from the calcaneus to the navicular. It provides support to the medial side of the longitudinal arch. The longest of the tarsal ligaments is the long plantar ligament. It is more superficial than the spring ligament and runs from the posterior calcaneus forward to the cuboid and bases of the third, fourth, and fifth metatarsals. This ligament's job is to provide support to the lateral longitudinal arch.

The last of the tarsal ligaments is the short plantar ligament. It also runs from the calcaneus to the cuboid and assists the long plantar ligament in supporting the lateral longitudinal arch.

Supporting Structures

The two other important structures that play a role in the functioning of the ankle and foot are the arches and the plantar aponeurosis. To help offset the effects of being in constant contact with the ground, the bones of the foot are strategically arranged to form three arches to help absorb the continuous stresses placed upon it. This domelike formation distributes half the weight of the body when standing or walking to the heel bones and the other half to the heads of the metatarsals. The main weight-bearing surfaces of the foot form a triangle with the base point at the calcaneus and the other two points at the head of the first and fifth metatarsals. The supporting arches of the foot run between these three points and are upheld by the shape of the bones, the surrounding muscles, the plantar ligaments, and the aponeurosis.

There are two longitudinal arches and one transverse arch. The medial longitudinal arch provides support to the foot medially, runs from the calcaneus up to the talus, and descends past the three cuneiforms to the first three metatarsal heads. The talus is known as the keystone. Like the keystone of an arch, it is an important and central portion of the arch of the foot because it receives the weight of the body. The lateral longitudinal arch supports the foot laterally and is much lower than the medial arch. It runs from the calcaneus through the cuboid to the fourth and fifth metatarsals.

The cuboid is the keystone in this arch and helps with weight bearing by elevating the lateral part of the foot, which aids in the redistribution of the weight to the calcaneus and the fifth metatarsal head. The two longitudinal arches act as posts for the transverse arch. This arch runs from one side of the foot to the other through the three cuneiforms to the cuboid with the second cuneiform acting as the keystone (see Figure 4-10).

The plantar aponeurosis plays a role in supporting the longitudinal arch. It is a flat band of connective tissue covering the width of the foot and is found on the plantar surface of the foot (see Figure 4-9). It provides strength and stability to the bottom of the foot by securing the calcaneus and talus to the anterior tarsals and metatarsal heads.

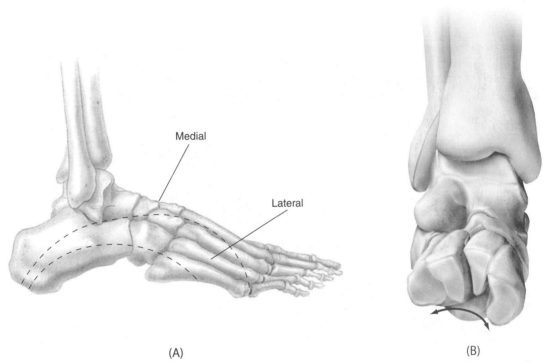

(A) (B)

Figure 4-10 Arches of the foot: (A) Longitudinal arches of the foot, (B) Transverse arch of the foot *(See color plate).*

Source: Delmar/Cengage Learning

MUSCLE TESTING OF THE ANKLE AND FOOT

Although there are no true planar movements at the ankle joint, for the purpose of this text, the MMT instructions for the ankle will discuss testing the motions of dorsiflexion, plantar flexion, inversion, and eversion as straight planar movements. These motions, as well as great toe and the four lesser toes' flexion and extension, will be covered in this section. Because it is important to review the muscles associated with the movement, each test starts with a table of the muscles responsible for the movement being tested, followed by a drawing of the primary muscles.

Ankle Dorsiflexion

The primary and accessory muscles responsible for ankle dorsiflexion are shown in Table 4-1. The tibialis anterior muscle is the prime mover for ankle dorsiflexion (see Figure 4-11).

TABLE 4-1 — MUSCLES RESPONSIBLE FOR ANKLE DORSIFLEXION

PRIMARY MUSCLES	ORIGIN	INSERTION	INNERVATIONS
Tibialis anterior	Lateral tibia and interosseous membrane	First cuneiform and metatarsal	Deep peroneal (L4, L5, S1)

ACCESSORY MUSCLES	ORIGIN	INSERTION	INNERVATIONS
Peroneus tertius	Distal medial fibula	Base fifth metatarsal	Deep peroneal (L4, L5, S1)
Extensor digitorum longus	Fibula, tibia, interosseous membrane	Distal phalanx of four lesser toes	Deep peroneal (L4, L5, S1)
Extensor hallucis longus	Fibula and interosseous membrane	Distal phalanx of great toe	Deep peroneal (L4, L5, S1)

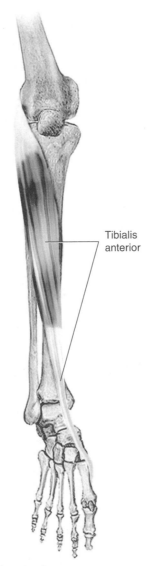

Tibialis
anterior

Figure 4-11 Tibialis anterior muscle *(See color plate).* Source: Delmar/Cengage Learning

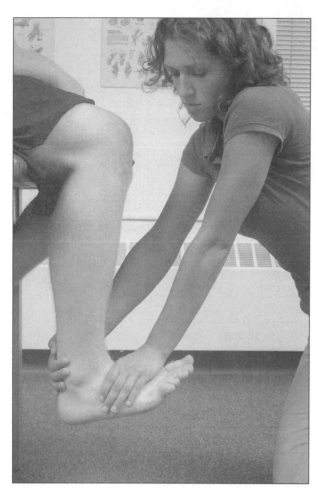

Figure 4-12 Proper positioning for ankle dorsiflexion grades 5–3. Source: Delmar/Cengage Learning

Testing for Ankle Dorsiflexion Grades 5, 4, 3 (Normal, Good, Fair) Gravity Resisted

POSITION OF PATIENT: Short sitting with ankle at neutral.

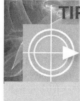

TIPS of the Trade

Having the knee flexed during this test puts the gastrocnemius on slack. A tight gastrocnemius results in the patient's inability to dorsiflex the ankle through full ROM.

POSITION OF THERAPIST: In front of patient with one hand around back of lower leg above the ankle and the other over the dorsomedial aspect of the foot to provide resistance (see Figure 4-12). Resistance is applied in a downward motion.

TEST: Patient dorsiflexes foot.

DIRECTIONS: Say to the patient, "While keeping the toes relaxed, bring your foot up and don't let me push it down."

TIPS of the Trade

Instructing the patient to keep the toes relaxed avoids substitution by the toe extensor muscles.

GRADING:

- **Grade 5 (Normal):** Patient dorsiflexes while holding against therapist's maximum resistance without breaking.
- **Grade 4 (Good):** Patient dorsiflexes foot and holds against therapist's strong to moderate resistance and then breaks.
- **Grade 3 (Fair):** Patient dorsiflexes ankle through full ROM and holds at end range but no resistance is tolerated.

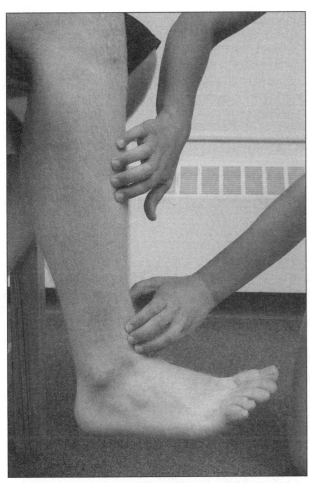

Figure 4-13 Proper positioning for palpation grades 2–0. Source: Delmar/Cengage Learning

Testing for Ankle Dorsiflexion Grades 2, 1, 0 (Poor, Trace, None) Gravity Minimal

POSITION OF PATIENT: Side-lying on test limb with the hip extended, the knee flexed, and the ankle in neutral or short sitting with ankle in neutral position.

POSITION OF THERAPIST: Next to patient with one hand stabilizing the lower leg above the ankle. No resistance is applied.

TEST: Patient is to dorsiflex the ankle without any resistance or assistance from the therapist.

DIRECTIONS: Say to the patient, "While keeping the toes relaxed, try to bring your foot up toward your shin."

GRADING:

- **Grade 2 (Poor):** Able to complete ankle dorsiflexion through full ROM with gravity minimized.

- **Grade 1 (Trace):** Tendon movement is palpable but there is no visible movement.

TIPS *of the* Trade

To palpate for muscle activity, place one hand over the muscle belly of the tibialis anterior just lateral to the shin. Place the other hand by the medial malleoli on the anteromedial aspect of the ankle to palpate tendon activity (see Figure 4-13).

- **Grade 0 (None):** Unable to palpate any contraction of the muscles or tendons.

Ankle Plantar Flexion

Table 4-2 details the primary and accessory muscles responsible for ankle plantar flexion. The gastroc-nemius and soleus muscles are the prime movers for ankle plantar flexion (see Figure 4-14).

TABLE 4-2	MUSCLES RESPONSIBLE FOR ANKLE PLANTAR FLEXION		
PRIMARY MUSCLES	**ORIGIN**	**INSERTION**	**INNERVATIONS**
Gastrocnemius	Medial head: medial condyle of femur Lateral head: Lateral condyle of femur	Posterior calcaneus	Tibial (S1, S2)
Soleus	Posterior tibia and fibula	Posterior calcaneus	Tibial (S1, S2)
ACCESSORY MUSCLES	**ORIGIN**	**INSERTION**	**INNERVATIONS**
Tibialis posterior	Interosseous membrane	Navicular, metatarsals, and most tarsals	Tibial (L5, S1)
Flexor hallucis longus	Posterior fibula and interosseous membrane	Distal phalanx of great toe	Tibial (L5, S1, S2)
Flexor digitorum longus	Posterior tibia	Distal phalanx of four lesser toes	Tibial (L5, S1)
Peroneus longus	Lateral proximal fibula and interosseous membrane	Plantar surface of first cuneiform and metatarsal	Superficial peroneal nerve (L4, L5, S1)
Peroneus brevis	Lateral distal fibula	Base of fifth metatarsal	Superficial peroneal nerve (L4, L5, S1)

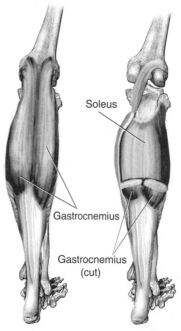

Figure 4-14 Gastrocnemius and soleus muscles *(See color plate).* Source: Delmar/Cengage Learning

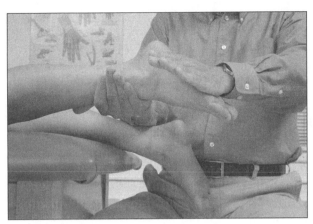

Figure 4-15 Proper positioning for ankle plantar flexion prone grades 5–3. Source: Delmar/Cengage Learning

Testing for Ankle Plantar Flexion Prone Grades 5, 4, 3 (Normal, Good, Fair) Gravity Resisted

POSITION OF PATIENT: Lying prone with feet hanging off end of table.

POSITION OF THERAPIST: Standing at end of table next to foot being tested. The stabilizing hand is around the front of the ankle while the testing hand is placed against the plantar surface of the foot by the metatarsal heads (see Figure 4-15). The heel of the testing palm provides resistance in a down and forward direction toward dorsiflexion.

TEST: Patient plantar flexes the ankle by pointing the toes.

DIRECTIONS: Say to the patient, "Point your toes down and do not let me push them up."

GRADING:

- **Grade 5 (Normal):** Patient plantar flexes ankle while holding against therapist's maximum resistance without breaking.
- **Grade 4 (Good):** Patient plantar flexes ankle and holds against therapist's strong to moderate resistance and then breaks.
- **Grade 3 (Fair):** Patient plantar flexes ankle through full ROM and holds at end range but no resistance is tolerated.

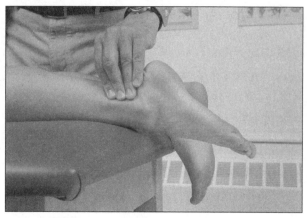

Figure 4-16 Proper positioning for ankle plantar flexion prone grades 2–0. Source: Delmar/Cengage Learning

Testing for Ankle Plantar Flexion Prone Grades 2, 1, 0 (Poor, Trace, None) Gravity Minimal

POSITION OF PATIENT: Lying prone with feet hanging off end of table.

POSITION OF THERAPIST: Standing at end of table next to foot being tested. No resistance is applied (see Figure 4-16).

TEST: Patient is to try to plantar flex the ankle without any resistance or assistance from the therapist.

DIRECTIONS: Say to the patient, "Try to point your toes."

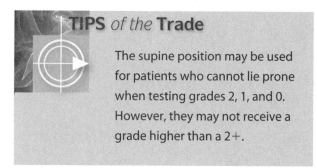

TIPS *of the* **Trade**

The supine position may be used for patients who cannot lie prone when testing grades 2, 1, and 0. However, they may not receive a grade higher than a 2+.

GRADING:

- **Grade 2 (Poor):** Able to complete plantar flexion through full ROM.
- **Grade 1 (Trace):** Tendon movement is palpable but there is no visible movement.

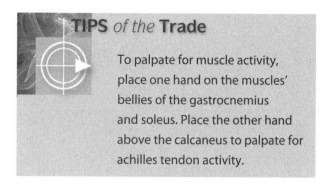

TIPS *of the* **Trade**

To palpate for muscle activity, place one hand on the muscles' bellies of the gastrocnemius and soleus. Place the other hand above the calcaneus to palpate for achilles tendon activity.

- **Grade 0 (None):** Unable to palpate any contraction of the muscles or tendons.

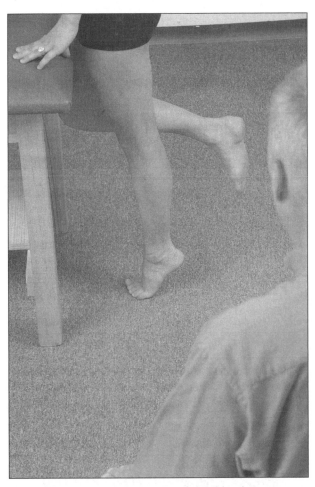

Figure 4-17 Proper positioning for ankle plantar flexion standing grades 5–3. Source: Delmar/Cengage Learning

Testing for Ankle Plantar Flexion Standing Grades 5, 4, 3 (Normal, Good, Fair) Gravity Resisted

POSITION OF PATIENT: Standing on test foot with knee extended and nontest knee flexed. To assist with balance, the patient is allowed to lightly place one or two fingers on table (see Figure 4-17).

POSITION OF THERAPIST: Standing next to patient to observe test limb.

TEST: Patient fully plantar flexes ankle by raising heel off floor.

DIRECTIONS: After demonstrating the correct form for a heel raise, say to the patient, "Stand on one leg and go up on your tip toes and then down. Please repeat this 20 times."

GRADING:

- **Grade 5 (Normal):** Patient is able to complete at least 20 heel raises correctly without rest or fatigue. According to Hislop and Montgomery (2002), "Twenty heel raises represent over 60 percent of maximum electromyographic activity of the plantar flexors" (p. 228).

- **Grade 4 (Good):** Patient is able to correctly complete 10 to 19 heel raises without rest, fatigue, or a break in form. If there is a break in form for even one repetition, the patient must receive a grade 3.

- **Grade 3 (Fair):** Patient is able to complete between one and nine heel raises correctly without rest, fatigue, or a break in form. A patient must be able to complete at least one correct full range heel raise to receive a grade 3.

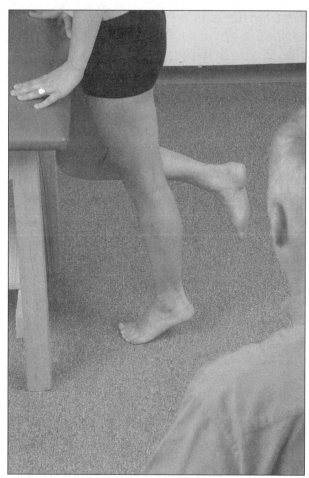

Figure 4-18 Proper positioning for ankle plantar flexion standing grade 2. Source: Delmar/Cengage Learning

Testing for Ankle Plantar Flexion Standing Grade 2+ (Poor+) Gravity Minimal

POSITION OF PATIENT: Standing on test foot with knee extended and nontest knee flexed. To assist with balance, the patient is allowed to lightly place one or two fingers on table (see Figure 4-18).

POSITION OF THERAPIST: Standing next to patient to observe test limb.

TEST: Patient is to attempt to perform a heel raise through full range of motion.

DIRECTIONS: After demonstrating the correct form for a heel raise, say to the patient, "Stand on one leg and try to go up on your tip toes and then down."

GRADING:

- Grade 2+ (Poor+): The use of 2+ is appropriate in this situation because there is no straight grade 2 (Hislop & Montgomery, 2002). Patient scores a 2+ if the heel is able to just clear the floor, but the patient is unable to get up on the toes.

Testing for Ankle Plantar Flexion Standing Grades 1, 0 (Trace, None) Gravity Minimal

For grades 1 and 0, follow the previous instructions and grading for these grades in the previous section for ankle plantar flexion in the prone position. There is not a test for these grades in the standing position.

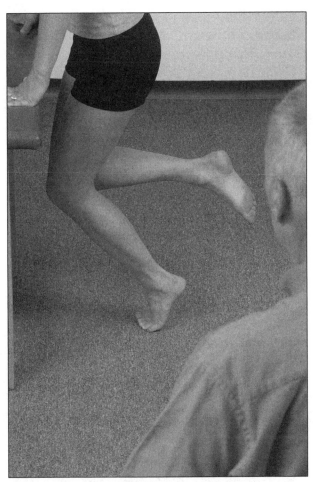

Figure 4-19 Proper positioning for ankle plantar flexion soleus only grades 5–3. Source: Delmar/Cengage Learning

Testing for Ankle Plantar Flexion Standing Soleus Only Grades 5, 4, 3 (Normal, Good, Fair) Gravity Resisted

POSITION OF PATIENT: Standing on test foot with knee slightly flexed and nontest knee flexed. Slightly flexing the test limb knee isolates the soleus muscle. The patient is allowed to lightly place one or two fingers on table to help with balance (see Figure 4-19).

POSITION OF THERAPIST: Standing next to patient to observe test limb.

TEST: Patient fully plantar flexes ankle by raising heel off floor and keeping test limb knee slightly flexed.

DIRECTIONS: After demonstrating the correct form for a heel raise, say to the patient, "Stand on one leg, bend your knee a little, and go up on your tip toes and then down. Please repeat this 20 times."

GRADING:

- **Grade 5 (Normal):** Patient is able to complete at least 20 heel raises correctly without rest or fatigue.
- **Grade 4 (Good):** Patient is able to correctly complete 10 to 19 heel raises without rest, fatigue, or a break in form. If there is a break in form for even one repetition, the patient must receive a grade 3.
- **Grade 3 (Fair):** Patient is able to complete between one and nine heel raises correctly without rest, fatigue, or a break in form. A patient must be able to complete at least one correct full range heel raise to receive a grade 3. Patient receives a 2+ if able to complete a partial heel raise.

Testing for Ankle Plantar Flexion Standing Soleus Only Grades 2, 1, 0 (Poor, Trace, None) Gravity Minimal

POSITION OF PATIENT: Lying prone with test limb knee flexed 90°.

POSITION OF THERAPIST: Standing at end of table next to foot being tested. No resistance is applied.

TEST: Patient is to try to plantar flex the ankle without any resistance or assistance from the therapist.

DIRECTIONS: Say to the patient, "Try to point your toes."

GRADING:

- **Grade 2 (Poor):** Able to complete ankle plantar flexion through full ROM.

- **Grade 1 (Trace):** Tendon movement is palpable but there is no visible movement.

TIPS *of the* **Trade**

To palpate for muscle activity, place one hand on the muscle belly of the soleus. Place the other hand above the calcaneus to palpate for achilles tendon activity.

- **Grade 0 (None):** Unable to palpate any contraction of the muscles or tendons.

Ankle Inversion

Table 4-3 lists the primary and accessory muscles responsible for ankle inversion. The tibialis posterior muscle is the primary mover for ankle inversion (see Figure 4-20).

TABLE 4-3	MUSCLES RESPONSIBLE FOR ANKLE INVERSION		
PRIMARY MUSCLES	**ORIGIN**	**INSERTION**	**INNERVATIONS**
Tibialis posterior	Interosseous membrane	Navicular, metatarsals, and most tarsals	Tibial (L5, S1)
ACCESSORY MUSCLES	**ORIGIN**	**INSERTION**	**INNERVATIONS**
Flexor hallucis longus	Posterior fibula and interosseous membrane	Distal phalanx of great toe	Tibial (L5, S1, S2)
Flexor digitorum longus	Posterior tibia	Distal phalanx of four lesser toes	Tibial (L5, S1)
Tibialis anterior	Lateral tibia and interosseous membrane	First cuneiform and metatarsal	Deep peroneal (L4, L5, S1)
Extensor hallucis longus	Fibula and interosseous membrane	Distal phalanx of great toe	Deep peroneal (L4, L5, S1)

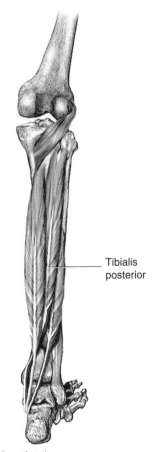

Tibialis posterior

Figure 4-20 Tibialis posterior muscle *(See color plate).* Source: Delmar/Cengage Learning

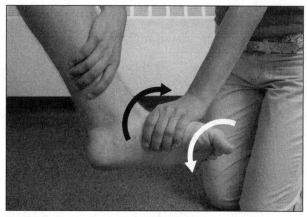

Figure 4-21 Proper positioning for inversion grades 5–3. Source: Delmar/Cengage Learning

Testing for Ankle Inversion Grades 5, 4, 3 (Normal, Good, Fair) Gravity Resisted

POSITION OF PATIENT: Short sitting with ankle at neutral position or 90°.

POSITION OF THERAPIST: In front of patient with stabilizing hand behind ankle above the malleoli. Testing hand placed by the metatarsal heads over the dorsum and medial side of the foot and applies resistance toward eversion (see Figure 4-21).

TEST: Patient inverts foot.

DIRECTIONS: Say to the patient, "Turn your foot in and do not let me pull you out of this position."

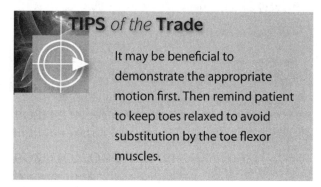

TIPS *of the* **Trade**

It may be beneficial to demonstrate the appropriate motion first. Then remind patient to keep toes relaxed to avoid substitution by the toe flexor muscles.

GRADING:

- **Grade 5 (Normal):** Patient inverts foot through full ROM while holding against therapist's maximum resistance without breaking.
- **Grade 4 (Good):** Patient inverts foot through available ROM and holds against therapist's strong to moderate resistance and then breaks.
- **Grade 3 (Fair):** Patient inverts foot through full ROM and holds at end range but no resistance is tolerated.

Testing for Ankle Inversion Grade 2 (Poor) Gravity Minimal

POSITION OF PATIENT: Supine with ankle flexed at 90°.

POSITION OF THERAPIST: Next to patient on a stool. No resistance is applied.

TEST: Patient is to invert foot without any resistance or assistance from the therapist.

DIRECTIONS: Say to the patient, "Try and turn your foot inward."

GRADING:

- **Grade 2 (Poor):** Able to complete ankle inversion through full ROM with gravity minimized.

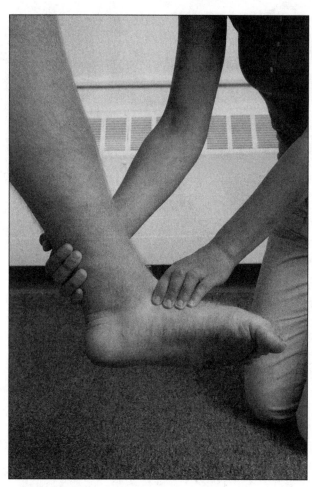

Figure 4-22 Proper positioning for inversion grades 1–0. Source: Delmar/Cengage Learning

Ankle Inversion Grades 1, 0 (Trace, None) Gravity Minimal

POSITION OF PATIENT: Short sitting with ankle flexed at 90°.

POSITION OF THERAPIST: Next to patient with one hand contoured behind ankle for support while the other hand palpates the tendon of the tibialis posterior between the navicular bone and the medial malleolus (see Figure 4-22).

TEST: Patient attempts to invert foot.

DIRECTIONS: Say to the patient, "Try to turn your foot inward."

GRADING:

- **Grade 1 (Trace):** Tendon movement is palpable but there is no visible movement.
- **Grade 0 (None):** Unable to palpate any contraction of the muscles or tendons.

Ankle Eversion

The primary and accessory muscles responsible for ankle eversion are listed in Table 4-4. The peroneus brevis and peroneus longus muscles are the primary movers for ankle eversion (see Figure 4-23).

TABLE 4-4	MUSCLES RESPONSIBLE FOR ANKLE EVERSION		
PRIMARY MUSCLES	**ORIGIN**	**INSERTION**	**INNERVATIONS**
Peroneus longus	Lateral proximal fibula and interosseous membrane	Plantar surface of first cuneiform and metatarsal	Superficial peroneal nerve (L4, L5, S1)
Peroneus brevis	Lateral distal fibula	Base of fifth metatarsal	Superficial peroneal nerve (L4, L5, S1)
ACCESSORY MUSCLES	**ORIGIN**	**INSERTION**	**INNERVATIONS**
Peroneus tertius	Distal medial fibula	Base fifth metatarsal	Deep peroneal (L4, L5, S1)

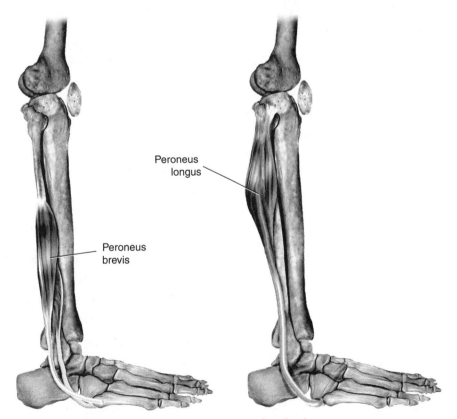

Figure 4-23 Peroneus longus and peroneus brevis muscles *(See color plate).* Source: Delmar/Cengage Learning

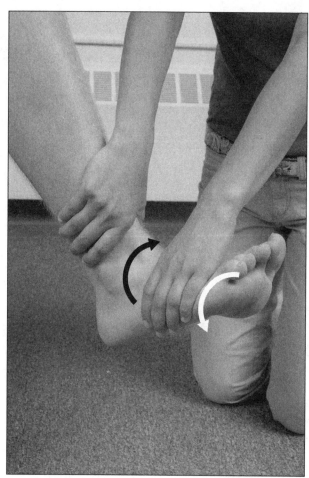

Figure 4-24 Proper positioning for eversion grades 5–3.

Source: Delmar/Cengage Learning

Testing for Ankle Eversion Grades 5, 4, 3 (Normal, Good, Fair) Gravity Resisted

POSITION OF PATIENT: Short sitting with ankle at neutral position or 90°.

POSITION OF THERAPIST: In front of patient on a stool with stabilizing hand behind ankle above the malleoli or around the anterior surface of the shin. Testing hand placed around the dorsum and lateral side of the foot and applies resistance toward inversion (see Figure 4-24).

TEST: Patient everts foot.

DIRECTIONS: Say to the patient, "Turn your foot out and do not let me pull you out of this position."

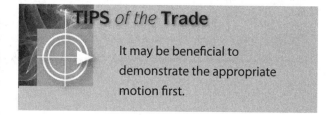

TIPS *of the* **Trade**

It may be beneficial to demonstrate the appropriate motion first.

GRADING:

- **Grade 5 (Normal):** Patient everts foot through full ROM while holding against therapist's maximum resistance without breaking.
- **Grade 4 (Good):** Patient everts foot through available ROM and holds against therapist's strong to moderate resistance and then breaks.
- **Grade 3 (Fair):** Patient everts foot through full ROM and holds at end range but no resistance is tolerated.

Testing for Ankle Eversion Grade 2 (Poor) Gravity Minimal

POSITION OF PATIENT: Supine with ankle flexed at 90°.

POSITION OF THERAPIST: Next to patient on a stool. No resistance is applied.

TEST: Patient is to evert foot without any resistance or assistance from the therapist.

DIRECTIONS: Say to the patient, "Try to turn your foot outward."

GRADING:

- **Grade 2 (Poor):** Able to complete ankle eversion through full ROM with gravity minimized.

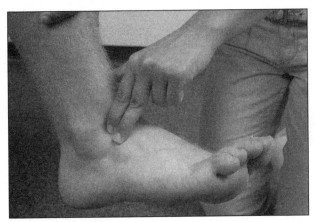

Figure 4-25 Proper positioning for palpation grades 1–0.

Source: Delmar/Cengage Learning

Testing for Ankle Eversion Grades 1, 0 (Trace, None) Gravity Minimal

POSITION OF PATIENT: Supine with ankle flexed at 90°.

POSITION OF THERAPIST: Next to patient with one hand contoured behind ankle for support while the other hand palpates the tendon of the peroneus longus or peroneus brevis.

> **TIPS** *of the* **Trade**
>
> Place the fingers just below the head of the fibula and posterior to the lateral malleolus to palpate the tendon of the peroneus longus. To palpate the peroneus brevis, place the fingers proximal to the fifth metatarsal and inferior to the middle of the lateral malleoli (see Figure 4-25).

TEST: Patient attempts to evert foot.

DIRECTIONS: Say to the patient, "Try to turn your foot outward."

GRADING:

- **Grade 1 (Trace):** Tendon movement is palpable but there is no visible movement.
- **Grade 0 (None):** Unable to palpate any contraction of the muscles or tendons.

Hallux and Toe MTP Flexion

Table 4-5 describes the primary and accessory muscles responsible for flexing the toes. The flexor hallucis longus and flexor digitorum longus muscles are the primary movers for toe flexion (see Figure 4-26).

TABLE 4-5	MUSCLES RESPONSIBLE FOR HALLUX AND TOE MTP FLEXION		
PRIMARY MUSCLES	**ORIGIN**	**INSERTION**	**INNERVATIONS**
Flexor hallucis longus	Posterior fibula and interosseous membrane	Distal phalanx of great toe	Tibial (L5, S1, S2)
Flexor digitorum longus	Posterior tibia	Distal phalanx of four lesser toes	Tibial (L5, S1)
ACCESSORY MUSCLES (INTRINSIC)	**ORIGIN**	**INSERTION**	**INNERVATIONS**
Flexor hallucis brevis	Plantar surface of cuboid bone	Both sides of base of proximal phalanx of great toe	Tibial (medial plantar branch) (L4-S1)
Lumbricales	From each tendon of flexor digitorum longus	Toes 2–5 on the proximal phalanges and the dorsal expansions of the extensor digitorum longus tendons	Tibial (L4-S2) (Medial plantar 1st lumbricale) (Lateral plantar lumbricales 2–4)

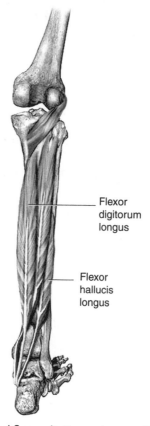

Flexor digitorum longus

Flexor hallucis longus

Figure 4-26 Flexor hallucis longus muscle and flexor digitorum longus *(See color plate).* Source: Delmar/Cengage Learning

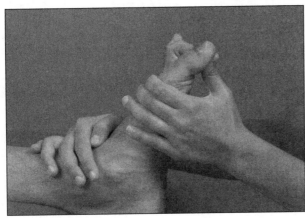

Figure 4-27 Proper positioning for great toe flexion grades 5–0. Source: Delmar/Cengage Learning

Testing for Hallux MTP Flexion Grades 5–0 (Normal to None)

POSITION OF PATIENT: Supine with ankle at neutral position or 90°.

POSITION OF THERAPIST: In front of patient with stabilizing hand placed around the dorsum of the forefoot. The index finger of the testing hand is placed under the proximal phalanx of great toe and applies resistance toward extension (see Figure 4-27).

TEST: Patient flexes great toe.

DIRECTIONS: Say to the patient, "Bend your big toe and do not let me straighten it."

GRADING:

- **Grade 5 (Normal):** Patient flexes great toe through full ROM while holding against therapist's maximum resistance without breaking.
- **Grade 4 (Good):** Patient flexes great toe through available ROM and holds against therapist's strong to moderate resistance and then breaks.
- **Grade 3 (Fair):** Patient flexes great toe through full ROM and holds at end range but no resistance is tolerated.
- **Grade 2 (Poor):** Partial ROM is completed.
- **Grade 1 (Trace):** No toe motion observed but contractile activity may be noted.
- **Grade 0 (None):** No contractile activity.

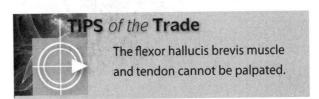

TIPS *of the* **Trade**

The flexor hallucis brevis muscle and tendon cannot be palpated.

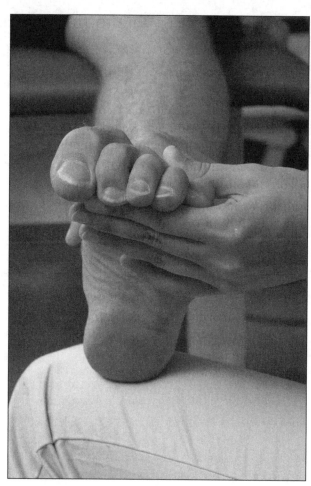

Figure 4-28 Proper positioning for lesser toes flexion grades 5–0. Source: Delmar/Cengage Learning

Testing for Toe MTP Flexion Grades 5–0 (Normal to None)

POSITION OF PATIENT: Supine with ankle at neutral position or 90°.

POSITION OF THERAPIST: In front of patient on a stool with patient's foot resting on therapist's lap. Stabilizing hand is placed around the dorsum of the forefoot. The index finger of the testing hand is placed under the MTP joints of four lesser toes and applies resistance toward extension (see Figure 4-28).

TEST: Patient flexes MTP joints of four lesser toes.

DIRECTIONS: Say to the patient, "Bend your toes and do not let me straighten them."

GRADING:

- **Grade 5 (Normal):** Patient flexes toes through full ROM while holding against therapist's maximum resistance without breaking.
- **Grade 4 (Good):** Patient flexes toes through available ROM and holds against therapist's strong to moderate resistance and then breaks.
- **Grade 3 (Fair):** Patient flexes toes through full ROM and holds at end range but no resistance is tolerated.
- **Grade 2 (Poor):** Partial ROM is completed.
- **Grade 1 (Trace):** No toe motion observed but contractile activity may be noted.
- **Grade 0 (None):** No contractile activity noted.

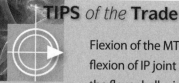

TIPS *of the* **Trade**

Flexion of the MTP joint without flexion of IP joint is observed when the flexor hallucis brevis takes over due to an improperly functioning flexor hallucis longus muscle. Conversely, IP joint flexion and MTP hyperextension is observed when the flexor hallucis longus muscle takes over for a poorly functioning flexor hallucis brevis muscle. When this becomes a chronic condition, it is known as hammer toes.

Hallux and Toe MTP Extension

Table 4-6 shows the primary and accessory muscles responsible for extending the toes. The extensor hallucis longus and extensor digitorum longus muscles are the primary movers for toe extension (see Figure 4-29).

TABLE 4-6	MUSCLES RESPONSIBLE FOR HALLUX AND TOE MTP EXTENSION		
PRIMARY MUSCLES	**ORIGIN**	**INSERTION**	**INNERVATIONS**
Extensor hallucis longus	Fibula and interosseous membrane	Distal phalanx of great toe	Deep peroneal (L4, L5, S1)
Extensor digitorum longus	Fibula, tibia, and interosseous membrane	Distal phalanx of four lesser toes	Deep peroneal (L4, L5, S1)

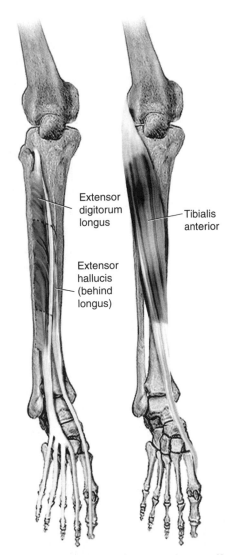

Figure 4-29 Extensor hallucis longus muscle and extensor digitorum longus *(See color plate).* Source: Delmar/Cengage Learning

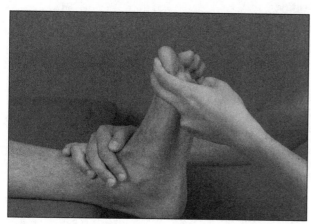

Figure 4-30   Proper positioning for great toe extension grades 5–0. Source: Delmar/Cengage Learning

Testing for Hallux MTP Extension Grades 5–0 (Normal to None)

POSITION OF PATIENT: Supine with ankle at neutral position or 90°.

POSITION OF THERAPIST: In front of patient with the stabilizing hand placed around the heel. The fingers of the testing hand are placed around the plantar surface of the metatarsal heads with the thumb curving around the base of the great toe and resting on the dorsal surface to apply resistance in a downward motion (see Figure 4-30).

TEST: Patient extends great toe.

DIRECTIONS: Say to the patient, "Bring your big toe up toward the ceiling and do not let me bend it down."

GRADING:

- **Grade 5 (Normal):** Patient extends great toe through full ROM while holding against therapist's maximum resistance without breaking.

- **Grade 4 (Good):** Patient extends great toe through available ROM and holds against therapist's strong to moderate resistance and then breaks.

- **Grade 3 (Fair):** Patient extends great toe through full ROM and holds at end range but no resistance is tolerated.

- **Grade 2 (Poor):** Partial ROM is completed.

- **Grade 1 (Trace):** No toe motion observed but contractile activity may be noted.

- **Grade 0 (None):** No contractile activity noted.

Testing for Lesser Toes MTP Extension Grades 5–0 (Normal to None)

POSITION OF PATIENT: Short sitting with ankle at neutral position or 90°.

POSITION OF THERAPIST: In front of patient on a stool with patient's foot resting on therapist's lap. The fingers of both hands stabilize the metatarsals on the plantar surface of the foot. The thumbs are placed on the dorsal surface of the proximal phalanges to apply resistance in a downward motion (see Figure 4-31).

TEST: Patient extends MTP joints of four lesser toes.

DIRECTIONS: Say to the patient, "Bring your toes up to the ceiling and do not let me push them down."

GRADING:

- **Grade 5 (Normal):** Patient extends toes through full ROM while holding against therapist's maximum resistance without breaking.
- **Grade 4 (Good):** Patient extends toes through available ROM and holds against therapist's strong to moderate resistance and then breaks.
- **Grade 3 (Fair):** Patient extends toes through full ROM and holds at end range but no resistance is tolerated.
- **Grade 2 (Poor):** Partial ROM is completed.
- **Grade 1 (Trace):** Palpable activity is noted of the extensor digitorum longus by placing the fingers over the dorsum of the metatarsals.
- **Grade 0 (None):** No contractile activity noted.

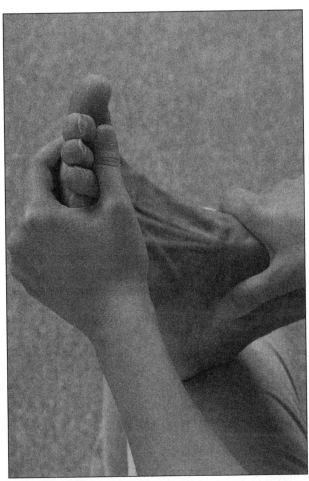

Figure 4-31 Proper positioning for lesser toe extension grades 5–0. Source: Delmar/Cengage Learning

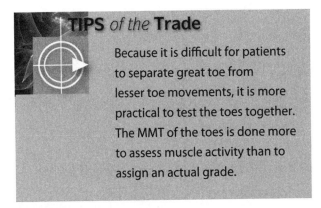

TIPS *of the* **Trade**

Because it is difficult for patients to separate great toe from lesser toe movements, it is more practical to test the toes together. The MMT of the toes is done more to assess muscle activity than to assign an actual grade.

Testing for Hallux IP and Lesser Toes DIP and PIP Flexion and Extension

It is possible to perform MMT on the IP joint of the great toe and the PIP and DIP joints of the four lesser toes. However, it is not very practical, so it will not be covered in detail in this text. Refer to the MMT of the MTP joints of the foot for proper procedure.

Testing for Abduction of Hallux and Four Lesser Toes

Because it is difficult for patients to isolate the abductor hallucis muscle, abduction of the great toe is not usually tested. However, the procedure is similar to abduction testing of the thumb. Refer to Chapter 9 on the hand for details. As for the four lesser toes, it is more practical to perform a functional test by asking the patient to spread the toes apart and observe if they can complete this motion.

Substitutions

Important substitutions to watch for during MMT of the ankle and foot are as follows:

- In the prone position, foot eversion during plantar flexion testing means substitution by the peroneus longus and brevis.
- Foot inversion during plantar flexion while prone signifies substitution by the tibialis posterior.
- Plantar flexion of the forefoot instead of the ankle during prone plantar flexion signifies substitution by the tibialis posterior, peroneus longus, and peroneus brevis together.
- Incomplete calcaneal movement and plantar flexion of the forefoot during prone plantar flexion signifies substitution by the flexor hallucis longus and flexor digitorum longus muscles.
- Extension of the toes during dorsiflexion testing signifies substitution by the extensor digitorum longus and the extensor hallucis longus muscles.
- Toe flexion during ankle inversion results in substitution by the flexor digitorum longus and flexor hallucis longus.

RANGE OF MOTION

Ankle Dorsiflexion

Ankle dorsiflexion occurs in the sagittal plane around the medial-lateral axis. The primary muscle involved is the anterior tibialis. According to the American Academy of Orthopaedic Surgeons (1965), normal ROM for this motion is 0°–20°. The end-feel for ankle dorsiflexion should be firm due to the tension in the posterior joint capsule, achilles tendon, and surrounding ligaments.

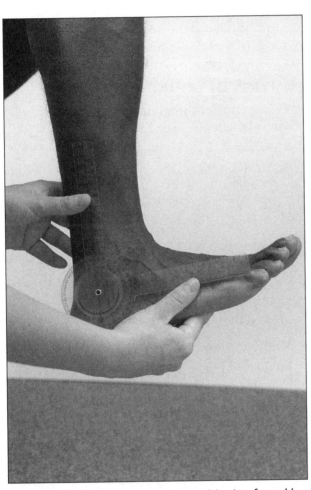

Figure 4-32 Proper goniometer positioning for ankle dorsiflexion. Source: Delmar/Cengage Learning

POSITION OF PATIENT: Supine or short sitting with ankle in neutral.

POSITION OF THERAPIST: Sitting on a stool next to patient by test limb. One hand is placed above and behind the ankle to prevent knee movement and the other pushes upward on the plantar surface of the foot for dorsiflexion.

POSITION OF GONIOMETER:

- **Fulcrum:** Slightly lateral and posterior to lateral malleolus (see Figure 4-32)

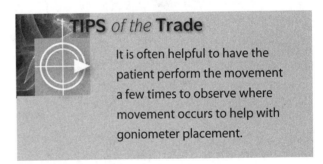

TIPS *of the* **Trade**

It is often helpful to have the patient perform the movement a few times to observe where movement occurs to help with goniometer placement.

- **Stationary arm:** Up toward head of fibula parallel to lateral midline of fibula
- **Movable arm:** Parallel to the fifth metatarsal

Ankle Plantar Flexion

Ankle plantar flexion occurs in the sagittal plane around the medial-lateral axis. As previously mentioned, the primary muscles involved are the gastrocnemius and soleus. According to the American Academy of Orthopaedic Surgeons (1965), normal ROM for this motion is 0°–50°. The end-feel for ankle plantar flexion should be firm due to the tension in the anterior joint capsule and the surrounding muscles and ligaments.

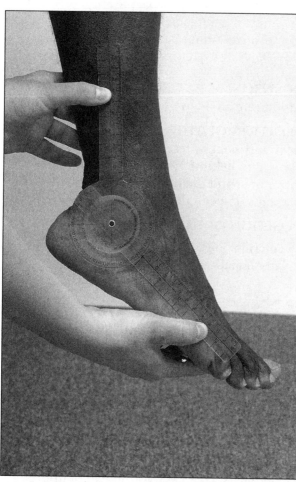

Figure 4-33 Proper goniometer positioning for ankle plantar flexion. Source: Delmar/Cengage Learning

POSITION OF PATIENT: Supine or short sitting with ankle in neutral.

POSITION OF THERAPIST: Sitting on a stool next to patient by test limb. One hand above and behind the ankle to prevent knee movement and the other on the dorsal surface of the foot facilitate plantar flexion.

POSITION OF GONIOMETER:

- **Fulcrum:** Slightly lateral and posterior to lateral malleolus (see Figure 4-33)

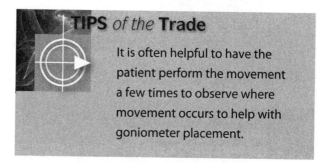

TIPS *of the* **Trade**

It is often helpful to have the patient perform the movement a few times to observe where movement occurs to help with goniometer placement.

- **Stationary arm:** Up toward head of fibula parallel to lateral midline of fibula
- **Movable arm:** Parallel to the fifth metatarsal

Ankle Forefoot Inversion

Ankle forefoot inversion is a combination of motions; therefore, it occurs around an oblique axis and is not a true plane motion. The primary muscle involved is the tibialis posterior. According to the American Academy of Orthopaedic Surgeons (1965), normal ROM for this motion is 0°–35°. The end-feel for inversion should be firm due to the tension in the joint capsules and the surrounding muscles and ligaments.

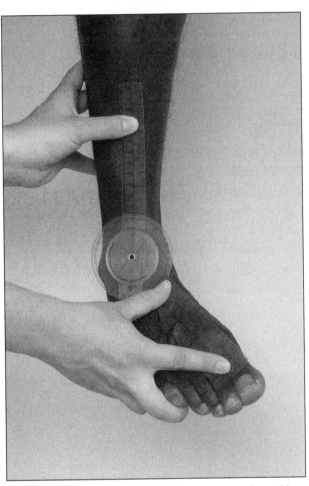

Figure 4-34 Proper goniometer positioning for ankle inversion. Source: Delmar/Cengage Learning

POSITION OF PATIENT: Supine or short sitting with ankle in neutral.

POSITION OF THERAPIST: Sitting on a stool next to patient by test limb. One hand is above and behind the ankle to prevent knee movement and the other contoured around the lateral surface of the forefoot to maintain inversion.

POSITION OF GONIOMETER:

- **Fulcrum:** On the dorsal ankle crease midway between the two malleoli on the anterior side (see Figure 4-34)
- **Stationary arm:** Toward the tibial tuberosity
- **Movable arm:** Anterior midline of second metatarsal head

Ankle Forefoot Eversion

Like inversion, ankle forefoot eversion occurs around an oblique axis and is not a true plane motion. The primary muscles involved are the peroneus longus and peroneus brevis. According to the American Academy of Orthopaedic Surgeons (1965), normal ROM for this motion is 0°–15°. The end-feel for inversion can be hard due to the contact between the calcaneus and the floor of the sinus tarsi or firm due to the tension in the joint capsules and the surrounding muscles and ligaments.

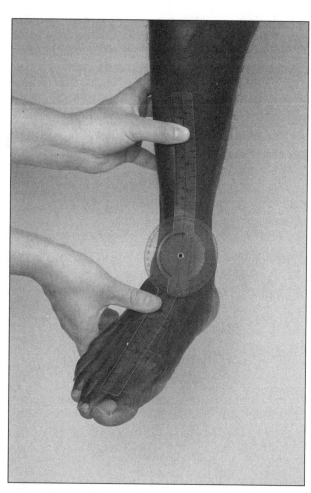

Figure 4-35 Proper goniometer positioning for ankle eversion. Source: Delmar/Cengage Learning

POSITION OF PATIENT: Supine or short sitting with ankle in neutral.

POSITION OF THERAPIST: Sitting on a stool next to patient by test limb. One hand above and behind the ankle to prevent knee movement and the other contoured around the medial surface of the forefoot to maintain eversion.

POSITION OF GONIOMETER:

- **Fulcrum:** On the dorsal ankle crease midway between the two malleoli on the anterior side (see Figure 4-35)
- **Stationary arm:** Toward the tibial tuberosity
- **Movable arm:** Anterior midline of second metatarsal head

Ankle Hindfoot/Subtalar Inversion

Because of the combination of motions that occur during hindfoot inversion, this motion also occurs around an oblique axis and is not a true plane motion. According to the American Academy of Orthopaedic Surgeons (1965), normal ROM for this motion is 0°–5°. The end-feel for hindfoot inversion is firm due to the tension in the lateral joint capsule and the surrounding ligaments.

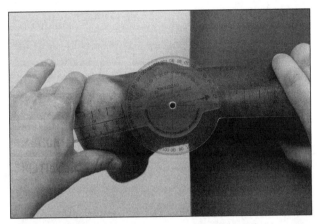

Figure 4-36 Proper goniometer positioning for hindfoot/subtalar inversion. Source: Delmar/Cengage Learning

POSITION OF PATIENT: Prone with foot over the edge in subtalar neutral.

POSITION OF THERAPIST: Sitting on a stool next to patient by test limb. One hand is contoured over posterior lower leg for stabilization. The other hand is around the plantar aspect of the hindfoot and pulls the calcaneus medially into subtalar inversion.

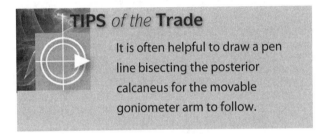

TIPS *of the* **Trade**

It is often helpful to draw a pen line bisecting the posterior calcaneus for the movable goniometer arm to follow.

POSITION OF GONIOMETER:

- **Fulcrum:** Midway between the two malleoli on the posterior side (see Figure 4-36)
- **Static arm:** Midline up the lower leg
- **Movable arm:** Follows pen line along the posterior midline of the calcaneus

Ankle Hindfoot/Subtalar Eversion

Like hindfoot inversion, hindfoot eversion also occurs around an oblique axis and is not a true plane motion. According to the American Academy of Orthopaedic Surgeons (1965), normal ROM for this motion is 0°–5°. The end-feel for hindfoot eversion can be hard due to the contact between the calcaneus and the floor of the sinus tarsi or firm due to the tension in the surrounding muscles and ligaments.

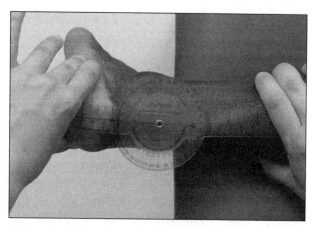

Figure 4-37 Proper goniometer positioning for hindfoot/subtalar eversion. Source: Delmar/Cengage Learning

POSITION OF PATIENT: Prone with foot over the edge in subtalar neutral.

POSITION OF THERAPIST: Sitting on a stool next to patient by test limb. One hand is contoured over posterior lower leg for stabilization. The other hand is around the plantar aspect of the hindfoot and pulls the calcaneus laterally into subtalar eversion.

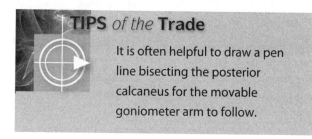

TIPS *of the* **Trade**

It is often helpful to draw a pen line bisecting the posterior calcaneus for the movable goniometer arm to follow.

POSITION OF GONIOMETER:

- **Fulcrum:** Midway between the two malleoli on the posterior side (see Figure 4-37)
- **Stationary arm:** Midline up the lower leg
- **Movable arm:** Follows pen line along the posterior midline of the calcaneus

MTP Flexion of the Great and Lesser Toes

MTP flexion occurs in the sagittal plane around the medial-lateral axis. The primary muscles involved are the flexor hallucis longus and flexor digitorum longus. According to the American Academy of Orthopaedic Surgeons (1965), normal ROM for the great toe flexion is 0°–45° and for the lesser toes 0°–40°. The end-feel for MTP flexion is firm due to the tension in the dorsal joint capsule, collateral ligaments, and surrounding muscles.

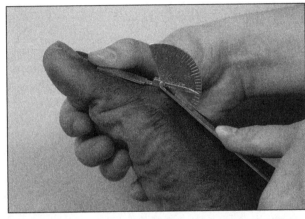

Figure 4-38 Proper goniometer positioning for MTP flexion. Source: Delmar/Cengage Learning

POSITION OF PATIENT: Supine with ankle in neutral.

POSITION OF THERAPIST: Sitting on a stool next to patient by test limb. One hand is placed around the metatarsals for stabilization, and the other moves MTP joint of the testing toe into flexion.

POSITION OF GONIOMETER:

- **Fulcrum:** Dorsal surface of MTP joint (see Figure 4-38)
- **Stationary arm:** Midline of metatarsal being tested
- **Movable arm:** Midline over proximal phalange of toe being tested

MTP Extension of the Great and Lesser Toes

MTP extension occurs in the sagittal plane around the medial-lateral axis. As previously mentioned, the primary muscles involved are the extensor hallucis longus and extensor digitorum longus. According to the American Academy of Orthopaedic Surgeons (1965), normal ROM for the great toe extension is 0°–70° and for the lesser toes 0°–40°. The end-feel for MTP extension is firm due to the tension in the plantar joint capsule and surrounding muscles.

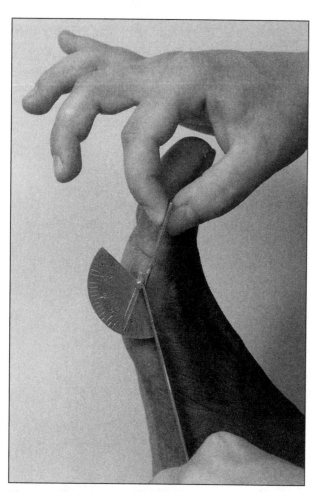

Figure 4-39 Proper goniometer positioning for MTP extension. Source: Delmar/Cengage Learning

POSITION OF PATIENT: Supine with ankle in neutral.

POSITION OF THERAPIST: Sitting on a stool next to patient by test limb. One hand is placed around the metatarsals for stabilization and the other moves MTP joint of the testing toe into extension.

POSITION OF GONIOMETER:

- **Fulcrum:** Dorsal surface of MTP joint (see Figure 4-39)
- **Stationary arm:** Midline of metatarsal being tested
- **Movable arm:** Midline over proximal phalange of toe being tested

MTP Abduction and DIP and PIP Flexion and Extension

Because it is not typically performed, MTP abduction, as well as DIP and PIP flexion and extension, are not covered in depth here. Measuring abduction of the MTP joints of the foot is similar to measuring MTP abduction in the hand. Refer to Chapter 9 for details. As for flexion and extension of the DIP and PIP joints in the foot, follow the same procedure previously outlined for measuring flexion and extension of the MTP joints of the foot.

⦿ FUNCTIONAL APPLICATION

Like the hip and knee, normal strength and ROM of the ankle joint are necessary for completing many daily mobility tasks like walking and ambulating stairs. To walk on level surfaces, the ankle joint needs 15° of dorsiflexion and 20° of plantar flexion, according to the *Observational Gait Analysis Handbook* of the Professional Staff Association, Rancho Los Amigos Medical Center (1989). Livingston, Stevenson, and Olney (1991) studied stair ambulation and found 14°–27° of ankle dorsiflexion and 23°–30° of ankle plantar flexion is needed for ambulating up stairs. They also found 20°–35° of ankle dorsiflexion and 20°–30° of ankle plantar flexion are required to ambulate down stairs. Limitations or pathologies in the ankle and foot can result in disabling consequences because they play such a crucial role in distributing the weight-bearing forces, helping maintain balance, and providing a stable base of support during ambulation. Symptoms in the ankle and foot can result in pain or other problems up into the knee, hip, and back. It is not uncommon for a patient presenting with back pain to find out the real culprit is improper footwear resulting in ankle and foot problems. It is easy to see why it is so important to take good care of the feet.

⦿ LEARNER CHALLENGE

1. List all the ankle and foot motions. Then identify the plane and axis in which they occur.
2. Palpate the following landmarks significant to the ankle and foot: medial and lateral malleoli; fibular head; calcaneus; metatarsals 1–5; proximal, middle, and distal phalanges of the toes; proximal and distal phalanges of great toe; and MTP, DIP, PIP, and IP joints of the phalanges.
3. On a lab partner, use a wax marker to shade in the following muscles of the anklet: tibialis anterior, gastrocnemius, soleus, tibialis posterior, peroneus longus, and peroneus brevis. Instruct your lab partner to perform ankle dorsiflexion, plantar flexion, eversion, and inversion, and observe/palpate the movements under the shaded areas. Then switch places and have the other lab partner use the wax marker to shade in the following muscles of the foot: flexor hallucis longus, flexor digitorum longus, extensor hallucis longus, and extensor digitorum longus. Instruct your lab partner to perform great toe and lesser toes flexion and extension while observing/palpating the movements under the shaded areas.
4. To practice manual muscle testing (MMT), one lab partner acts as the therapist and performs MMT of the ankle, including dorsiflexion, plantar flexion, eversion, and inversion grades 5–0. Then switch roles and the other lab partner performs MMT for the toes, including hallux and toe MTP flexion and hallux and toe MTP extension.
5. Using a goniometer, measure ROM on your lab partner for ankle dorsiflexion, plantar flexion, forefoot inversion, forefoot eversion, hindfoot/subtalar inversion, and hindfoot/subtalar eversion, as well as MTP flexion and extension of the toes. Switch roles and have the other partner use the goniometer to measure the same. Double-check for proper goniometer placement and compare your findings to normal ROM for each movement.
6. Fill in the following tables summarizing MMT and ROM measurements of the ankle and foot.

A) Manual Muscle Testing for Grades 5, 4, 3 Gravity Resisted

MOTION	TESTING POSITION	STABILIZING HAND	RESISTANCE HAND
Ankle Dorsiflexion			
Ankle Plantar Flexion Prone			
Ankle Plantar Flexion Standing			
Ankle Plantar Flexion Standing Soleus Only			
Ankle Inversion			
Ankle Eversion			
Hallux and Toe MTP Flexion			
Hallux and Toe MTP Extension			

B) Manual Muscle Testing for Grades 2, 1, 0 Gravity Minimal

MOTION	TESTING POSITION	STABILIZING HAND	RESISTANCE HAND	PALPATION
Ankle Dorsiflexion				
Ankle Plantar Flexion Prone				
Ankle Plantar Flexion Standing				
Ankle Plantar Flexion Standing Soleus Only				

continues

B) Manual Muscle Testing for Grades 2, 1, 0 Gravity Minimal *(continued)*

MOTION	TESTING POSITION	STABILIZING HAND	RESISTANCE HAND	PALPATION
Ankle Inversion				
Ankle Eversion				
Hallux and Toe MTP Flexion				
Hallux and Toe MTP Extension				

C) Range of Motion

MOTION	MOVABLE ARM	STATIONARY ARM	FULCRUM	NORMAL ROM
Ankle Dorsiflexion				
Ankle Plantar Flexion				
Ankle Forefoot Inversion				
Ankle Forefoot Eversion				
Ankle Hindfoot Inversion				
Ankle Hindfoot Eversion				
MTP Flexion of the Great and Lesser Toes				
MTP Extension of the Great and Lesser Toes				

NOTES

THE SHOULDER GIRDLE

CHAPTER **5**

OBJECTIVES

Upon completion of this chapter, the reader will be able to:

- Describe the shoulder girdle.

- Identify the bony landmarks of the scapula.

- Name the major ligaments.

- Describe the major motions of the shoulder girdle and name the muscles that perform them.

- Become familiar with the origins, insertions, and innervations of the muscles of the shoulder girdle.

- Perform proper manual muscle testing on the major muscles of the shoulder girdle grades 5–0.

- Be aware of possible substitutions during manual muscle testing on the shoulder girdle.

MUSCULOSKELETAL OVERVIEW

Scapular motion exists for the primary purpose of allowing us to place the hand in functional positions. It works in tandem with the shoulder joint, which will be discussed in Chapter 6, and the two together are often referred to as the *shoulder complex.* The scapula is located superficially on the posterior side of the thorax. It is triangular in shape and slightly concave in order to glide over the **convex** ribs located directly underneath it. The only bony structure to which the scapula is attached via ligaments is the clavicle. The scapula serves as an insertion point for a great number of muscles that also connect it to the spine.

Joints

The motions performed by the scapula are **elevation, depression, protraction, retraction,** and **upward** and **downward rotation.** Elevation/depression and protraction/retraction are essentially up/down and side/side motions, respectively. Upward and downward rotations are more angular motions and describe the movement of the scapula going up and away from the vertebral column or downward and toward the vertebral column.

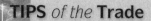

TIPS *of the* **Trade**

When trying to identify upward and downward rotation, picture the scapula "pinned" onto the skeleton at the superior angle and rotating around that pin. When the acromion goes up, upward rotation occurs. When the acromion goes down, downward rotation occurs.

The scapula works in tandem with the shoulder joint. The term *scapulohumeral rhythm* refers to this concept and occurs in a 2:1 ratio, meaning that for every 2° of shoulder motion after 30° of flexion or abduction, the scapula must rotate upward 1°. The beginning of glenohumeral motion is pure, but later on the scapula must work in conjunction with the glenohumeral joint. For example, from 0° to 30° of flexion or abduction, shoulder motion occurs with no scapular involvement. From 30° flexion or abduction, shoulder motion occurs in conjunction with scapular motion (Lippert, 2000).

TIPS *of the* **Trade**

When glenohumeral restriction is present, scapular movement may occur immediately as a compensatory movement. As a result, both of these structures should be assessed when there is limitation.

Bones

Bony landmarks on the scapula (see Figure 5-1) include:

- **Superior angle:** Superior medial aspect of scapula
- **Vertebral border:** The medial edge of the scapula (closest to the spine)
- **Inferior angle:** Inferior point of the scapula where the vertebral border and the axillary border meet
- **Axillary border:** The lateral edge of the scapula from the glenoid fossa to the inferior angle
- **Spine:** Runs mediolaterally across the upper portion of the scapula from border to border
- **Coracoid process:** Anterior projection found inferior to the clavicle
- **Acromion process:** Broad flat surface on the superior/lateral surface of the scapula
- **Glenoid fossa:** Concave surface that articulates with the humerus and is inferior to the acromion process

TIPS *of the* **Trade**

The inferior angle of the scapula should be found in line with the T7 vertebra.

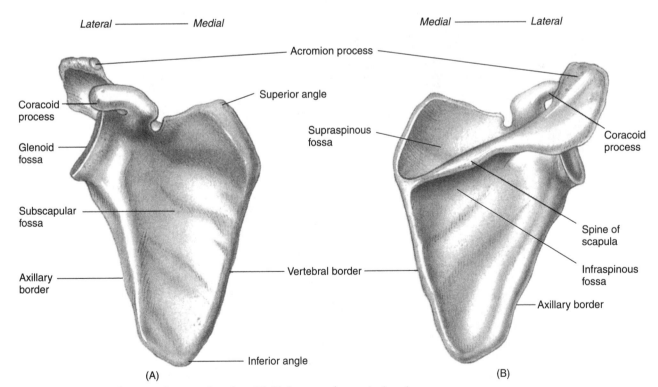

Figure 5-1 (A) Right scapula, anterior view (B) Right scapula, posterior view. Source: Delmar/Cengage Learning

Ligaments

Three major ligaments provide support to the scapula: the coracoclavicular, acromioclavicular, and the coracoacromial ligaments (see Figure 5-2).

TIPS *of the* **Trade**

Notice how the names of the ligaments help you locate each ligament by the attachment points on the bony structures.

The coracoclavicular ligament allows suspension and prevents backward motion of the scapula from the clavicle while the acromioclavicular ligament connects the acromion process of the scapula with the lateral end of the clavicle. The coracoacromial ligament arches over the head of the humerus forming a superior support when the head of the humerus responds to an upward force.

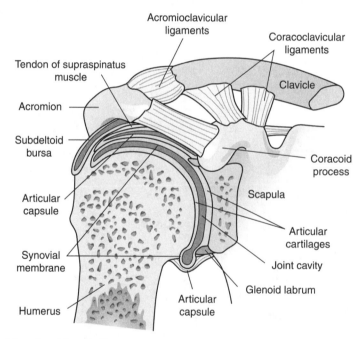

Figure 5-2 Ligaments of the shoulder girdle. Source: Delmar/Cengage Learning

MUSCLE TESTING OF THE SHOULDER GIRDLE

The techniques for muscle testing the scapular motions of elevation, depression, protraction, retraction, and upward and downward rotation will be discussed in depth.

Scapular Protraction and Upward Rotation

Table 5-1 presents the primary and accessory muscles responsible for scapular protraction and upward rotation. The serratus anterior muscle is the primary mover for these motions (see Figure 5-3).

TABLE 5-1	MUSCLES RESPONSIBLE FOR SCAPULAR PROTRACTION AND UPWARD ROTATION		
PRIMARY MUSCLES	**ORIGIN**	**INSERTION**	**INNERVATIONS**
Serratus anterior	Ribs 1–8, intercostal fascia, aponeurosis of intercostals	Scapula (ventral surface of vertebral border)	Long thoracic nerve (C5, C6, C7)
ACCESSORY MUSCLES	**ORIGIN**	**INSERTION**	**INNERVATIONS**
Pectoralis minor	Anterior surface of 3–5 ribs	Coracoid process of the scapula	Medial pectoral nerve

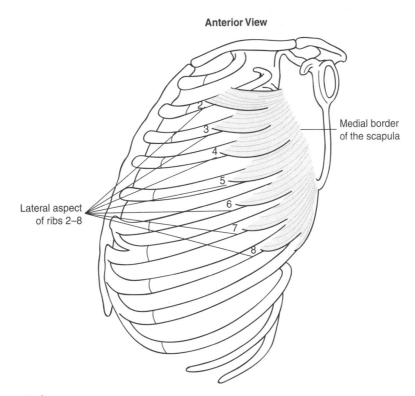

Anterior View

Medial border of the scapula

Lateral aspect of ribs 2–8

Figure 5-3 Serratus anterior. Source: Delmar/Cengage Learning

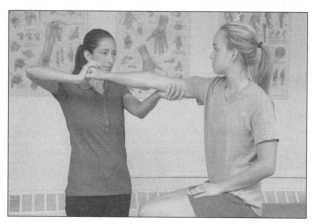

Figure 5-4 Proper positioning for scapular protraction grades 3–5. Source: Delmar/Cengage Learning

Testing for Scapular Protraction and Upward Rotation Grades 5, 4, 3 (Normal, Good, Fair) Gravity Resisted

POSITION OF PATIENT: Short sitting.

POSITION OF THERAPIST: Standing at test side of patient with testing hand on patient's raised fist and stabilizing hand resting on lateral ribs with fingers on the scapula (see Figure 5-4).

TEST: Instruct patient to raise arm to 130° **scaption** (midway between flexion and abduction), make a fist, and punch upward. Therapist pushes back against the motion.

DIRECTIONS: Say to patient "Punch and hold your position. Don't let me push you back."

GRADING:

- **Grade 5 (Normal):** Patient lifts to position and holds against maximum resistance.

- **Grade 4 (Good):** Patient lifts to position and holds against strong (but not full) resistance.

- **Grade 3 (Fair):** Patient lifts to position but tolerates no resistance.

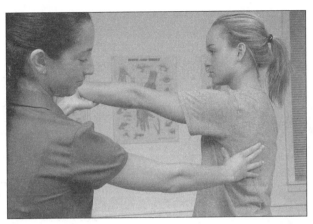

Figure 5-5 Proper positioning for scapular protraction grades 0–2. Source: Delmar/Cengage Learning

Testing for Scapular Protraction and Upward Rotation Grades 2, 1, 0 (Poor, Trace, None) Gravity Minimal

POSITION OF PATIENT: Short sitting.

POSITION OF THERAPIST: Standing at test side of patient with testing hand supporting arm in position and stabilizing hand palpating scapula (see Figure 5-5).

TEST: Therapist notes scapula's ability to maintain abducted and upwardly rotated position as therapist removes some support.

DIRECTIONS: Say to patient, "Hold your arm in this position."

GRADING:

- **Grade 2 (Poor):** Scapula maintains position.
- **Grade 1 (Trace):** Muscle contraction is noted but unable to maintain position.
- **Grade 0 (None):** No contraction noted.

Scapular Elevation

Table 5-2 shows the primary and accessory muscles responsible for scapular elevation. The upper trapezius (see Figure 5-6) and levator scapula (see Figure 5-7) are the primary movers for scapula elevation.

TABLE 5-2	MUSCLES RESPONSIBLE FOR SCAPULAR ELEVATION		
PRIMARY MUSCLES	**ORIGIN**	**INSERTION**	**INNERVATIONS**
Upper trapezius	Occiput (external protruberance), ligamentum nuchae, and C7 (spinous process)	Clavicle (posterior, lateral 1/3)	Spinal accessory, C3 and C4 sensory component
Levator scapula	C1–C4 vertebrae (transverse process)	Scapula (vertebral border between superior angle and root of scapular spine)	3rd and 4th cervical nerves, dorsal scapular nerve (C5)
ACCESSORY MUSCLES	**ORIGIN**	**INSERTION**	**INNERVATIONS**
Rhomboid major	T2–T5 spinous processes and supraspinous ligaments	Mid-portion of the vertebral border of the scapula	Dorsal scapular nerve
Rhomboid minor	C7–T1 spinous processes and ligamentum nuchae	Root of the spine of the scapula	Dorsal scapular nerve

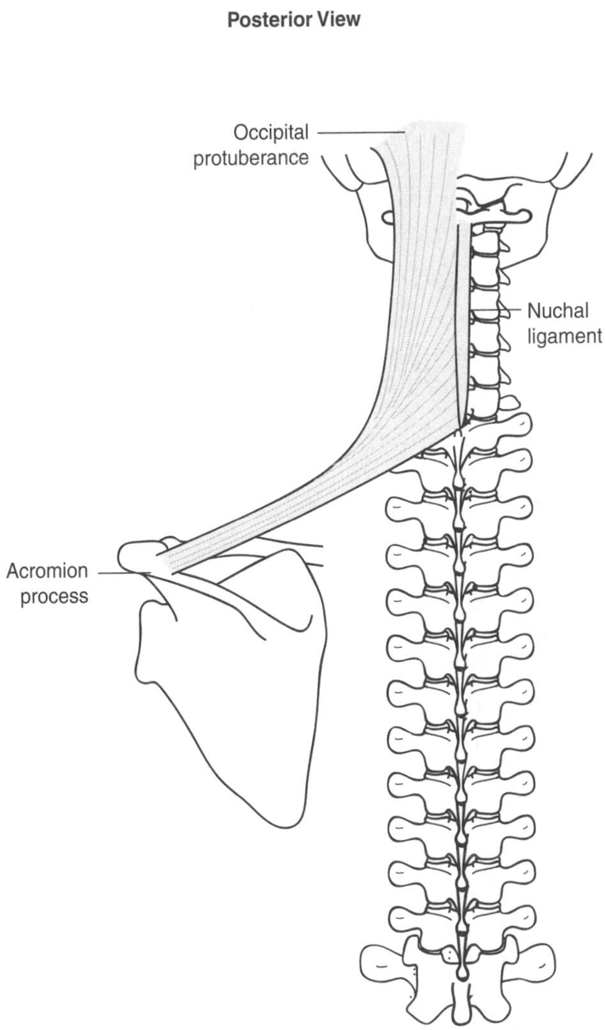

Posterior View

Occipital protuberance

Nuchal ligament

Acromion process

Figure 5-6 Upper trapezius. Source: Delmar/Cengage Learning

Posterior View

Transverse processes of C1–C4

Superior angle

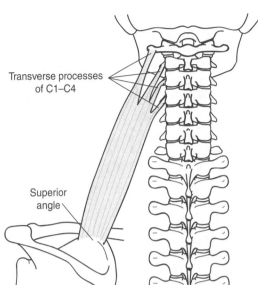

Figure 5-7 Levator scapula. Source: Delmar/Cengage Learning

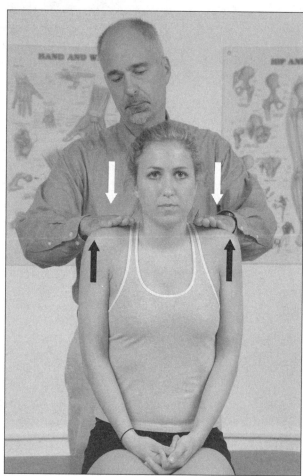

Figure 5-8 Proper positioning for scapular elevation grades 3–5. Source: Delmar/Cengage Learning

Testing for Scapular Elevation Grades 5, 4, 3 (Normal, Good, Fair) Gravity Resisted

POSITION OF PATIENT: Short sitting.

POSITION OF THERAPIST: Standing behind patient with hands resting on top of shoulders to apply downward pressure (see Figure 5-8).

TEST: Patient elevates shoulders bilaterally. Patient holds position as therapist applies downward resistance.

DIRECTIONS: Say to patient. "Lift your shoulders toward your ears" or "shrug your shoulders." "Hold your position and don't let me push your shoulders down."

GRADING:

- **Grade 5 (Normal):** Patient shrugs shoulders and holds against maximum resistance.
- **Grade 4 (Good):** Patient shrugs shoulders and holds against strong (but not full) resistance.
- **Grade 3 (Fair):** Patient shrugs shoulders but tolerates no resistance.

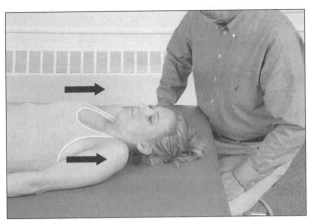

Figure 5-9 Proper positioning for scapular elevation grades 0–2. Source: Delmar/Cengage Learning

Scapular Elevation Grades 2, 1, 0 (Poor, Trace, None) Gravity Minimal

POSITION OF PATIENT: Patient lying supine or prone.

POSITION OF THERAPIST: Test side of patient with one hand supporting under the shoulder and the other hand over muscles to be palpated (see Figure 5-9).

TEST: Patient elevates shoulder toward ear (usually unilaterally).

DIRECTIONS: Say to patient. "Raise your shoulder toward your ear."

GRADING:

- **Grade 2 (Poor):** Patient is able to complete full motion.
- **Grade 1 (Trace):** Partial or no shoulder movement noted but muscle movement can be palpated.
- **Grade 0 (None):** No muscle movement noted.

Scapular Retraction

The primary and accessory muscles responsible for scapular retraction are shown in Table 5-3. The middle trapezius (see Figure 5-10) and the rhomboid major muscles (see Figure 5-11) are the primary movers for scapular retraction.

TABLE 5-3 — MUSCLES RESPONSIBLE FOR SCAPULAR RETRACTION

PRIMARY MUSCLES	ORIGIN	INSERTION	INNERVATIONS
Middle trapezius	T1–T5 vertebrae (spinous process)	Scapula (acromion)	Spinal accessory, C3 and C4 sensory component
Rhomboid major	T2–T5 vertebrae (spinous process)	Scapula (vertebral border)	Dorsal scapular nerve (C5)

ACCESSORY MUSCLES	ORIGIN	INSERTION	INNERVATIONS
Rhomboid minor	C7–T1 spinous processes and ligamentum nuchae	Root of the spine of the scapula	Dorsal scapular nerve
Trapezius (upper and lower)	Occiput (external protruberance), Ligamentum nuchae, C7 (spinous process)	Clavicle (posterior, lateral 1/3)	Spinal accessory, C3 and C4 sensory component
	T6–T12 vertebrae (spinous processes)	Scapula (spine)	
Levator scapulae	C1–C4 vertebrae (transverse process)	Scapula (vertebral border between superior angle and root of scapular spine)	3rd and 4th cervical nerves, dorsal scapular nerve (C5)

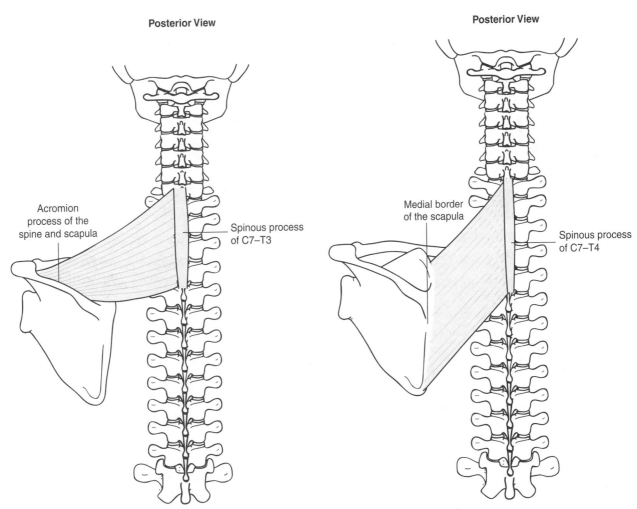

Posterior View

Acromion process of the spine and scapula

Spinous process of C7–T3

Figure 5-10 Middle trapezius. Source: Delmar/Cengage Learning

Posterior View

Medial border of the scapula

Spinous process of C7–T4

Figure 5-11 Rhomboids. Source: Delmar/Cengage Learning

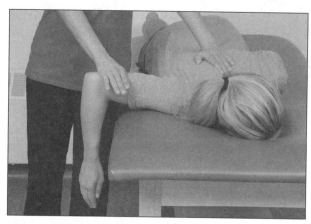

Figure 5-12 Proper positioning for scapular retraction grades 3–5. Source: Delmar/Cengage Learning

Testing for Scapular Retraction Grades 5, 4, 3 (Normal, Good, Fair) Gravity Resisted

POSITION OF PATIENT: Prone with shoulder abducted to 90° and resting over edge of table. Elbow is flexed at 90°.

POSITION OF THERAPIST: Standing at test side with testing hand on upper arm just above elbow to apply downward resistance. The stabilizing hand is placed on scapula to provide support (see Figure 5-12).

TEST: Patient performs horizontal abduction, thus retracting the scapula. Patient holds position while therapist applies downward pressure.

DIRECTIONS: Say to patient, "Raise your elbow toward the ceiling. Hold the position and don't let me push your arm down."

GRADING:

- **Grade 5 (Normal):** Completes motion and holds against maximum resistance.
- **Grade 4 (Good):** Completes motion and holds against strong (but not full) resistance.
- **Grade 3 (Fair):** Completes motion but tolerates no resistance.

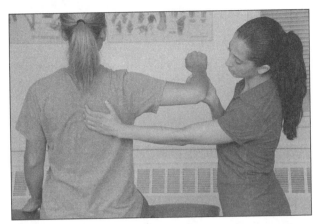

Figure 5-13 Proper positioning for scapular retraction grades 0–2. Source: Delmar/Cengage Learning

Testing for Scapular Retraction Grades 2, 1, 0 (Poor, Trace, None) Gravity Minimal

POSITION OF PATIENT: Short sitting.

POSITION OF THERAPIST: Standing at test side with testing hand supporting patient's arm in shoulder abduction (90°) and elbow flexion (90°). Stabilizing hand is placed over the scapula to palpate muscle movement (see Figure 5-13).

TEST: Patient performs horizontal abduction.

DIRECTIONS: Say to patient, "Move your elbow back as far as you can."

GRADING:

- **Grade 2 (Poor):** Patient is able to complete full motion.
- **Grade 1 (Trace):** Partial or no shoulder movement noted but muscle movement can be palpated.
- **Grade 0 (None):** No muscle movement noted.

Scapular Retraction and Downward Rotation

Table 5-4 lists the primary and accessory muscles responsible for scapular retraction and downward rotation. The rhomboid major and minor muscles are the primary muscles responsible for these two motions (refer to Figure 5-11).

TABLE 5-4	MUSCLES RESPONSIBLE FOR SCAPULAR RETRACTION AND DOWNWARD ROTATION		
PRIMARY MUSCLES	**ORIGIN**	**INSERTION**	**INNERVATIONS**
Rhomboid major	T2–T5 vertebrae (spinous processes)	Scapula (vertebral border)	Dorsal scapular nerve (C5)
Rhomboid minor	C7–T1 vertebrae (spinous processes), ligamentum nuchae	Scapula (root of spine)	Dorsal scapular nerve (C5)
ACCESSORY MUSCLES	**ORIGIN**	**INSERTION**	**INNERVATIONS**
Levator scapulae	C1–C4 vertebrae (transverse process)	Scapula (vertebral border between superior angle and root of scapular spine)	3rd and 4th cervical nerves, dorsal scapular nerve (C5)

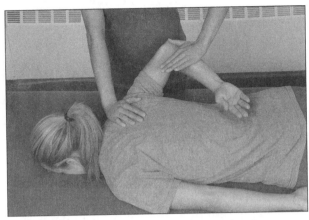

Figure 5-14 Proper positioning for rhomboids grades 3–5. Source: Delmar/Cengage Learning

Testing for Scapular Retraction and Downward Rotation Grades 5, 4, 3 (Normal, Good, Fair) Gravity Resisted

There is much debate about the individual testing of the rhomboid musculature and positioning for this test. To avoid confusion, only one method is discussed here with the understanding that others are also used.

POSITION OF PATIENT: Prone with arm positioned so that the back of the hand is resting on the small of the back.

POSITION OF THERAPIST: Standing at test side with testing hand on the upper arm just above the elbow to apply downward resistance and stabilizing hand placed over scapula to support (see Figure 5-14).

TEST: Patient lifts the hand off the back, and the therapist applies downward resistance.

DIRECTIONS: Say to patient, "Raise your hand off your back. Hold that position and don't let me push you down."

GRADING:

- **Grade 5 (Normal):** Completes motion and holds against maximum resistance.
- **Grade 4 (Good):** Completes motion and holds against strong (but not full) resistance.
- **Grade 3 (Fair):** Completes motion but tolerates no resistance.

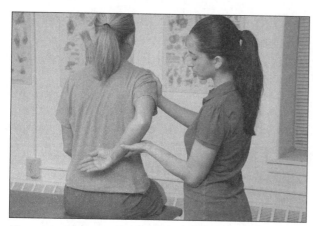

Figure 5-15 Proper positioning for rhomboids grades 0–2. Source: Delmar/Cengage Learning

Testing for Scapular Retraction and Downward Rotation Grades 2, 1, 0 (Poor, Trace, None) Gravity Minimal

POSITION OF PATIENT: Short sitting with arm in same position behind the back as stated for grades 3–5.

POSITION OF THERAPIST: Standing at test side with one hand supporting the patient's hand as needed and the other hand palpating over scapula (see Figure 5-15).

TEST: Patient moves hand away from back.

DIRECTIONS: Say to patient, "Lift hand away from your back."

GRADING:

- **Grade 2 (Poor):** Patient is able to complete full motion.
- **Grade 1 (Trace):** Partial or no shoulder movement noted but muscle movement can be palpated.
- **Grade 0 (None):** No muscle movement noted.

Scapular Depression

The primary and accessory muscles responsible for scapular depression are detailed in Table 5-5. The lower trapezius muscle is the primary mover for scapular depression (see Figure 5-16).

TABLE 5-5	MUSCLES RESPONSIBLE FOR SCAPULAR DEPRESSION		
PRIMARY MUSCLES	**ORIGIN**	**INSERTION**	**INNERVATIONS**
Lower trapezius	T6–T12 vertebrae (spinous processes)	Scapula (spine)	Spinal accessory, C3 and C4 sensory component
ACCESSORY MUSCLES	**ORIGIN**	**INSERTION**	**INNERVATIONS**
Middle trapezius	Spinous processes C7–T3	Spine of scapula	Spinal accessory, C3 and C4 sensory component
Latissimus dorsi	Spinous processes of T7–L5	Medial lip of bicipital groove of the humerous	Thoracodorsal nerve
Pectoralis minor	Anterior surface of 3–5 ribs	Coracoid process of the scapula	Medial pectoral nerve

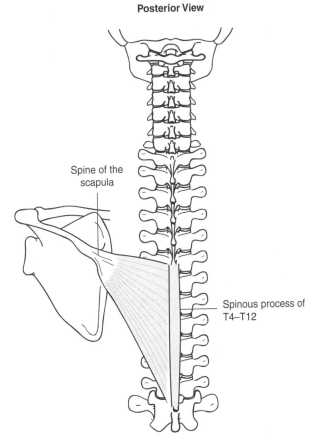

Posterior View

Spine of the scapula

Spinous process of T4–T12

Figure 5-16 Lower trapezius. Source: Delmar/Cengage Learning

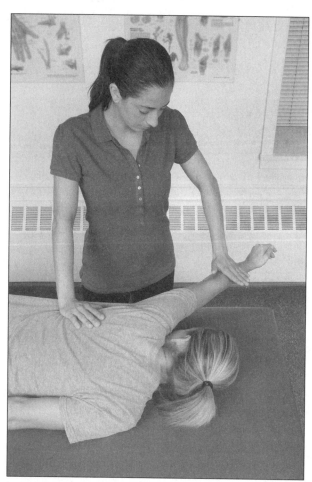

Figure 5-17 Proper positioning for scapular depression grades 3–5. Source: Delmar/Cengage Learning

Testing for Scapular Depression Grades 5, 4, 3 (Normal, Good, Fair) Gravity Resisted

POSITION OF PATIENT: Prone with arm ready to be raised into scaption to about 130°.

POSITION OF THERAPIST: Standing at test side of patient with testing hand on upper arm just above elbow and stabilizing hand resting on scapula for support (see Figure 5-17).

TEST: Patient raises arm as described; then therapist applies downward resistance.

DIRECTIONS: Say to patient, "Raise your arm off the table and hold it. Don't let me push you back down."

GRADING:

- **Grade 5 (Normal):** Completes motion and holds against maximum resistance.
- **Grade 4 (Good):** Completes motion and holds against strong (but not full) resistance.
- **Grade 3 (Fair):** Completes motion but tolerates no resistance.

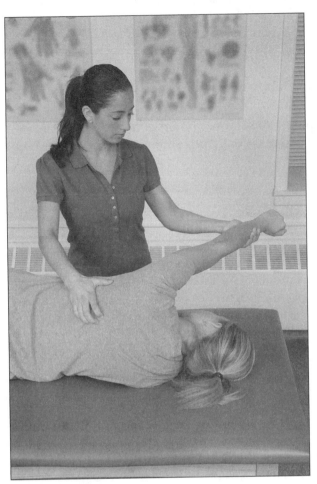

Figure 5-18 Proper positioning for scapular depression grades 0–2. Source: Delmar/Cengage Learning

Testing for Scapular Depression
Grade 2, 1, 0 (Poor, Trace, None)
Gravity Minimal

POSITION OF PATIENT: Side-lying with arm ready to be raised as described previously.

POSITION OF THERAPIST: Standing at test side of patient with one hand supporting arm as needed and other hand over scapula to palpate (see Figure 5-18).

TEST: Patient attempts to move arm through motion.

DIRECTIONS: Say to patient as you demonstrate, "Try to lift your arm in this direction."

GRADING:

- **Grade 2 (Poor):** Patient is able to complete full motion.
- **Grade 1 (Trace):** Partial or no shoulder movement noted but muscle movement can be palpated.
- **Grade 0 (None):** No muscle movement noted.

Substitutions

Important substitutions to watch for during MMT of the shoulder girdle are as follows:

- If shoulder elevators are weak, the rhomboids may try to take on more than their usual role of assisting in the motion. You will know this is happening if, during an unsuccessful attempt to elevate the shoulders, the scapula also adducts and downwardly rotates.
- During normal shoulder adduction, the scapula will upwardly rotate as the trapezius kicks in. If the rhomboids are substituting, the upward rotation component will be absent and the rhomboids will cause downward rotation instead.

FUNCTIONAL APPLICATION

The shoulder girdle is unlike the other joints discussed in this text. As the scapula glides around the rib cage, it is capable of both angular and linear movements. As the upper quadrant is assessed, it is important to remember how vital scapular function is to the function of the entire upper extremity. It is very unusual for activity occurring at the shoulder joint to happen without scapular movement.

LEARNER CHALLENGE

1. Given the distinct, almost triangular, shape of the scapula, how can you determine if its rotational direction is upward or downward?
2. Palpate the following bony landmarks of the scapula: spine of scapula, inferior angle, vertebral border, medial border, coracoid process, acromion process.
3. On a lab partner, use a china marker to shade in the supraspinatus and infraspinatus muscles on one side of the back and the rhomboids and the levator scapula on the other. Instruct lab partner to perform scapular motions and observe/palpate the movement under your shaded areas.
4. Fill in the following tables summarizing MMT and ROM measurements of the shoulder girdle.

A)   Manual Muscle Testing for Grades 5, 4, 3 Gravity Resisted

MOTION	TESTING POSITION	STABILIZING HAND	RESISTANCE HAND
Scapular Protraction and Upward Rotation			
Scapular Elevation			
Scapular Retraction			

continues

A) Manual Muscle Testing for Grades 5, 4, 3 Gravity Resisted (continued)

MOTION	TESTING POSITION	STABILIZING HAND	RESISTANCE HAND
Scapular Retraction and Downward Rotation			
Scapular Depression			

B) Manual Muscle Testing for Grades 2, 1, 0 Gravity Minimal

MOTION	TESTING POSITION	STABILIZING HAND	RESISTANCE HAND	PALPATION
Scapular Protraction and Upward Rotation				
Scapular Elevation				
Scapular Retraction				
Scapular Retraction and Downward Rotation				
Scapular Depression				

NOTES

THE SHOULDER

CHAPTER **6**

OBJECTIVES

Upon completion of this chapter, the reader will be able to:

- Describe the shoulder joint.

- Identify the bony landmarks significant to the shoulder joint.

- Name the major ligaments and their purpose.

- Describe any supporting structures important to the shoulder.

- Describe the major motions of the shoulder and name the muscles that perform them.

- Become familiar with the origins, insertions, and innervations of the muscles of the shoulder.

- Perform proper manual muscle testing on the major muscles of the shoulder grades 5–0.

- Be aware of possible substitutions during manual muscle testing on the shoulder.

- Accurately perform range of motion testing using the goniometer on the shoulder joint.

163

MUSCULOSKELETAL OVERVIEW

The shoulder joint moves in numerous ways to allow us to place the hand in a multitude of functional positions. This mobility comes at a price, however, in that the joint is less stable and more susceptible to injury. This joint actually works in conjunction with the scapula (see Chapter 6), thus proving an important assessment point: You should *never* assess an individual joint without also examining the joints above and below it to note limitations.

Joints

The shoulder joint is formed by the articulation between the glenoid fossa of the scapula and the head of the humerus. We have previously discussed the scapular landmarks, so we will focus in this chapter on the bony landmarks and palpation points of the humerus (see Figure 6-1).

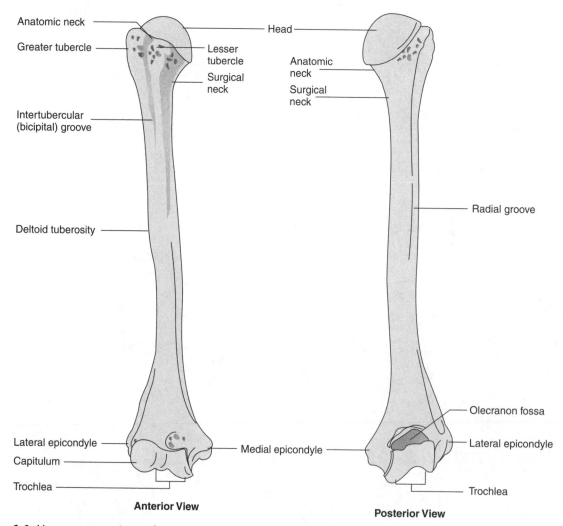

Figure 6-1 Humerus, anterior and posterior views. Source: Delmar/Cengage Learning

Bones

The following list identifies bony landmarks of the humerus:

- **Head:** Articulates with the scapula at the glenoid fossa; gently rounded proximal end
- **Anatomical neck:** The groove around the circumference between the head and the tubercles
- **Greater tubercle:** The larger, more lateral protuberance
- **Lesser tubercle:** Smaller protuberance located on the anterior surface between the greater tubercle and the head
- **Bicipital groove:** The longitudinal groove that separates the tubercles
- **Surgical neck:** Slightly narrowed area where the head meets the shaft of the bone just below the tubercles
- **Shaft:** The long body of the bone that extends from the surgical head distally to the epicondyles
- **Deltoid tuberosity:** About midshaft on the lateral surface

TIPS *of the* **Trade**

The deltoid tuberosity is not a well-defined palpation point but is often tender to the touch and therefore easy to locate.

- **Medial epicondyle:** Rounded protuberance located on the medial side of the distal shaft of the humerus
- **Lateral epicondyle:** Rounded protuberance located on the lateral side of the distal shaft of the humerus
- **Trochlea:** The articulation point with the ulna; located at the distal end on the medial side
- **Capitulum:** The articulation point with the radius; located at the distal end on the lateral side
- **Olecranon fossa:** Located on the posterior surface between the epicondyles; provides an articulation with the olecranon process of the ulna

Ligaments

Three ligamentous structures surround the shoulder joint. The three glenohumeral ligaments are named for their location in relationship to each other (superior, middle, and inferior). These structures are not well defined and appear to be a part of the actual capsule. These structures attach to the rim of the glenoid fossa and the anatomical neck of the humerus. The coracohumeral ligament runs from the lateral side of the coracoid process across the anterior surface of the joint to the medial side of the greater tubercle. The coracoacromial ligament is an indirect superior support for the joint (see Figure 6-2).

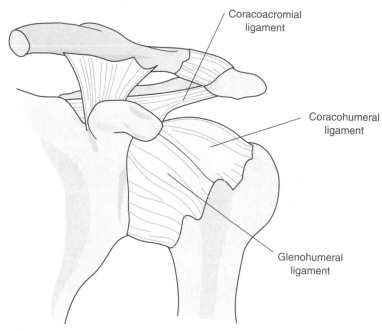

Coracoacromial
ligament

Coracohumeral
ligament

Glenohumeral
ligament

Figure 6-2 Ligaments of the shoulder. Source: Delmar/Cengage Learning

Supporting Structures

The pure movements possible at the shoulder joint include flexion/extension, medial/lateral (internal/external) rotation, and abduction/adduction. By combining the flexion/extension actions with abduction/adduction, the joint also has available movement in **horizontal abduction/adduction** and **circumduction.** Many functional **activities of daily living (ADLs)** require shoulder ROM, but it is important to note that the movements achieved by this joint require associated movements by the scapula and clavicle.

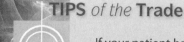

TIPS *of the* **Trade**

> If your patient has limited shoulder ROM, it is imperative that you assess ADLs and provide adaptations and assistive devices as needed as part of a well-rounded home program.

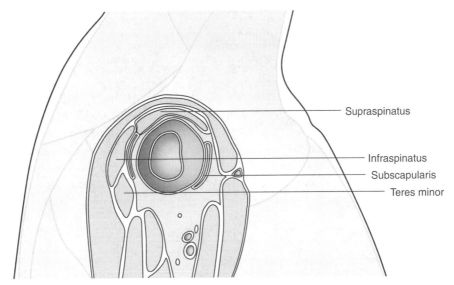

Figure 6-3 Muscles of the rotator cuff (lateral view of shoulder). Source: Delmar/Cengage Learning

The shoulder joint could not be discussed without mentioning the rotator cuff. The rotator cuff is responsible for providing stability to the shoulder joint. It is made up of the tendinous insertions of several muscles into the joint capsule. These muscles are the supraspinatus, providing support superiorly; the infraspinatus and the teres minor, providing support posteriorly; and the subscapularis, providing support anteriorly (see Figure 6-3).

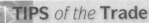
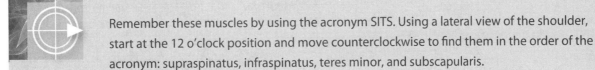

TIPS *of the* **Trade**

Remember these muscles by using the acronym SITS. Using a lateral view of the shoulder, start at the 12 o'clock position and move counterclockwise to find them in the order of the acronym: supraspinatus, infraspinatus, teres minor, and subscapularis.

These relatively small muscles are often required to participate in strenuous activities such as pitching a baseball. They can be injured easily if not maintained at the proper level of strength. There is also a propensity toward impingement, especially in the supraspinatus if proper body mechanics and/or frequent rest breaks are not imposed, especially during activities involving horizontal abduction and adduction, such as window washing or painting.

MUSCLE TESTING OF THE SHOULDER

Eight pure motions are available at the shoulder: flexion, extension, abduction, adduction, internal (medial) rotation, external (lateral) rotation, horizontal abduction, and horizontal adduction. These motions are tested individually. Because the shoulder joint allows such freedom of movement, there is also a combination of these pure motions called *circumduction*. There are no specific tests for this motion as it uses a coordinated combination of the previously mentioned motions. Because it is important to review the muscles associated with these movements, each section begins with a table of the muscles responsible for the movement being tested, followed by a depiction of the primary muscles.

Shoulder Flexion

Table 6-1 describes the primary and accessory muscles responsible for shoulder flexion. The deltoid muscle is the prime mover for shoulder flexion (see Figure 6-4).

TABLE 6-1	MUSCLES RESPONSIBLE FOR SHOULDER FLEXION		
PRIMARY MUSCLES	**ORIGIN**	**INSERTION**	**INNERVATION**
Deltoid, anterior fibers	Lateral 1/3 of clavicle, anterior superior surface	Deltoid tuberosity of the humerus	Axillary nerve
ACCESSORY MUSCLES	**ORIGIN**	**INSERTION**	**INNERVATION**
Corcacobrachialis	Coracoid process of the scapula	Midpoint of the medial surface of the humerus	Musculocutaneous nerve
Pectoralis major (upper)	Medial third of the clavicle	Lateral lip of the bicipital groove of the humerus	Lateral and medial pectoral nerve
Deltoid	Acromion process	Deltoid tuberosity of humerus	Axillary
Serratus anterior	Ribs 1–8, intercostal fascia, aponeurosis of intercostals	Scapula (ventral surface of vertebral border)	Long thoracic nerve (C5, C6, C7)

Anterior View

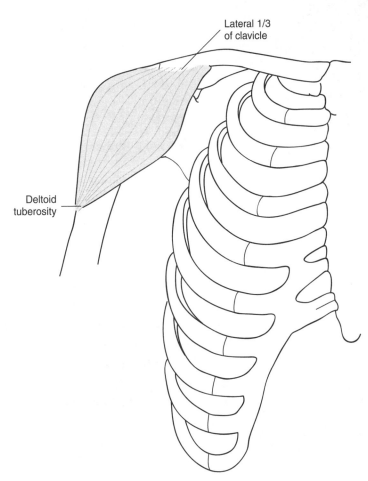

Lateral 1/3
of clavicle

Deltoid
tuberosity

Figure 6-4 Anterior deltoid. Source: Delmar/Cengage Learning

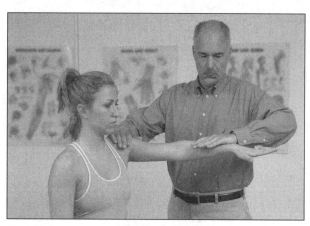

Figure 6-5 Proper positioning for shoulder flexion grades 5–0. Source: Delmar/Cengage Learning

Testing for Shoulder Flexion Grades 5–0 (Normal to None)

POSITION OF PATIENT: Short sitting.

POSITION OF THERAPIST: Standing on test side. Hand giving resistance is placed over the distal humerus, taking care to stay above the elbow. Pressure is applied in a downward direction (see Figure 6-5).

TEST: Patient raises the arm to 90° of pure flexion and is instructed to hold that position against resistance.

DIRECTIONS: Say to the patient, "Raise your arm straight out in front of you and hold it. Don't let me push it down."

GRADING:

- **Grade 5 (Normal):** Patient lifts to position and holds against maximum resistance.
- **Grade 4 (Good):** Patient lifts to position and holds against strong (but not full) resistance.
- **Grade 3 (Fair):** Patient lifts to position but tolerates no resistance.
- **Grade 2 (Poor):** Patient lifts through partial range.
- **Grade 1 (Trace):** Therapist notes contraction but no actual motion.
- **Grade 0 (None):** No contraction noted.

Shoulder Extension

The primary and accessory muscles responsible for shoulder extension are presented in Table 6-2. The latissimus dorsi (see Figure 6-6), deltoid (see Figure 6-7), and teres minor (see Figure 6-8) muscles are the prime movers for shoulder extension.

TABLE 6-2	MUSCLES RESPONSIBLE FOR SHOULDER EXTENSION		
PRIMARY MUSCLES	**ORIGIN**	**INSERTION**	**INNERVATION**
Latissimus dorsi	Spinous processes of T7–L5, posterior surface of the sacrum, iliac crest, and lower three ribs	Medial lip of the bicipital groove of the humerus	Thoracodorsal
Deltoid, posterior fibers	Spine of the scapula	Deltoid tuberosity of the humerus	Axillary
Teres minor	Axillary border of scapula	Greater tubercle of humerus	Axillary
ACCESSORY MUSCLES	**ORIGIN**	**INSERTION**	**INNERVATION**
Triceps brachii (long head)	Infraglenoid tubercle of scapula	Olecranon process of ulna	Radial

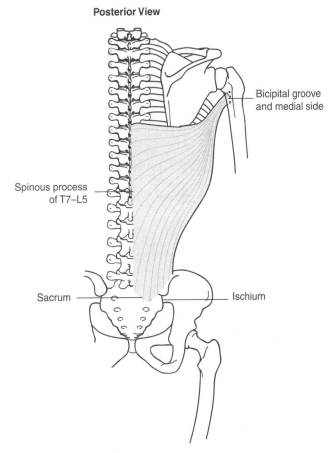

Posterior View

Bicipital groove and medial side

Spinous process of T7–L5

Sacrum

Ischium

Figure 6-6 Latissimus dorsi. Source: Delmar/Cengage Learning

Posterior View

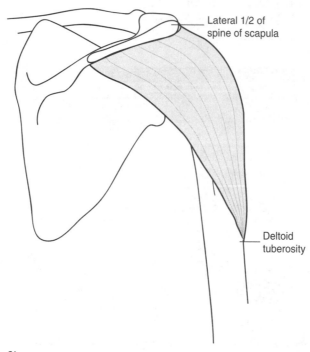

Figure 6-7 Deltoid, posterior fibers. Source: Delmar/Cengage Learning

Posterior View

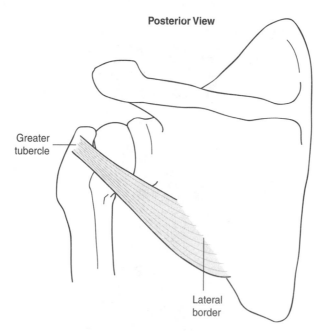

Figure 6-8 Teres minor. Source: Delmar/Cengage Learning

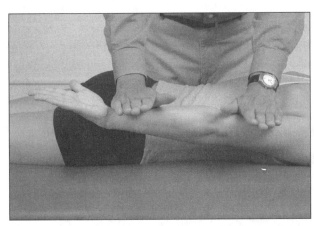

Figure 6-9 Proper positioning for shoulder extension grades 5–0. Source: Delmar/Cengage Learning

Testing for Shoulder Extension Grades 5–0 (Normal to None)

POSITION OF PATIENT: Prone with arms at sides, palm up.

POSITION OF THERAPIST: Stand at test side with resistance hand placed just above the elbow (see Figure 6-9).

TEST: With elbow straight, patient lifts arm off the table and is instructed to hold that position against resistance.

DIRECTIONS: Say to the patient, "Raise your arm up and hold it. Don't let me push it down."

GRADING:

- **Grade 5 (Normal):** Patient lifts to position and holds against maximum resistance.
- **Grade 4 (Good):** Patient lifts to position and holds against strong (but not full) resistance.
- **Grade 3 (Fair):** Patient lifts to position but tolerates no resistance.
- **Grade 2 (Poor):** Patient lifts through partial range.
- **Grade 1 (Trace):** Therapist notes contraction but no actual motion.
- **Grade 0 (None):** No contraction noted.

Shoulder Scaption

Table 6-3 lists the primary and accessory muscles responsible for shoulder scaption. The deltoid (see Figures 6-4 and 6-10) and supraspinatus (see Figure 6-11) muscles are the prime movers for shoulder scaption.

TABLE 6-3	MUSCLES RESPONSIBLE FOR SHOULDER SCAPTION		
PRIMARY MUSCLES	**ORIGIN**	**INSERTION**	**INNERVATION**
Deltoid, anterior and middle fibers	Lateral 1/3 clavicle Acromion process	Deltoid tuberosity	Axillary
Supraspinatus	Supraspinatus fossa, scapula	Greater tubercle of humerus	Suprascapular

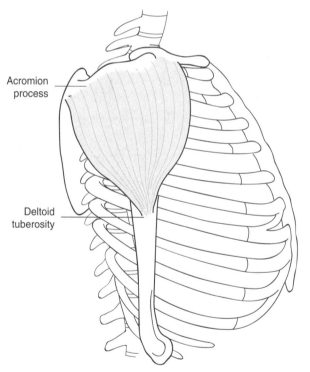

Figure 6-10 Deltoid, middle fibers. Source: Delmar/Cengage Learning

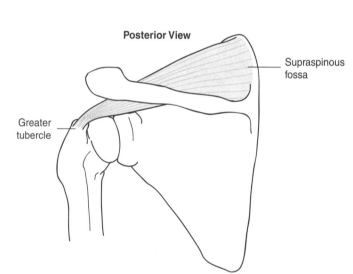

Figure 6-11 Supraspinatus. Source: Delmar/Cengage Learning

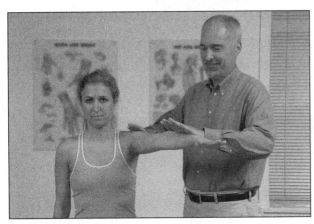

Figure 6-12 Proper positioning for shoulder scaption grades 5–0. Source: Delmar/Cengage Learning

Testing for Shoulder Scaption Grades 5–0 (Normal to None)

POSITION OF PATIENT: Short sitting

POSITION OF THERAPIST: Standing on test side, slightly in front of patient with resistance hand placed just above the elbow (see Figure 6-12).

TEST: Patient lifts arm in a plane halfway between flexion and abduction (about 45° anterior to the frontal plane) and is instructed to hold that position against resistance.

DIRECTIONS: Say to the patient, "Lift your arm and hold the position. Don't let me push it down."

GRADING:

- **Grade 5 (Normal):** Patient lifts to position and holds against maximum resistance.
- **Grade 4 (Good):** Patient lifts to position and holds against strong (but not full) resistance.
- **Grade 3 (Fair):** Patient lifts to position but tolerates no resistance.
- **Grade 2 (Poor):** Patient lifts through partial range.
- **Grade 1 (Trace):** Therapist notes contraction but no actual motion.
- **Grade 0 (None):** No contraction noted.

Shoulder Abduction

Table 6-4 presents the primary and accessory muscles responsible for shoulder abduction. The deltoid and supraspinatus muscles are the prime movers for shoulder abduction (refer to Figures 6-10 and 6-11).

TABLE 6-4	MUSCLES RESPONSIBLE FOR SHOULDER ABDUCTION		
PRIMARY MUSCLES	**ORIGIN**	**INSERTION**	**INNERVATION**
Deltoid middle fibers	Acromion process	Deltoid tuberosity of humerus	Axillary
Supraspinatus	Supraspinatus fossa of scapula	Greater tubercle of humerus	Suprascapular

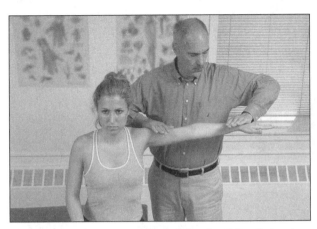

Figure 6-13 Proper positioning for shoulder abduction grades 5–0. Source: Delmar/Cengage Learning

Testing for Shoulder Abduction Grades 5–0 (Normal to None)

POSITION OF PATIENT: Short sitting.

POSITION OF THERAPIST: Standing behind patient with resistance hand placed just above the elbow (see Figure 6-13).

TEST: Patient lifts arm to 90° of abduction and is instructed to hold that position against resistance.

DIRECTIONS: Say to the patient, "With your thumb leading, raise your arm out to the side and hold it. Don't let me push it down."

GRADING:

- **Grade 5 (Normal):** Patient lifts to position and holds against maximum resistance.
- **Grade 4 (Good):** Patient lifts to position and holds against strong (but not full) resistance.
- **Grade 3 (Fair):** Patient lifts to position but tolerates no resistance.
- **Grade 2 (Poor):** Patient lifts through partial range.
- **Grade 1 (Trace):** Therapist notes contraction but no actual motion.
- **Grade 0 (None):** No contraction noted.

Shoulder Horizontal Abduction

Table 6-5 lists the primary and accessory muscles responsible for shoulder horizontal abduction. The posterior deltoid muscle is the prime mover for shoulder horizontal abduction (see Figure 6-7).

TABLE 6-5	MUSCLES RESPONSIBLE FOR SHOULDER HORIZONTAL ABDUCTION		
PRIMARY MUSCLES	**ORIGIN**	**INSERTION**	**INNERVATION**
Deltoid posterior fibers	Spine of scapula	Deltoid tuberosity of humerus	Axillary
ACCESSORY MUSCLES	**ORIGIN**	**INSERTION**	**INNERVATION**
Infraspinatus	Infraspinatus fossa of the scapula	Greater tubercle of humerus	Suprascapular
Teres minor	Axillary border of scapula	Greater tubercle of humerus	Axillary

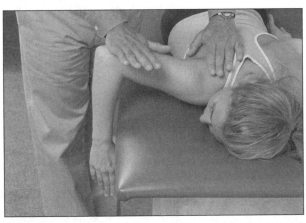

Figure 6-14 Proper positioning for shoulder horizontal abduction grades 5–3. Source: Delmar/Cengage Learning

Testing for Shoulder Horizontal Abduction Grades 5, 4, 3 (Normal, Good, Fair) Gravity Resisted

POSITION OF PATIENT: Prone with shoulder abducted to 90° and elbow flexed over the edge of the table.

POSITION OF THERAPIST: Standing at test side with resistance hand placed just above the elbow (see Figure 6-14).

TEST: Patient lifts elbow toward the ceiling and is instructed to hold that position against resistance.

DIRECTIONS: Say to the patient, "Raise your elbow toward the ceiling and hold it. Don't let me push it down."

GRADING:

- **Grade 5 (Normal):** Patient lifts to position and holds against maximum resistance.
- **Grade 4 (Good):** Patient lifts to position and holds against strong (but not full) resistance.
- **Grade 3 (Fair):** Patient lifts to position but tolerates no resistance.

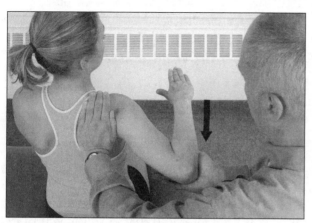

Figure 6-15 Proper positioning for shoulder horizontal abduction grades 2–0. Source: Delmar/Cengage Learning

Testing for Shoulder Horizontal Abduction Grades 2, 1, 0 (Poor, Trace, None) Gravity Minimal

POSITION OF PATIENT: Short sitting with shoulder abducted to 90° and elbow slightly flexed.

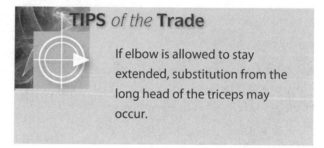

TIPS *of the* **Trade**

If elbow is allowed to stay extended, substitution from the long head of the triceps may occur.

POSITION OF THERAPIST: Standing on test side supporting the forearm with one hand. The other hand is positioned over the posterior deltoid to palpate as necessary (see Figure 6-15).

TEST: Patient instructed to move the arm in the horizontal plane.

DIRECTIONS: Say to the patient, "Move your elbow back."

GRADING:

- **Grade 2 (Poor):** Patient moves through partial range.
- **Grade 1 (Trace):** Therapist notes contraction but no actual motion.
- **Grade 0 (None):** No contraction noted.

Shoulder Horizontal Adduction

The primary and accessory muscles responsible for shoulder horizontal adduction are listed in Table 6-6. The pectoralis major muscle is the prime mover for shoulder horizontal adduction (see Figure 6-16).

TABLE 6-6	MUSCLES RESPONSIBLE FOR SHOULDER HORIZONTAL ADDUCTION		
PRIMARY MUSCLES	**ORIGIN**	**INSERTION**	**INNERVATION**
Pectoralis major, clavicular part	Medial 1/3 of clavicle	Lateral lip of the bicipital groove of the humerus	Lateral and medial pectoral nerve
Pectoralis major, sternal part	Sternum, ribs 2–7	Same as above	Same as above
ACCESSORY MUSCLES	**ORIGIN**	**INSERTION**	**INNERVATION**
Deltoid, anterior fibers	Lateral 1/3 of clavicle, anterior superior surface	Deltoid tuberosity of the humerus	Axillary nerve

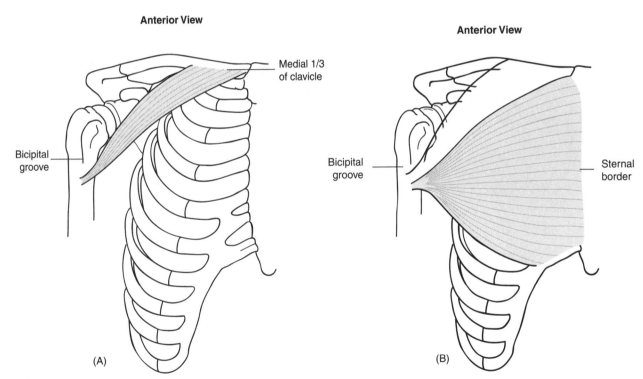

Figure 6-16 (A) Pectoralis major, clavicular position (B) Pectoralis major, sternal portion. Source: Delmar/Cengage Learning

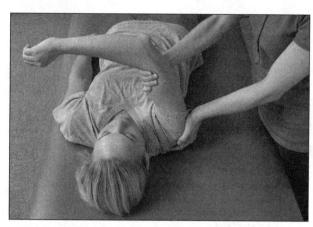

Figure 6-17 Proper positioning for shoulder horizontal adduction grades 5–3. Source: Delmar/Cengage Learning

Testing for Shoulder Horizontal Adduction Grades 5, 4, 3 (Normal, Good, Fair) Gravity Resisted

POSITION OF PATIENT: Supine with shoulder abducted to 90° and elbow flexed to 90°.

POSITION OF THERAPIST: Standing at test side with hand providing resistance placed just above the elbow. The resistance provided will be opposite of the movement the patient is trying to achieve. The other hand may stabilize at the shoulder or palpate the muscle as needed (see Figure 6-17).

TEST: Patient instructed to move arm across the chest and hold the position against resistance.

DIRECTIONS: Say to the patient, "Raise your arm across your body and hold it. Don't let me pull it back."

GRADING:

- **Grade 5 (Normal):** Patient lifts to position and holds against maximum resistance.
- **Grade 4 (Good):** Patient lifts to position and holds against strong (but not full) resistance.
- **Grade 3 (Fair):** Patient lifts to position but tolerates no resistance.

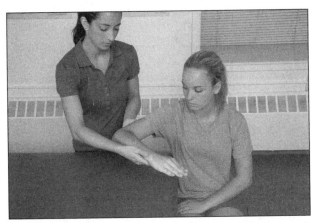

Figure 6-18 Proper positioning for shoulder horizontal adduction grades 2–0. Source: Delmar/Cengage Learning

Testing for Shoulder Horizontal Adduction Grades 2, 1, 0 (Poor, Trace, None) Gravity Minimal

POSITION OF PATIENT: Supine with arm supported. Shoulder abducted 90° and elbow flexed 90°.

POSITION OF THERAPIST: Standing at test side supporting arm as needed (see Figure 6-18).

TEST: Patient is instructed to move arm across chest.

DIRECTIONS: Say to the patient, "Move your arm in front of your body."

GRADING:

- **Grade 2 (Poor):** Patient moves through partial range.
- **Grade 1 (Trace):** Therapist notes contraction but no actual motion.
- **Grade 0 (None):** No contraction noted.

Shoulder External Rotation

Table 6-7 lists the primary and accessory muscles responsible for shoulder external rotation. The infraspinatus and teres minor muscles are the prime movers for shoulder external rotation (see Figure 6-19).

TABLE 6-7	MUSCLES RESPONSIBLE FOR SHOULDER EXTERNAL ROTATION		
PRIMARY MUSCLES	**ORIGIN**	**INSERTION**	**INNERVATION**
Infraspinatus	Infraspinatus fossa of the scapula	Greater tubercle of humerus	Suprascapular
Teres minor	Axillary border of the scapula	Greater tubercle of the humerus	Axillary
ACCESSORY MUSCLES	**ORIGIN**	**INSERTION**	**INNERVATION**
Deltoid posterior fibers	Spine of scapula	Deltoid tuberosity of humerus	Axillary

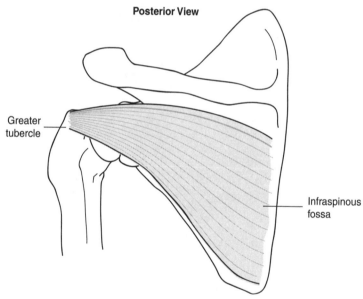

Posterior View

Greater tubercle

Infraspinous fossa

Figure 6-19 Infraspinatus. Source: Delmar/Cengage Learning

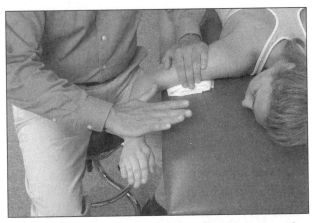

Figure 6-20 Proper positioning for shoulder external rotation grades 5–3. Source: Delmar/Cengage Learning

Testing for Shoulder External Rotation Grades 5, 4, 3 (Normal, Good, Fair) Gravity Resisted

POSITION OF PATIENT: Prone with shoulder abducted to 90° with upper arm supported on table. Elbow flexed to 90° over edge of table.

POSITION OF THERAPIST: Standing at test side with resistance hand placed on forearm above wrist and support hand placed against humerus just above the elbow (see Figure 6-20).

TEST: Patient instructed to rotate forearm forward and upward and to hold that position against resistance.

DIRECTIONS: Say to the patient, "Lift the back of your hand toward the ceiling and hold it. Don't let me push it down."

GRADING:

- **Grade 5 (Normal):** Patient lifts to position and holds against maximum resistance.
- **Grade 4 (Good):** Patient lifts to position and holds against strong (but not full) resistance.
- **Grade 3 (Fair):** Patient lifts to position but tolerates no resistance.

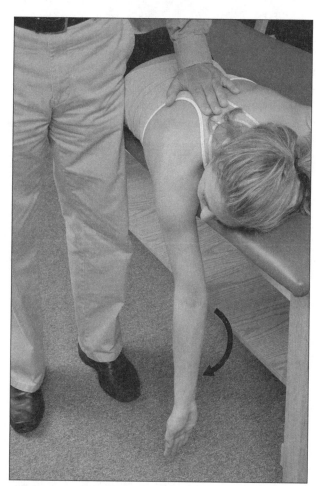

Figure 6-21 Proper positioning for shoulder external rotation grades 2–0. Source: Delmar/Cengage Learning

Testing for Shoulder External Rotation Grades 2, 1, 0 (Poor, Trace, None) Gravity Minimal

POSITION OF PATIENT: Prone with entire arm hanging loosely over edge of table.

POSITION OF THERAPIST: Standing on test side with hand placed to palpate the teres minor (see Figure 6-21).

TEST: Patient instructed to externally rotate shoulder.

DIRECTIONS: Say to the patient, "Rotate your arm clockwise."

GRADING:

- **Grade 2 (Poor):** Patient moves through partial range.
- **Grade 1 (Trace):** Therapist notes contraction but no actual motion.
- **Grade 0 (None):** No contraction noted.

Shoulder Internal Rotation

The primary and accessory muscles responsible for shoulder internal rotation are described in Table 6-8. The subscapularis (see Figure 6-22), pectoralis major, latissimus dorsi, and teres major (see Figure 6-23) muscles are the prime movers for shoulder internal rotation.

TABLE 6-8	MUSCLES RESPONSIBLE FOR SHOULDER INTERNAL ROTATION		
PRIMARY MUSCLES	**ORIGIN**	**INSERTION**	**INNERVATION**
Subscapularis	Subscapular fossa of the scapula	Tubercle of the humerus	Subscapular
Pectoralis major, clavicular part	Medial 1/3 of clavicle	Lateral lip of the bicipital groove of the humerus	Lateral and medial pectoral nerve
Pectoralis major, sternal part	Sternum, ribs 2–7	Same as above	Same as above
Latissimus dorsi	Spinous processes of T7–L5, posterior surface of sacrum, iliac crest, and lower three ribs	Medial lip of bicipital groove of the humerus	Thoracodorsal
Teres major	Axillary border of scapula near the inferior angle	Crest below lesser tubercle, next to latissimus	Subscapular
ACCESSORY MUSCLES	**ORIGIN**	**INSERTION**	**INNERVATION**
Deltoid, anterior fibers	Lateral 1/3 of clavicle, anterior superior surface	Deltoid tuberosity of the humerus	Axillary nerve

Anterior View

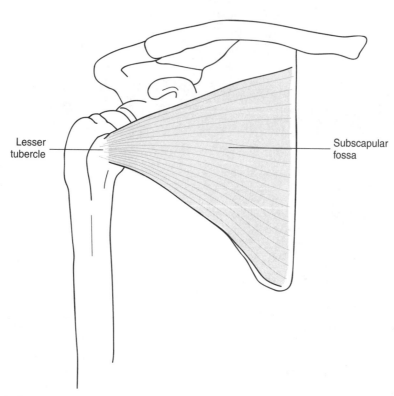

Figure 6-22 Subscapularis. Source: Delmar/Cengage Learning

Posterior View

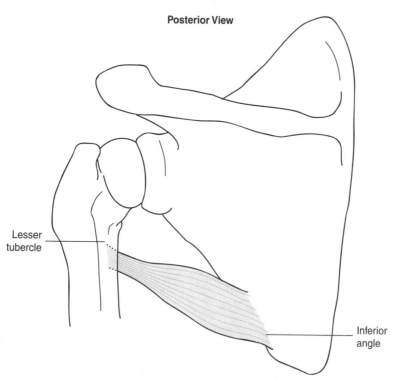

Figure 6-23 Teres major. Source: Delmar/Cengage Learning

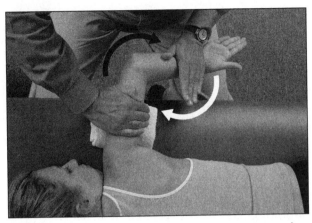

Figure 6-24 Proper positioning for shoulder internal rotation grades 5–3. Source: Delmar/Cengage Learning

Testing for Shoulder Internal Rotation Grades 5, 4, 3 (Normal, Good, Fair) Gravity Resisted

POSITION OF PATIENT: Prone with shoulder abducted to 90° with upper arm supported on table. Elbow flexed to 90° over edge of table.

POSITION OF THERAPIST: Standing at test side with resistance hand placed on forearm above wrist and support hand placed against humerus just above the elbow (see Figure 6-24).

TEST: Patient instructed to rotate forearm backward and upward and to hold that position against resistance.

DIRECTIONS: Say to the patient, "Lift your palm toward the ceiling and hold it. Don't let me push it down."

GRADING:

- **Grade 5 (Normal):** Patient lifts to position and holds against maximum resistance.
- **Grade 4 (Good):** Patient lifts to position and holds against strong (but not full) resistance.
- **Grade 3 (Fair):** Patient lifts to position but tolerates no resistance.

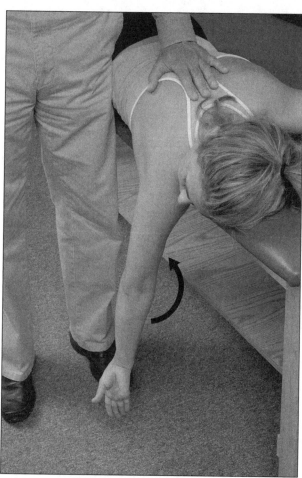

Figure 6-25 Proper positioning for shoulder internal rotation grades 2–0. Source: Delmar/Cengage Learning

Testing for Shoulder Internal Rotation Grades 2, 1, 0 (Poor, Trace, None) Gravity Minimal

POSITION OF PATIENT: Prone with entire arm hanging loosely over edge of table.

POSITION OF THERAPIST: Standing on test side with hand placed to palpate the subscapular tendon where it lies deep in the central axilla (see Figure 6-25).

TEST: Patient instructed to internally rotate shoulder.

DIRECTIONS: Say to the patient, "Rotate your arm counterclockwise."

GRADING:

- **Grade 2 (Poor):** Patient moves through partial range.
- **Grade 1 (Trace):** Therapist notes contraction but no actual motion.
- **Grade 0 (None):** No contraction noted.

Substitutions

Important substitutions to watch for during MMT of the shoulder are as follows:

- Keep the arm in a position midpoint between internal and external rotation during testing of shoulder flexion. If the deltoid is absent or weak, the biceps brachii will attempt to kick in by externally rotating the shoulder prior to flexing.
- During flexion, if the shoulder girdle elevates, the upper trapezius is kicking in.
- During flexion, if the pectoralis major kicks in, the arm will begin to horizontally abduct.
- When assessing horizontal abduction, keep the elbow flexed to avoid substitution by the long head of the triceps.

RANGE OF MOTION

The following section discusses measuring ROM for the eight motions available at the shoulder joint: flexion, extension, abduction, adduction, medial rotation, lateral rotation, horizontal abduction, and horizontal adduction.

Shoulder Flexion

Shoulder flexion occurs in the sagittal plane around the medial/lateral (frontal) axis. Overall, normal active range of motion (AROM) for shoulder flexion is 0°–180°, according to the American Academy of Orthopaedic Surgeons (1965). The end-feel for shoulder flexion is firm due to tension felt in the various muscles, ligaments, and joint capsule during this action.

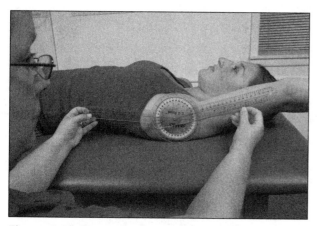

Figure 6-26 Proper positioning for shoulder flexion ROM. Source: Delmar/Cengage Learning

POSITION OF PATIENT: Comfortable supine position with arm resting comfortably in a neutral position alongside the body. Patient lifts the arm overhead through the flexion motion to end range.

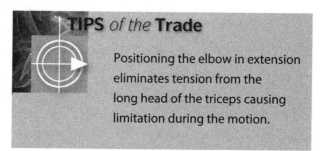

TIPS *of the* **Trade**

Positioning the elbow in extension eliminates tension from the long head of the triceps causing limitation during the motion.

POSITION OF THERAPIST: Standing or sitting at test side to provide support as patient moves and then to position the goniometer. One hand stabilizes the scapula to prevent excessive scapular movement.

POSITION OF GONIOMETER:

- **Fulcrum:** Placed over the lateral aspect of the greater tubercle (see Figure 6-26)
- **Stationary arm:** Aligned with the midline of the trunk
- **Movable arm:** Aligned along the midline of the humerus with the lateral epicondyle as the reference point

Shoulder Extension

Shoulder extension occurs in the sagittal plane around a medial/lateral or frontal axis. Normal AROM is 0°–60°, according to the American Academy of Orthopaedic Surgeons (1965). The end-feel for shoulder extension is firm due to tension felt in the various muscles and ligaments as well as the joint capsule during this action.

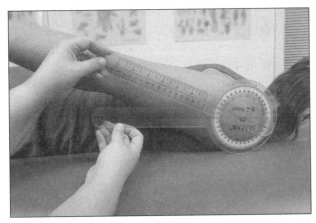

Figure 6-27 Proper position for shoulder extension ROM. Source: Delmar/Cengage Learning

POSITION OF PATIENT: Prone with the arm resting comfortably in a neutral position at the side of the body. With elbow slightly flexed, the arm is then extended above the body.

POSITION OF THERAPIST: Standing or sitting at test side to provide support as patient moves and then to position the goniometer. One hand stabilizes the scapula to prevent elevation.

POSITION OF GONIOMETER:

- **Fulcrum:** Placed over the lateral aspect of the greater tubercle (see Figure 6-27)
- **Stationary arm:** Aligned with the midline of the trunk
- **Movable arm:** Aligned along the midline of the humerus with the lateral epicondyle as the reference point

Shoulder Abduction

Shoulder abduction/adduction occurs in the frontal plane around an anterior/posterior or sagittal axis. Normal AROM is 0°–180°, according to the American Academy of Orthopaedic Surgeons (1965). Adduction is not usually measured or recorded since it is simply the returning to the starting position for abduction. For abduction, the end-feel is firm due to tension felt in the various muscles ligaments as well as the joint capsule during this action.

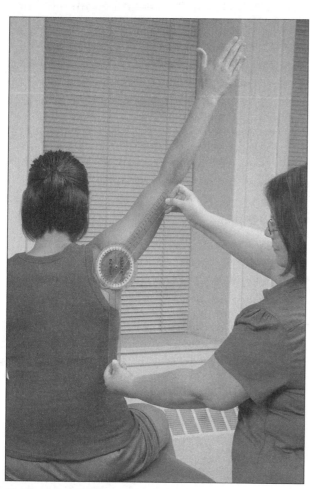

Figure 6-28 Proper position for shoulder abduction ROM. Source: Delmar/Cengage Learning

POSITION OF PATIENT: Supine with arm alongside the body. The palm should be facing upward. Patient moves the arm laterally away from the body using the abduction motion.

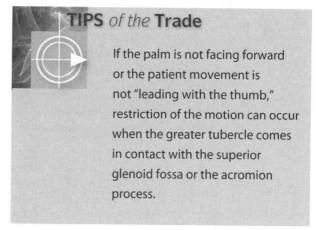

TIPS *of the* **Trade**

If the palm is not facing forward or the patient movement is not "leading with the thumb," restriction of the motion can occur when the greater tubercle comes in contact with the superior glenoid fossa or the acromion process.

POSITION OF THERAPIST: Sitting or standing on test side to provide support as patient moves and then to position the goniometer. One hand stabilizes the scapula to prevent elevation and upward rotation.

POSITION OF GONIOMETER:

- **Fulcrum:** Just lateral to the acromion process (see Figure 6-28)

- **Stationary arm:** Parallel with the anterior surface of the trunk

- **Movable arm:** Aligned along the midline of the humerus with the medial epicondyle as the reference point

Shoulder Medial Rotation

The motion of medial (internal) rotation occurs in a transverse plane around a vertical axis when the body is in the anatomical position. The position of the arm during the actual testing process makes this somewhat difficult to visualize. Normal AROM is 0°–70°, according to the American Academy of Orthopaedic Surgeons (1965). The end-feel for medial rotation is firm due to tension felt in the various muscles ligaments as well as the joint capsule during this action.

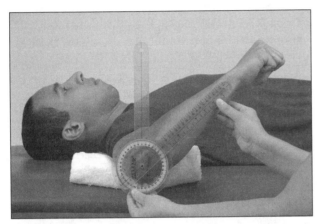

Figure 6-29 Proper position for shoulder medial rotation ROM. Source: Delmar/Cengage Learning

POSITION OF PATIENT: Supine with the shoulder abducted to 90° and the elbow flexed to 90°. Maintaining this position, the patient then rotates the shoulder, moving the palm of the hand toward the floor.

POSITION OF THERAPIST: Sitting at test side. One hand should be ready to stabilize as needed either at the distal end of the humerus to maintain the original position of the shoulder and elbow at 90° or to stabilize at the shoulder to prevent tilting of the clavicle or the anterior portions of the scapula.

POSITION OF GONIOMETER:

- **Fulcrum:** Centered on the olecranon (see Figure 6-29)
- **Stationary arm:** Perpendicular to the floor
- **Movable arm:** Aligned with the ulna using the ulnar styloid process as the reference point

Shoulder Lateral Rotation

As with medial rotation, lateral (external) rotation occurs in a transverse plane around a vertical axis when the body is in the anatomical position. The position of the arm during the actual testing process makes this somewhat difficult to visualize. Normal AROM is 90°, according to the American Academy of Orthopaedic Surgeons (1965). The end-feel for medial rotation is firm due to tension felt in the various muscles, ligaments, and joint capsule during this action.

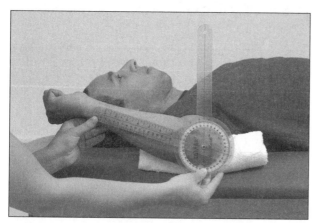

Figure 6-30 Proper position for shoulder lateral rotation ROM. Source: Delmar/Cengage Learning

POSITION OF PATIENT: Supine with the shoulder abducted to 90° and the elbow flexed to 90°. Maintaining this position, the patient then rotates the shoulder, moving the dorsal surface of the hand toward the floor.

POSITION OF THERAPIST: Sitting at test side. One hand should be ready to stabilize as needed either at the distal end of the humerus to maintain the original position of the shoulder and elbow at 90° or to stabilize at the shoulder to prevent posterior tilting of the scapula.

POSITION OF GONIOMETER:

- **Fulcrum:** Centered on the olecranon (see Figure 6-30)
- **Stationary arm:** Perpendicular to the floor
- **Movable arm:** Aligned with the ulna using the ulnar styloid process as the reference point

Horizontal Abduction

Horizontal abduction occurs in a transverse plane around a vertical axis. The normal AROM is 0°–90°, according to the American Academy of Orthopaedic Surgeons (1965). The end-feel for horizontal abduction is firm due to tension felt in the various muscles and ligaments as well as the joint capsule during this action.

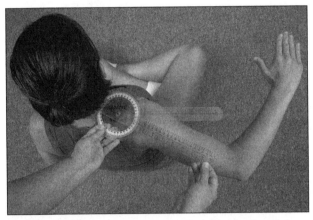

Figure 6-31 Proper position for shoulder horizontal abduction ROM. Source: Delmar/Cengage Learning

POSITION OF PATIENT: Short sitting with shoulder abducted to 90° and medially rotated so palm faces the floor. Elbow flexed to 90°. Maintaining this position, the patient then pulls elbow back.

POSITION OF THERAPIST: Standing on test side. One hand placed to stabilize the scapula.

POSITION OF GONIOMETER:

- **Fulcrum:** Superior aspect of the acromion process (see Figure 6-31)
- **Stationary arm:** Aligned with the frontal plane

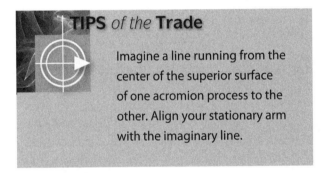

TIPS *of the* Trade

Imagine a line running from the center of the superior surface of one acromion process to the other. Align your stationary arm with the imaginary line.

- **Movable arm:** Aligned along the midline of the humerus with the lateral epicondyle as the reference point

Shoulder Horizontal Adduction

Shoulder horizontal adduction occurs in a transverse plane around a vertical axis. The normal AROM is 0°–40°, according to the American Academy of Orthopaedic Surgeons (1965). The end-feel for horizontal adduction is firm due to tension felt in the various muscles ligaments as well as the joint capsule during this action.

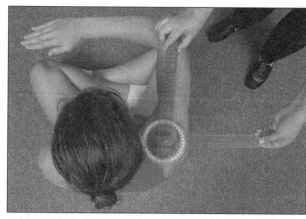

Figure 6-32 Proper position for shoulder horizontal adduction ROM. Source: Delmar/Cengage Learning

POSITION OF PATIENT: Short sitting with shoulder abducted to 90° and medially rotated so palm faces the floor. Elbow flexed to 90°. Maintaining this position, the patient moves arm across in front of the body as if trying to touch the opposite shoulder.

POSITION OF THERAPIST: Standing on test side. One hand placed to stabilize the scapula.

POSITION OF GONIOMETER:

- **Fulcrum:** Superior aspect of the acromion process (see Figure 6-32)
- **Stationary arm:** Aligned with the frontal plane

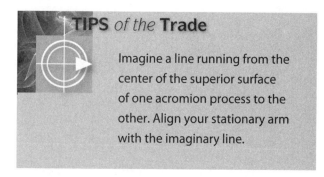

TIPS *of the* **Trade**

Imagine a line running from the center of the superior surface of one acromion process to the other. Align your stationary arm with the imaginary line.

- **Movable arm:** Aligned along the midline of the humerus with the lateral epicondyle as the reference point

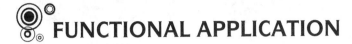

FUNCTIONAL APPLICATION

Good function of the entire upper extremity requires availability of both strength and mobility at the shoulder joint. For example, Matsen and colleagues (1994) report that flexion of 52° and horizontal adduction of 104° are needed for washing the axilla. Matsen and colleagues note that combing one's hair requires abduction of 112° and horizontal adduction of 54°. When adding the component of strength to this equation, you can see that at least a grade 3 would be required. As you conduct assessments, it is imperative to tie your findings back to patient function.

LEARNER CHALLENGE

1. List shoulder joint motions. Then identify the plane and axis in which they occur.
2. List the rotator cuff muscles.
3. Palpate the following landmarks of the shoulder: greater tubercle of the humerus, bicipital groove, and deltoid tuberosity.
4. On a lab partner, use a china marker to shade in the three parts of the deltoid muscle. Instruct your lab partner to perform shoulder motions such as flexion, abduction, and horizontal abduction and observe/palpate the movement under your shaded areas.
5. Fill in the following tables summarizing MMT and ROM measurements of the shoulder.

A) Manual Muscle Testing for Grades 5, 4, 3 Gravity Resisted

MOTION	TESTING POSITION	STABILIZING HAND	RESISTANCE HAND
Shoulder Flexion			
Shoulder Extension			
Shoulder Scaption			
Shoulder Abduction			
Horizontal Abduction			
Horizontal Adduction			

continues

A) Manual Muscle Testing for Grades 5, 4, 3 Gravity Resisted *(continued)*

MOTION	TESTING POSITION	STABILIZING HAND	RESISTANCE HAND
Shoulder External Rotation			
Shoulder Internal Rotation			

B) Manual Muscle Testing for Grades 2, 1, 0 Gravity Minimal

MOTION	TESTING POSITION	STABILIZING HAND	RESISTANCE HAND	PALPATION
Shoulder Flexion				
Shoulder Extension				
Shoulder Scaption				
Shoulder Abduction				
Horizontal Abduction				
Horizontal Adduction				
Shoulder External Rotation				
Shoulder Internal Rotation				

C) Range of Motion

MOTION	MOVABLE ARM	STATIONARY ARM	FULCRUM	NORMAL ROM
Shoulder Flexion				
Shoulder Extension				
Shoulder Abduction				
Horizontal Abduction				
Horizontal Adduction				
Shoulder External Rotation				
Shoulder Internal Rotation				

NOTES

THE ELBOW AND FOREARM

OBJECTIVES

Upon completion of this chapter, the reader will be able to:

- Describe the elbow and forearm joints.

- Identify the bony landmarks significant to the elbow and forearm joints.

- Name the major ligaments and their purpose.

- Describe any supporting structures important to the elbow and forearm joints.

- Describe the major motions of the elbow and forearm and name the muscles that perform them.

- Become familiar with the origins, insertions, and innervations of the muscles of the elbow and forearm.

- Perform proper manual muscle testing on the major muscles of the elbow and forearm grades 5–0.

- Be aware of possible substitutions during manual muscle testing on the elbow and forearm.

- Accurately perform range of motion testing using the goniometer on the elbow and forearm joint.

MUSCULOSKELETAL OVERVIEW

Although professionals tend to loosely refer to this structure as a single joint, the elbow is really a complex consisting of three bones, two joints, three ligaments, and one capsule. Because muscles involved in this structure originate on the scapula, you will naturally review scapular landmarks as you palpate and study the musculature of the elbow. Also note that complete mobility of the elbow/forearm can only occur with a pivoting or rotational movement occurring between the ulna and the radius. As previously stated in Chapter 6, the flexibility of these more proximal joints allows the wrist and hand to accomplish a wide variety of tasks such as combing hair or turning a screwdriver.

Joints

The term *elbow joint* is the common reference to the articulation of the humerus with the radius and ulna. This joint allows the flexion and extension motions to occur at the elbow. The radius and ulna are unusual in that they have articulation points at both the superior (proximal) and the interior (distal) ends but are considered one joint. These articulations allow the bones to rotate around each other, thus allowing pronation and supination to occur.

Bones

Landmarks of the humerus listed in Chapter 6 are reiterated here for the convenience of quick reference as we proceed through the muscular and ligamentous attachments (refer to Figure 6-1).

Humerus

- **Head:** Articulates with the scapula at the glenoid fossa; gently rounded proximal end
- **Anatomical neck:** The groove around the circumference between the head and the tubercles
- **Greater tubercle:** The larger, more lateral protuberance
- **Lesser tubercle:** Smaller protuberance located on the anterior surface between the greater tubercle and the head
- **Bicipital groove:** The longitudinal groove that separates the tubercles
- **Surgical neck:** Slightly narrowed area where the head meets the shaft of the bone just below the tubercles
- **Shaft:** The long body of the bone that extends from the surgical head distally to the epicondyles
- **Deltoid tuberosity:** About midshaft on the lateral surface

TIPS *of the* **Trade**

The deltoid tuberosity is not a well-defined palpation point but is often a tender palpation point and therefore easy to locate.

- **Medial epicondyle:** Rounded protuberance located on the medial side of the distal shaft of the humerus

- **Lateral epicondyle:** Rounded protuberance located on the lateral side of the distal shaft of the humerus
- **Trochlea:** The articulation point with the ulna; located at the distal end on the medial side
- **Capitulum:** The articulation point with the radius; located at the distal end on the lateral side
- **Olecranon fossa:** Located on the posterior surface between the epicondyles; provides an articulation with the olecranon process of the ulna

When the body is placed in the anatomical position, the ulna is found on the medial side of the forearm parallel with the radius (see Figure 7-1). Of significance on this bone is the olecranon process. This hooklike structure at the proximal end of the ulna is the articulation point with the humerus and locks the elbow into full extension.

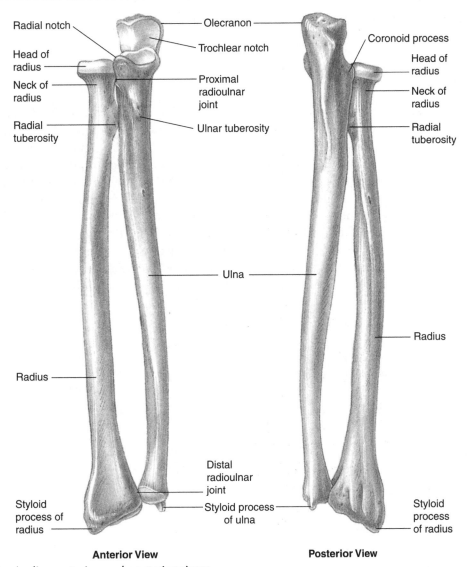

Anterior View   **Posterior View**

Figure 7-1 Ulna/radius, anterior, and posterior views. Source: Delmar/Cengage Learning

Ulna

- **Olecranon process:** Proximal end of the ulna on the posterior side
- **Trochlear notch:** Anterior surface of the proximal end of the ulna
- **Coronoid process:** Anterior surface of the proximal end of the ulna just distal to the trochlear notch

- **Radial notch:** Lateral surface of the proximal end of the ulna just distal to the trochlear notch
- **Ulnar tuberosity:** Anterior surface of the ulna just distal to the coronoid process
- **Styloid process:** Posterior/medial surface of the distal ulna
- **Head:** Lateral surface of the distal ulna

When the body is placed in the anatomical position, the radius is found on the lateral side of the forearm parallel with the ulna (refer to Figure 7-1). Again we find important attachment points for muscles and will review the bony landmarks.

Radius

- **Head:** Superior surface of the proximal end of the radius
- **Radial tuberosity:** Medial surface of the proximal end of the radius
- **Styloid process:** Posterior/lateral surface of the distal radius

Ligaments

The stability of the elbow is due largely to the three strong ligaments surrounding it (see Figure 7-2). The lateral collateral ligament is a triangular-shaped structure with a proximal attachment on the lateral epicondyle of the humerus and a distal attachment on the annular ligament and the lateral side of the ulna. On the medial side of the elbow is another triangular structure, the medial collateral ligament. This ligament runs on a diagonal from the proximal attachment point on the medial epicondyle of the humerus to the distal attachment on the coronoid and olecranon processes of the ulna. The final ligament stabilizing the elbow is the annular ligament. Its purpose is to hold the radius and the ulna together. This ligament attaches to the ulna anteriorly and posteriorly on the radial notch surrounding the head of the radius and holding it in place against the ulna.

The movements available at the humeroulnar and humeroradial joints are flexion/extension. The motions produced by the rotation of the radius and ulna are supination and pronation.

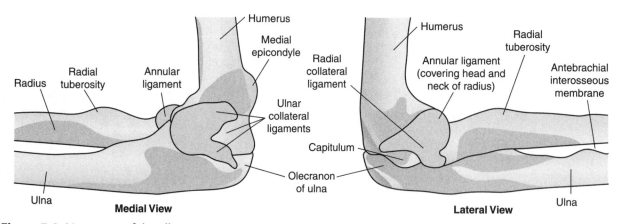

Figure 7-2 Ligaments of the elbow. Source: Delmar/Cengage Learning

MUSCLE TESTING OF THE ELBOW AND FOREARM

The motions at the elbow/forearm are flexion, extension, pronation, and supination. Because it is important to review the muscles associated with the movement, each section starts with a table of the muscles responsible for the movement being tested, followed by a depiction of the primary muscles.

Elbow Flexion

Table 7-1 lists the primary and accessory muscles responsible for elbow flexion. The biceps brachii (see Figure 7-3), brachialis (see Figure 7-4), and brachioradialis (see Figure 7-5) muscles are the prime movers for elbow flexion.

TABLE 7-1 — MUSCLES RESPONSIBLE FOR ELBOW FLEXION

PRIMARY MUSCLES	ORIGIN	INSERTION	INNERVATION
Biceps brachii, short head	Coracoid process of scapula	Radial tuberosity of radius	Musculocutaneous
Biceps brachii, long head	Supraglenoid tubercle of the scapula	Radial tuberosity of radius	Musculocutaneous
Brachialis	Anterior surface, distal half of humerus	Coronoid process, ulnar tuberosity of ulna	Musculocutaneous
Brachioradialis	Supracondylar ridge on the lateral humerus	Styloid process of radius	Radial nerve

ACCESSORY MUSCLES	ORIGIN	INSERTION	INNERVATION
Pronator teres	Medial epicondyle of humerus and coronoid process of ulna	Lateral surface of radius at midpoint	Median
Extensor carpi radialis longus	Supracondylar ridge of humerus	Base of second metacarpal	Radial
Flexor carpi radialis	Medial epicondyle of humerus	Base of second and third metacarpals	Median
Flexor carpi ulnaris	Medial epicondyle of humerus	Pisiform and base of fifth metacarpal	Ulnar

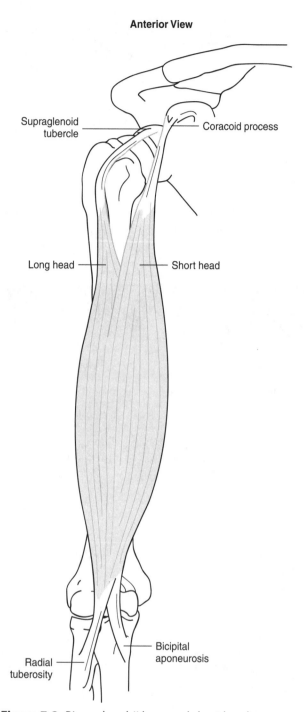

Anterior View

Supraglenoid tubercle

Coracoid process

Long head

Short head

Radial tuberosity

Bicipital aponeurosis

Figure 7-3 Biceps brachii long and short heads.

Source: Delmar/Cengage Learning

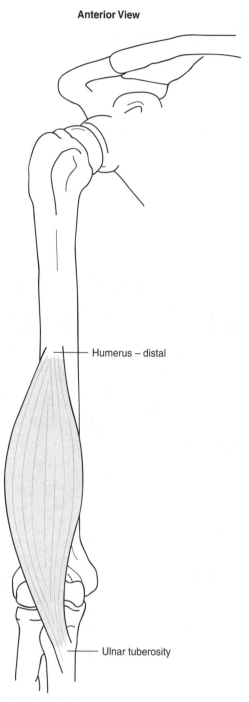

Anterior View

Humerus – distal

Ulnar tuberosity

Figure 7-4 Brachialis. Source: Delmar/Cengage Learning

Anterior View

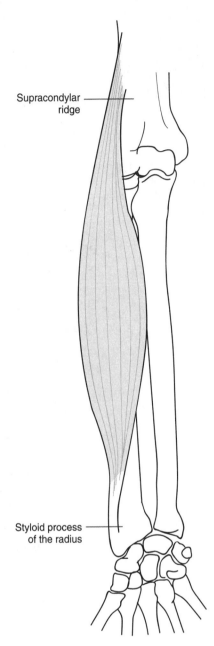

Supracondylar ridge

Styloid process of the radius

Figure 7-5 Brachioradialis. Source: Delmar/Cengage Learning

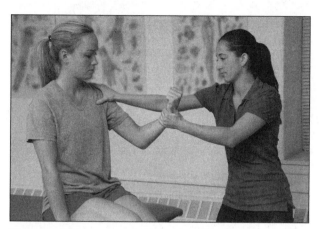

Figure 7-6 Proper positioning for elbow flexion grades 3–5. Source: Delmar/Cengage Learning

Testing for Elbow Flexion Grades 5, 4, 3 (Normal, Good, Fair) Gravity Resisted

Although therapists attempt to isolate each of the involved muscles by positioning of the forearm, there is some question whether these muscles can be isolated when strong effort is used. The specific positions are as follows:

- Biceps brachii: Forearm in supination
- Brachialis: Forearm in pronation
- Brachioradialis: Forearm in neutral position

POSITION OF PATIENT: Short sitting, arms at sides.

POSITION OF THERAPIST: Standing in front of patient on test side, with resistance hand on forearm proximal to wrist. Other hand stabilizes anterior shoulder (see Figure 7-6).

TEST: Patient flexes elbow through range.

DIRECTIONS: Say to the patient, "Bend your elbow and hold the position. Don't let me straighten your arm."

GRADING:

- **Grade 5 (Normal):** Patient flexes to position and holds against maximum resistance.
- **Grade 4 (Good):** Patient flexes to position and holds against strong (but not full) resistance.
- **Grade 3 (Fair):** Patient flexes to position but tolerates no resistance.

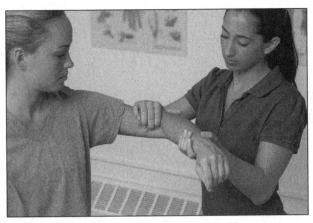

Figure 7-7 Proper positioning for elbow flexion grades 2–0. Source: Delmar/Cengage Learning

Elbow Flexion Grades 2, 1, 0 (Poor, Trace, None) Gravity Minimal

POSITION OF PATIENT: Short sitting with arm abducted to 90° (forearm position remains dependent on which muscle you wish to test) as therapist supports arm at elbow.

POSITION OF THERAPIST: Standing in front of patient on test side supporting abducted arm at the elbow (may also support at wrist if necessary) (see Figure 7-7).

TEST: Patient is instructed to flex elbow and hold against resistance.

DIRECTIONS: Say to the patient "Bend your elbow."

GRADING:

- **Grade 2 (Poor):** Patient moves through partial range.
- **Grade 1 (Trace):** Therapist notes contraction but no actual motion.
- **Grade 0 (None):** No contraction noted.

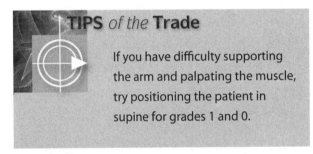

TIPS *of the* **Trade**

If you have difficulty supporting the arm and palpating the muscle, try positioning the patient in supine for grades 1 and 0.

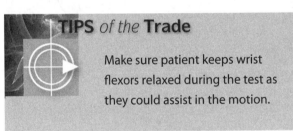

TIPS *of the* **Trade**

Make sure patient keeps wrist flexors relaxed during the test as they could assist in the motion.

Elbow Extension

Table 7-2 presents the primary and accessory muscles responsible for elbow extension. The triceps brachii muscle is the prime mover for elbow extension (see Figure 7-8).

TABLE 7-2	MUSCLES RESPONSIBLE FOR ELBOW EXTENSION		
PRIMARY MUSCLES	**ORIGIN**	**INSERTION**	**INNERVATION**
Triceps brachii, long head	Infraglenoid tubercle of scapula	Olecranon process of ulna	Radial
Triceps brachii, lateral head	Posterior humerus inferior to greater tubercle	Olecranon process of ulna	Radial
Triceps brachii, medial head	Posterior surface of humerus	Olecranon process of ulna	Radial
ACCESSORY MUSCLES	**ORIGIN**	**INSERTION**	**INNERVATION**
Anconeus	Lateral epicondyle of humerus	Lateral and inferior to olecranon process of ulna	Radial nerve

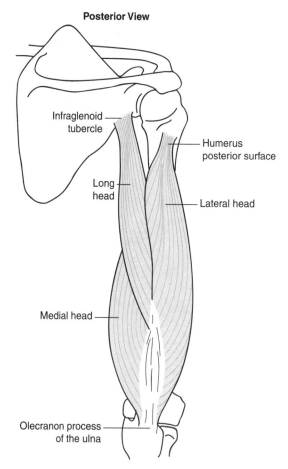

Posterior View

Infraglenoid tubercle

Humerus posterior surface

Long head

Lateral head

Medial head

Olecranon process of the ulna

Figure 7-8 Triceps. Source: Delmar/Cengage Learning

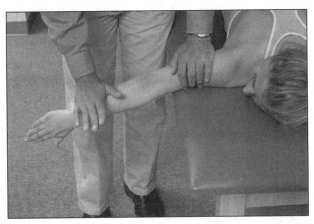

Figure 7-9 Proper positioning for elbow extension grades 5–3. Source: Delmar/Cengage Learning

Elbow Extension Grades 5, 4, 3 (Normal, Good, Fair) Gravity Minimal

POSITION OF PATIENT: Prone with shoulder abducted to 90° over edge of table and forearm hanging downward.

POSITION OF THERAPIST: Standing on test side with one hand supporting arm under the distal humerus. Other hand will provide downward resistance on the distal forearm just above the wrist (see Figure 7-9).

TEST: Patient is instructed to extend elbow and hold against resistance.

DIRECTIONS: Say to the patient, "Straighten your elbow and hold it. Don't let me bend it."

GRADING:

- **Grade 5 (Normal):** Patient extends to position and holds against maximum resistance.
- **Grade 4 (Good):** Patient extends to position and holds against strong (but not full) resistance.
- **Grade 3 (Fair):** Patient flexes to position but tolerates no resistance.

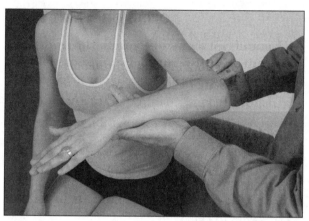

Figure 7-10 Proper positioning for elbow extension grades 2–0. Source: Delmar/Cengage Learning

Testing for Elbow Extension Grades 2, 1, 0 (Poor, Trace, None) Gravity Minimal

POSITION OF PATIENT: Short sitting with shoulder abducted to 90° and the entire extremity horizontal to the floor.

POSITION OF THERAPIST: Standing at test side supporting the arm at the elbow and wrist as needed (see Figure 7-10).

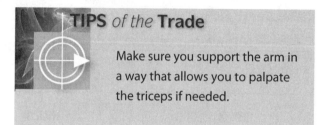

TIPS *of the* **Trade**

Make sure you support the arm in a way that allows you to palpate the triceps if needed.

TEST: Patient attempts to extend elbow.

DIRECTIONS: Say to the patient, "Straighten your elbow."

GRADING:

- **Grade 2 (Poor):** Patient moves through partial range.
- **Grade 1 (Trace):** Therapist notes contraction but no actual motion.
- **Grade 0 (None):** No contraction noted.

Forearm Supination

The primary and accessory muscles responsible for forearm supination are shown in Table 7-3. The supinator and biceps brachii muscles are the prime movers for forearm supination (see Figure 7-11).

TABLE 7-3	MUSCLES RESPONSIBLE FOR FOREARM SUPINATION		
PRIMARY MUSCLES	**ORIGIN**	**INSERTION**	**INNERVATION**
Supinator	Lateral epicondyle of humerus and supinator crest of ulna	Anterior surface, Proximal radius	Radial
Biceps brachii, short head	Coracoid process of scapula	Radial tuberosity of radius	Musculocutaneous
Biceps brachii, long head	Supraglenoid tubercle of the scapula	Radial tuberosity of radius	Musculocutaneous

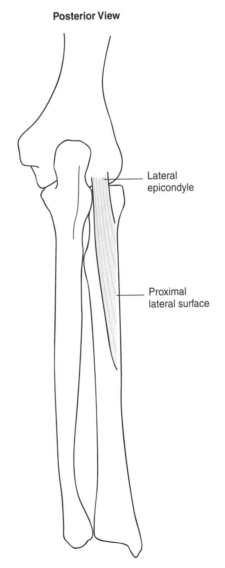

Posterior View

Lateral epicondyle

Proximal lateral surface

Figure 7-11 Supinator. Source: Delmar/Cengage Learning

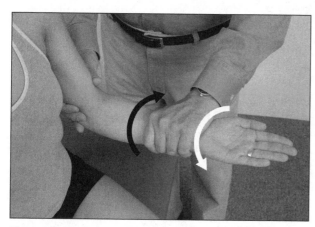

Figure 7-12 Proper positioning for forearm supination grades 3–5. Source: Delmar/Cengage Learning

Testing for Forearm Supination Grades 5, 4, 3 (Normal, Good, Fair) Gravity Resisted

POSITION OF PATIENT: Short sitting, arm at side with elbow flexed to 90° and forearm pronated.

POSITION OF THERAPIST: Standing in front or on test side. Supporting hand placed at the elbow. Resistance hand grasps the wrist on the palm side (see Figure 7-12).

TEST: Patient instructed to move forearm into supination and hold against resistance.

DIRECTIONS: Say to the patient, "Turn your palm up and hold it. Don't let me move it."

GRADING:

- **Grade 5 (Normal):** Patient moves to position and holds against maximum resistance.
- **Grade 4 (Good):** Patient moves to position and holds against strong (but not full) resistance.
- **Grade 3 (Fair):** Patient moves to position but tolerates no resistance.

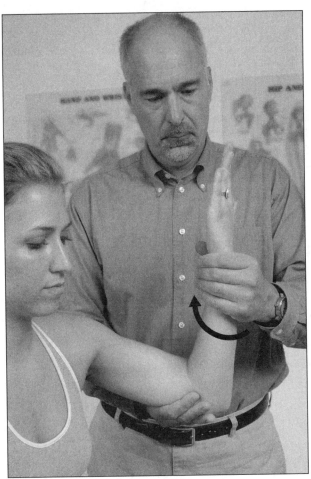

Figure 7-13 Proper positioning for forearm supination grades 2–0. Source: Delmar/Cengage Learning

Testing for Forearm Supination Grades 2, 1, 0 (Poor, Trace, None) Gravity Minimal

POSITION OF PATIENT: Short sitting with arm at side. Shoulder flexed about 45°, elbow flexed to 90°, forearm in neutral.

POSITION OF THERAPIST: Stand next to the patient, supporting the arm by cupping the elbow with fingers positioned to palpate as necessary (see Figure 7-13).

TEST: Patient attempts to move forearm into supination.

DIRECTIONS: Say to the patient, "Turn your palm toward your body."

GRADING:

- **Grade 2 (Poor):** Patient moves through partial range.
- **Grade 1 (Trace):** Therapist notes contraction but no actual motion.
- **Grade 0 (None):** No contraction noted.

Forearm Pronation

Table 7-4 lists the primary and accessory muscles responsible for forearm pronation. The pronator teres (see Figure 7-14) and pronator quadratus (see Figure 7-15) muscles are the prime movers for forearm pronation.

TABLE 7-4	MUSCLES RESPONSIBLE FOR FOREARM PRONATION		
PRIMARY MUSCLES	**ORIGIN**	**INSERTION**	**INNERVATION**
Pronator teres	Medial epicondyle of humerus and coronoid process of ulna	Lateral surface of radius at midpoint	Median
Pronator quadratus	Distal fourth of the ulna	Distal fourth of the radius	Median
ACCESSORY MUSCLES	**ORIGIN**	**INSERTION**	**INNERVATION**
Flexor carpi radialis	Medial epicondyle of humerus	Base of second and third metacarpals	Median

Posterior View

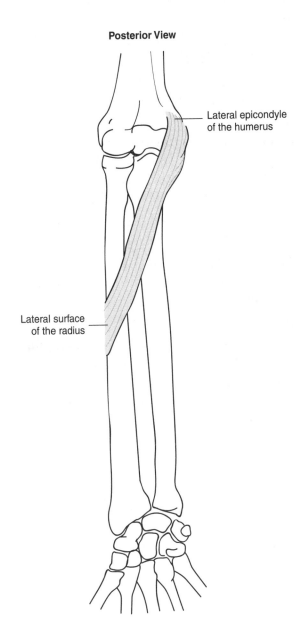

Lateral epicondyle
of the humerus

Lateral surface
of the radius

Figure 7-14 Pronator teres. Source: Delmar/Cengage Learning

Anterior View

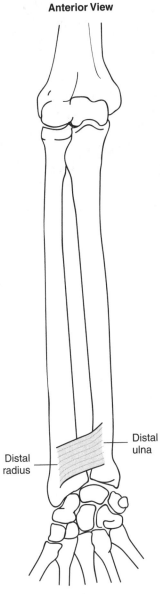

Distal
ulna

Distal
radius

Figure 7-15 Pronator quadratus. Source: Delmar/Cengage Learning

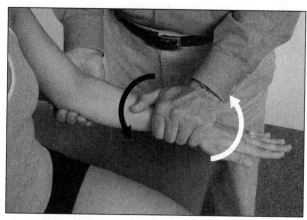

Figure 7-16 Proper positioning for forearm pronation grades 5–3. Source: Delmar/Cengage Learning

Testing for Forearm Pronation Grades 5, 4, 3 (Normal, Good, Fair) Gravity Minimal

POSITION OF PATIENT: Short sitting with arm at side, elbow flexed to 90° and forearm supinated.

POSITION OF THERAPIST: Standing in front of patient or on test side. Supporting hand placed at the elbow. Resistance hand grasps the wrist on the dorsal surface (see Figure 7-16).

TEST: Patient instructed to move forearm into pronation and hold against resistance.

DIRECTIONS: Say to the patient, "Turn your palm downward and hold the position. Don't let me move it."

GRADING:

- **Grade 5 (Normal):** Patient moves to position and holds against maximum resistance.
- **Grade 4 (Good):** Patient moves to position and holds against strong (but not full) resistance.
- **Grade 3 (Fair):** Patient moves to position but tolerates no resistance.

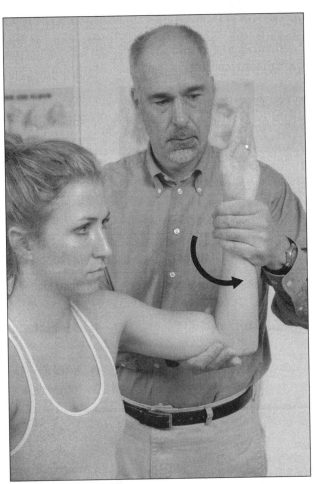

Figure 7-17 Proper positioning for forearm pronation grades 2–0. Source: Delmar/Cengage Learning

Testing for Forearm Pronation
Grades 2, 1, 0 (Poor, Trace, None)
Gravity Minimal

POSITION OF PATIENT: Short sitting with arm at side. Shoulder flexed about 45°, elbow flexed to 90°, forearm in neutral.

POSITION OF THERAPIST: Stand in front of patient supporting the arm by cupping the elbow with fingers positioned to palpate as necessary (see Figure 7-17).

TEST: Patient attempts to move forearm into pronation.

DIRECTIONS: Say to the patient, "Turn your palm away from you."

GRADING:

- **Grade 2 (Poor):** Patient moves through partial range.
- **Grade 1 (Trace):** Therapist notes contraction but no actual motion.
- **Grade 0 (None):** No contraction noted.

Substitutions

Important substitutions to watch for during MMT of the elbow/forearm are as follows:

- Elbow extension could occur with a grade 0 triceps if external rotation is allowed at the shoulder. When this occurs, the elbow will literally "fall" into extension.
- Patients should be instructed to relax wrist and fingers during supination to avoid substitution by the wrist extensors.
- Patients may internally rotate or abduct the shoulder while attempting pronation in which case gravity will cause the forearm to drop into pronation.

RANGE OF MOTION

The following text discusses range of motion for the elbow and forearm. The two motions available at the elbow are flexion and extension. The two motions available in the forearm are supination and pronation.

Elbow Flexion/Extension

Elbow flexion/extension occurs in the sagittal plane around a medial/lateral (frontal) axis. The normal AROM is from 0° to 150°, according to the American Academy of Orthopaedic Surgeons (1965).

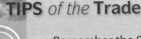

TIPS *of the* Trade

Remember the 0, or lower number of your reading, is your extension measurement and the 150, or higher number, is your flexion measurement.

The normal end-feel for elbow flexion is soft because the muscle bulk of the elbow flexors usually ends the motion. The normal end-feel for extension is hard because of the bony contact encountered between the humerus and the ulna at the end of this motion.

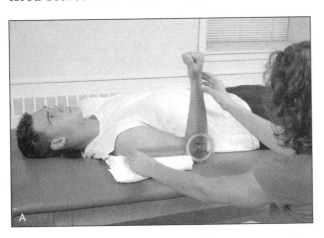

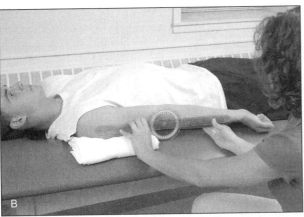

Figure 7-18 Proper positioning for (A) elbow flexion and (B) elbow extension. Source: Delmar/Cengage Learning

POSITION OF PATIENT: Supine with arm resting at side of body. A pad should be placed to facilitate the extension portion of this test. Arm begins motion from full extension with forearm supinated and flexes elbow to full range.

POSITION OF THERAPIST: Standing or sitting at test side to provide support as patient moves and then to position the goniometer. There may be a need to stabilize the shoulder during the action.

POSITION OF GONIOMETER:

- **Fulcrum:** Lateral epicondyle of the humerus (see Figure 7-18)
- **Stationary arm:** Aligned with the lateral midline of humerus with the acromion as a reference point
- **Movable arm:** Aligned with the lateral midline of the radius with the radial styloid as a reference point

Forearm Supination

Forearm supination occurs in a transverse plane around a vertical axis when the body is in anatomical position. The normal AROM is 0°–80°, according to the American Academy of Orthopaedic Surgeons (1965). The normal end-feel is firm due to the tension in the soft tissue of the area.

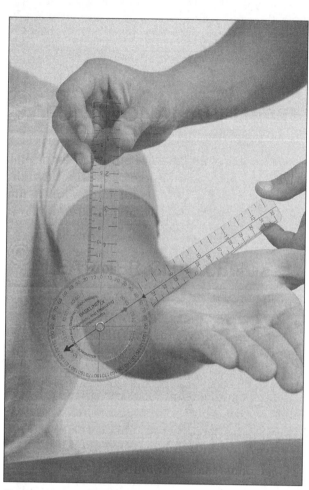

Figure 7-19 Proper positioning for forearm supination.

Source: Delmar/Cengage Learning

POSITION OF PATIENT: Short sitting with arm at side, elbow flexed to 90°, and forearm in a neutral position with the thumb pointing upward. From this position patient will supinate the forearm by turning the palm upward.

POSITION OF THERAPIST: Standing or sitting to the front of patient at test side to provide support as patient moves and then position the goniometer. There may be a need to stabilize the humerus during the action.

POSITION OF GONIOMETER:

- **Fulcrum:** Just medial and proximal to the ulnar styloid process (see Figure 7-19)
- **Stationary arm:** Aligned parallel to the midline of the humerus or perpendicular to the floor
- **Movable arm:** Across the palmar surface of the forearm proximal but parallel to the styloid processes of the ulna and radius where the forearm is most level

Forearm Pronation

Forearm pronation occurs in a transverse plane around a vertical axis when the body is in anatomical position. The normal AROM is 0°–80°. The normal end-feel may be hard due to bony contact between the ulna and radius or firm due to the tension in the soft tissue of the area.

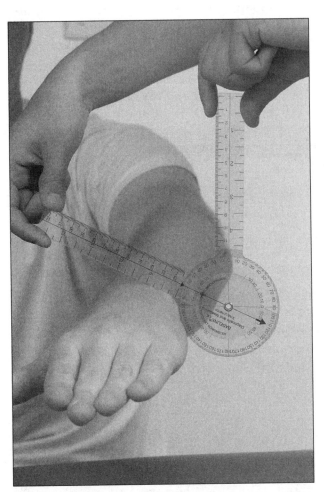

POSITION OF PATIENT: Short sitting with arm at side, elbow flexed to 90°, and forearm in a neutral position with the thumb pointing upward. From this position patient will pronate the forearm by turning the palm downward.

POSITION OF THERAPIST: Standing or sitting to the front of patient at test side to provide support as patient moves and then to position the goniometer. There may be a need to stabilize the humerus during the action.

POSITION OF GONIOMETER:

- **Fulcrum:** Just lateral and proximal to the ulnar styloid process (see Figure 7-20)
- **Stationary arm:** Aligned parallel to the midline of the humerus or perpendicular to the floor
- **Movable arm:** Across the dorsal surface of the forearm proximal but parallel to the styloid processes of the ulna and radius where the forearm is most level.

Figure 7-20 Proper positioning for forearm pronation.

Source: Delmar/Cengage Learning

FUNCTIONAL APPLICATION

Much research has been conducted on the functional activity required by the elbow and forearm in everyday activities. Statistics can also be found that would identify both strength and ROM requirements for athletes in various sports. Some conclusions can be drawn from these separate studies. Generally speaking, most activities of daily living occur within an arc of about 100° of elbow flexion. According to Norkin and White (1995), that arc occurs in a range from about 30° to 130°. They also state that a range of 100° of rotation is required from about 50° supination to 50° pronation. Activities such as holding a telephone or reaching the back of the head would require the most flexion. Cutting food on a plate would require more pronation, and lifting a fork to the mouth would require more supination. ADLs involving washing or clothing the lower part of the body would require more extension. Incorporating general questions regarding ADLs into your assessment could easily help identify areas of deficit that would warrant further testing.

LEARNER CHALLENGE

1. List elbow joint motions. Then identify the plane and axis in which they occur.
2. List forearm motions. Then identify the plane and axis in which they occur.
3. Palpate the following elbow forearm landmarks: medial epicondyle, lateral epicondyle, olecranon process, radial styloid process, ulnar styloid process, muscle belly of the triceps, and muscle belly of the biceps.
4. On a lab partner, use a china marker to shade in the elbow flexor and extensor muscles on one arm and the forearm supinator and pronator muscles on the other. Instruct a lab partner to perform appropriate motions with each arm and observe/palpate the movement under your shaded areas.
5. Fill in the following tables summarizing MMT and ROM measurements of the elbow and forearm.

A) Manual Muscle Testing for Grades 5, 4, 3 Gravity Resisted			
MOTION	**TESTING POSITION**	**STABILIZING HAND**	**RESISTANCE HAND**
Elbow Flexion			
Elbow Extension			
Forearm Supination			
Forearm Pronation			

B) Manual Muscle Testing for Grades 2, 1, 0 Gravity Minimal

MOTION	TESTING POSITION	STABILIZING HAND	RESISTANCE HAND	PALPATION
Elbow Flexion				
Elbow Extension				
Forearm Supination				
Forearm Pronation				

C) Range of Motion

MOTION	MOVABLE ARM	STATIONARY ARM	FULCRUM	NORMAL ROM
Elbow Flexion				
Elbow Extension				
Forearm Supination				
Forearm Pronation				

NOTES

THE WRIST

OBJECTIVES

Upon completion of this chapter, the reader will be able to:

- Describe the wrist joint.

- Identify the bony landmarks significant to the wrist joint.

- Name the major ligaments and their purpose.

- Describe supporting structures important to the wrist joint.

- Describe the major motions of the wrist and name the muscles that perform them.

- Identify the origins, insertions, and innervations of the muscles of the wrist.

- Perform proper manual muscle testing on the major muscles of the wrist grades 5–0.

- Be aware of possible substitutions during manual muscle testing on the wrist.

- Accurately perform range of motion testing using the goniometer on the wrist joint.

MUSCULOSKELETAL OVERVIEW

Although small in relation to other joints of the human body, the wrist plays a crucial part in a myriad of actions we do every day. In addition to ADLs, the wrist allows us to perform actions such as shooting a free throw in basketball, flipping a pancake while making breakfast, using a keyboard and mouse on the computer, and even something as simple as signing our name. From **gross motor movements** of the upper extremity to **fine motor movements** of the hand, the action of the wrist is essential.

Keep in mind that none of these upper extremity joints work alone. While one joint, such as the scapula, may provide stability, another, such as the forearm, offers mobility to allow the entire arm to be placed in position so an action can be completed. A thorough understanding of this interrelationship is essential when assessing a patient's overall functional ability.

This chapter focuses on this complex structure known as the *wrist*. It is easy to see why this joint is so flexible when you consider the bony structures involved. Aside from the forearm structures, there are numerous carpal bones of different sizes and shapes. The fact that the wrist is made up of these many small bones allows much more movement than would be seen if there were one large bone in this area. This can be more difficult for students as they learn initially, but as you become more comfortable correlating these structures with the movement they allow, it becomes easier to understand how the wrist works.

Joints

The wrist is made up of two joints. The first and largest is the radiocarpal joint (see Figure 8-1). This joint consists of the radius proximally and the carpal bones, specifically the scaphoid, lunate, and triquetrum, distally. The articular disk between the ulna and carpal bones is not considered a part of this joint. Due to its anterior location, the pisiform does not articulate with the disk either.

The mid-carpal joint is, just as the name implies, a collective joint between the two rows of carpal bones. The proximal row is made up of the scaphoid, lunate, triquetrum, and pisiform. The distal row contains the trapezium, trapezoid, capitate, and hamate.

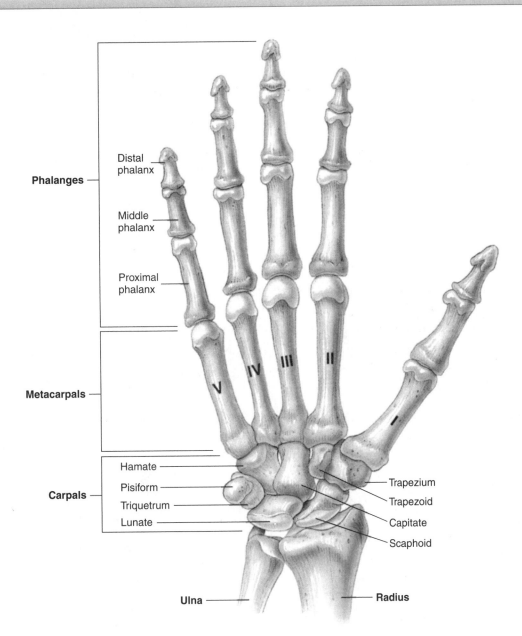

Phalanges

Distal phalanx

Middle phalanx

Proximal phalanx

Metacarpals

V IV III II I

Carpals

Hamate
Pisiform
Triquetrum
Lunate

Trapezium
Trapezoid
Capitate
Scaphoid

Ulna **Radius**

Figure 8-1 Carpal bones. Source: Delmar/Cengage Learning

Bones

Although discussed previously, the bony landmarks of the radius and ulna are presented here to correlate with the muscle attachments discussed later in this chapter (see Figure 8-2).

Radius

- **Head:** Superior surface of the proximal end of the radius
- **Radial tuberosity:** Medial surface of the proximal end of the radius
- **Styloid process:** Posterior/lateral surface of the distal radius

Ulna

- **Olecranon process:** Proximal end of the ulna on the posterior side
- **Trochlear notch:** Anterior surface of the proximal end of the ulna
- **Coronoid process:** Anterior surface of the proximal end of the ulna just distal to the trochlear notch
- **Radial notch:** Lateral surface of the proximal end of the ulna just distal to the trochlear notch
- **Ulnar tuberosity:** Anterior surface of the ulna just distal to the coronoid process
- **Styloid process:** Posterior/medial surface of the distal ulna
- **Head:** Lateral surface of the distal ulna

Even though there are no specific landmarks on the carpal bones (refer to Figure 8-1), each of the bones can be palpated.

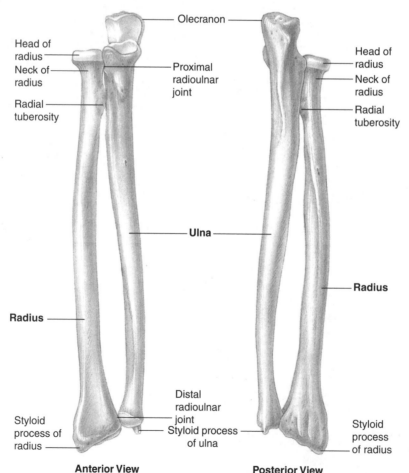

Figure 8-2 Ulna and radius anterior and posterior views. Source: Delmar/Cengage Learning

Ligaments

Stability of the wrist is primarily provided by four ligaments (see Figure 8-3). The radial collateral ligament originates on the radius and has insertion points on the scaphoid, trapezium, and first metacarpal. The ulnar collateral ligament originates on the ulna and inserts on the pisiform and triquetrum. These ligaments provide lateral support. Dorsal and ventral support is provided by the palmar and dorsal radiocarpal ligaments. The palmar radiocarpal ligament originates from the anterior surface of both the ulna and the radius and inserts on the anterior surfaces of the scaphoid, lunate, and triquetrum. The positioning of this ligament helps provide stability of the wrist by limiting extension. The dorsal radiocarpal ligament originates on the styloid process of the radius and inserts on the dorsal surfaces of the lunate and triquetrum.

Another structure of significance in this area is the palmar aponeurosis. This thick band of fascia is a relatively superficial structure that covers the palmar surface of the wrist and hand. The aponeurosis provides some muscular attachments but also serves the purpose of covering and protecting the deeper structures of the wrist and hand.

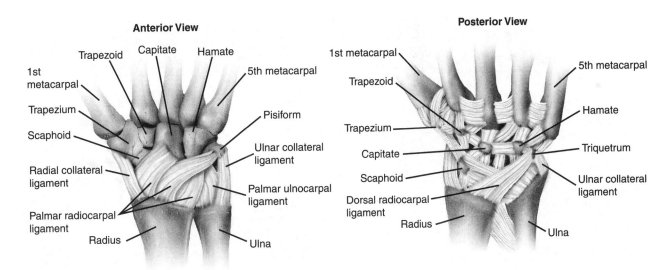

Figure 8-3 Ligaments of the wrist (*See color plate*). Source: Delmar/Cengage Learning

MUSCLE TESTING OF THE WRIST

The pure motions available at the wrist are flexion and extension. Combining these motions can produce **radial deviation** and **ulnar deviation** and a circumduction action that also increases mobility at this joint. Because it is important to review the muscles associated with the movement, each section begins with a table of the muscles responsible for the movement being tested, followed by a depiction of the primary muscles.

Wrist Flexion

Table 8-1 shows the primary and accessory muscles responsible for wrist flexion. The flexor carpi radialis (see Figure 8-4) and flexor carpi ulnaris (see Figure 8-5) muscles are the prime movers for wrist flexion.

TABLE 8-1   MUSCLES RESPONSIBLE FOR WRIST FLEXION

PRIMARY MUSCLES	ORIGIN	INSERTION	INNERVATION
Flexor carpi radialis	Medial epicondyle of humerus	Base of second and third metacarpals	Median
Flexor carpi ulnaris, two heads	Medial epicondyle of humerus	Pisiform and base of fifth metacarpal	Ulnar

ACCESSORY MUSCLES	ORIGIN	INSERTION	INNERVATION
Palmaris longus	Medial epicondyle of humerus	Palmar fascia	Median nerve
Flexor digitorum superficialis	Common flexor tendon, coronoid process, and radius	Sides of middle phalanx of the four fingers	Median
Flexor digitorum profundus	Upper 3/4 of the ulna	Distal phalanx of the four fingers	Median and ulnar
Abductor pollicis longus	Posterior surface of radius, interosseous membrane, and middle ulna	Base of first metacarpal	Radial
Flexor pollicis longus	Anterior surface of radius	Distal phalanx of thumb	Median nerve

Anterior View

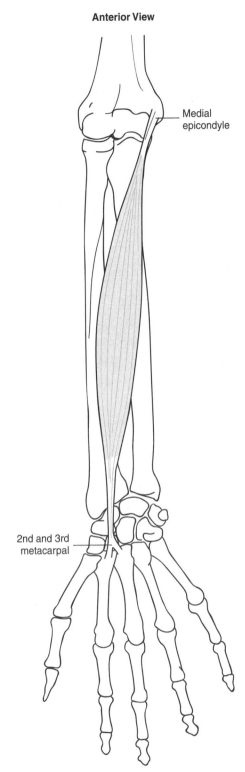

Medial epicondyle

2nd and 3rd metacarpal

Figure 8-4 Flexor carpi radialis. Source: Delmar/Cengage Learning

Anterior View

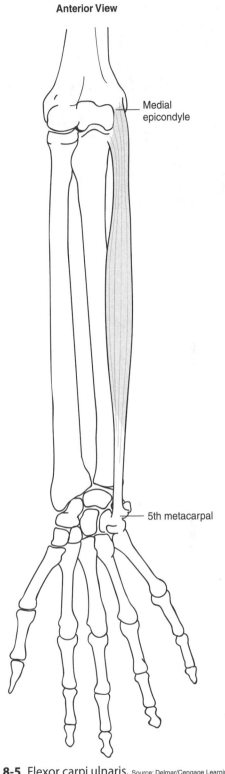

Medial epicondyle

5th metacarpal

Figure 8-5 Flexor carpi ulnaris. Source: Delmar/Cengage Learning

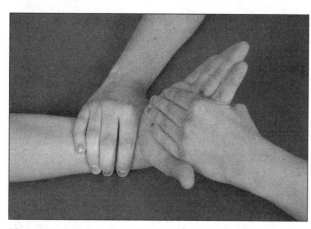

Figure 8-6 Proper positioning for wrist flexion grades 5–3. Source: Delmar/Cengage Learning

Testing for Wrist Flexion Grades 5, 4, 3 (Normal, Good, Fair) Gravity Resisted

POSITION OF PATIENT: Short sitting with forearm supported on a table and positioned in supination.

POSITION OF THERAPIST: In front of patient with supporting hand on forearm under wrist and resisting hand placed in patient's palm (see Figure 8-6).

TEST: Patient is instructed to move hand into flexion and hold against resistance.

DIRECTIONS: Say to the patient, "Bend your wrist upward and hold the position. Don't let me straighten it."

GRADING:

- **Grade 5 (Normal):** Patient flexes to position and holds against maximum resistance.
- **Grade 4 (Good):** Patient flexes to position and holds against strong (but not full) resistance.
- **Grade 3 (Fair):** Patient flexes to position but tolerates no resistance.

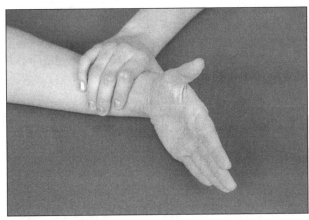

Figure 8-7 Proper positioning for wrist flexion grades 2–0. Source: Delmar/Cengage Learning

Testing for Wrist Flexion Grades 2, 1, 0 (Poor, Trace, None) Gravity Minimal

POSITION OF PATIENT: Short sitting with forearm supported on a table and in neutral position with ulnar border of the wrist on the table.

POSITION OF THERAPIST: In front of patient, supporting hand under forearm at the wrist with fingers placed over tendons to palpate if necessary (see Figure 8-7).

TEST: Patient attempts to flex wrist.

DIRECTIONS: Say to the patient, "Leading with your palm, bend your wrist."

GRADING:

- **Grade 2 (Poor):** Patient moves through partial range.
- **Grade 1 (Trace):** Therapist notes contraction but no actual motion.
- **Grade 0 (None):** No contraction noted.

Wrist Extension

Table 8-2 describes the primary and accessory muscles responsible for wrist extension. The extensor carpi radialis (see Figures 8-8 and 8-9) and extensor carpi ulnaris (see Figure 8-10) muscles are the prime movers for wrist extension.

TABLE 8-2	MUSCLES RESPONSIBLE FOR WRIST EXTENSION		
PRIMARY MUSCLES	**ORIGIN**	**INSERTION**	**INNERVATION**
Extensor carpi radialis, longus	Supracondylar ridge of humerus	Base of second metacarpal	Radial
Extensor carpi radialis, brevis	Lateral epicondyle of humerus	Base of third metacarpal	Radial
Extensor carpi ulnaris	Lateral epicondyle of humerus	Base of fifth metacarpal	Radial
ACCESSORY MUSCLES	**ORIGIN**	**INSERTION**	**INNERVATION**
Extensor digitorum	Lateral epicondyle of humerus	Base of distal phalanx digits 2–5	Radial
Extensor digiti minimi	Lateral epicondyle of humerus	Base of fifth distal phalanx	Radial
Extensor indicis	Distal ulna	Base of distal phalanx of second digit	Radial

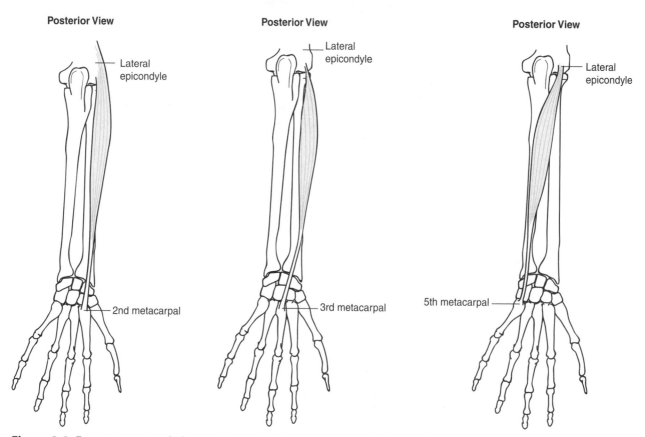

Figure 8-8 Extensor carpi radialis, longus. Source: Delmar/Cengage Learning

Figure 8-9 Extensor carpi radialis, brevis. Source: Delmar/Cengage Learning

Figure 8-10 Extensor carpi ulnaris. Source: Delmar/Cengage Learning

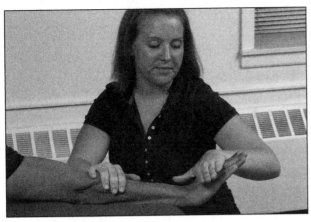

Figure 8-11 Proper positioning for wrist extension grades 5–3. Source: Delmar/Cengage Learning

Testing for Wrist Extension
Grades 5, 4, 3 (Normal, Good, Fair)
Gravity Resisted

POSITION OF PATIENT: Short sitting with forearm supported on a table and positioned in pronation.

POSITION OF THERAPIST: In front of patient with supporting hand on forearm under wrist and resisting hand placed on dorsal surface of hand (see Figure 8-11).

TEST: Patient is instructed to move hand into extension and hold against resistance.

DIRECTIONS: Say to the patient, "Bend your wrist and hold the position. Don't let me straighten it."

GRADING:

- **Grade 5 (Normal):** Patient extends to position and holds against maximum resistance.
- **Grade 4 (Good):** Patient extends to position and holds against strong (but not full) resistance.
- **Grade 3 (Fair):** Patient extends to position but tolerates no resistance.

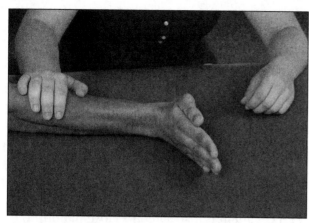

Figure 8-12 Proper positioning for wrist extension grades 2–0. Source: Delmar/Cengage Learning

Testing for Wrist Extension
Grades 2, 1, 0 (Poor, Trace, None)
Gravity Minimal

POSITION OF PATIENT: Short sitting with forearm is in neutral position with ulnar border of the wrist on the table.

POSITION OF THERAPIST: In front of patient, supporting hand on the forearm with fingers placed over tendons to palpate if necessary (see Figure 8-12).

TEST: Patient attempts to extend wrist.

DIRECTIONS: Say to the patient, "Leading with the back of your hand, bend your wrist."

GRADING:

- **Grade 2 (Poor):** Patient moves through partial range.
- **Grade 1 (Trace):** Therapist notes contraction but no actual motion.
- **Grade 0 (None):** No contraction noted.

Radial Deviation

The primary and accessory muscles responsible for radial deviation are described in Table 8-3. The flexor carpi radialis (refer to Figure 8-4) and extensor carpi radialis (refer to Figures 8-8 and 8-9) muscles are the prime movers for radial deviation.

TABLE 8-3 — MUSCLES RESPONSIBLE FOR RADIAL DEVIATION

PRIMARY MUSCLES	ORIGIN	INSERTION	INNERVATION
Flexor carpi radialis	Medial epicondyle of humerus	Base of second and third metacarpals	Median
Extensor carpi radialis, longus	Supracondylar ridge of humerus	Base of second metacarpal	Radial
Extensor carpi radialis, brevis	Lateral epicondyle of humerus	Base of third metacarpal	Radial

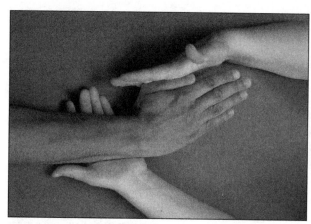

Figure 8-13 Proper positioning for radial deviation grades 5–3. Source: Delmar/Cengage Learning

Testing for Radial Deviation Grades 5, 4, 3 (Normal, Good, Fair) Gravity Resisted

POSITION OF PATIENT: Short sitting with hand resting on table, palm down.

POSITION OF THERAPIST: Standing in front of patient with supporting hand on forearm and resistance hand against the radial surface of the hand (see Figure 8-13).

TEST: Patient is instructed to move hand into radial deviation and hold against resistance.

DIRECTIONS: Say to the patient, "Leading with your thumb, bend your wrist to the side and hold the position. Don't let me straighten it."

GRADING:

- **Grade 5 (Normal):** Patient moves to position and holds against maximum resistance.
- **Grade 4 (Good):** Patient moves to position and holds against strong (but not full) resistance.
- **Grade 3 (Fair):** Patient moves to position but tolerates no resistance.

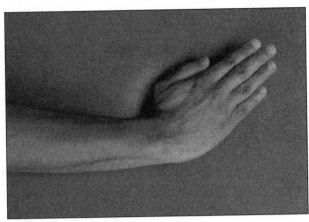

Figure 8-14 Proper positioning for radial deviation grades 2–0. Source: Delmar/Cengage Learning

Testing for Radial Deviation
Grades 2, 1, 0 (Poor, Trace, None)
Gravity Minimal

POSITION OF PATIENT: Short sitting with hand resting on table, forearm pronated.

POSITION OF THERAPIST: Standing in front of patient with one hand on distal forearm radial surface to palpate as necessary (see Figure 8-14).

TEST: Patient is instructed to move hand into radial deviation.

DIRECTIONS: Say to the patient, "Leading with your thumb, bend your wrist."

GRADING:

- **Grade 2 (Poor):** Patient moves through partial range.
- **Grade 1 (Trace):** Therapist notes contraction but no actual motion.
- **Grade 0 (None):** No contraction noted.

Ulnar Deviation

Table 8-4 lists the primary and accessory muscles responsible for ulnar deviation. The extensor carpi ulnaris (refer to Figure 8-10) and flexor carpi ulnaris (refer to Figure 8-5) muscles are the prime movers for ulnar deviation.

TABLE 8-4	MUSCLES RESPONSIBLE FOR ULNAR DEVIATION		
PRIMARY MUSCLES	**ORIGIN**	**INSERTION**	**INNERVATION**
Extensor carpi ulnaris	Lateral epicondyle of humerus	Base of fifth metacarpal	Radial
Flexor carpi ulnaris, two heads	Medial epicondyle of humerus	Pisiform and base of fifth metacarpal	Ulnar

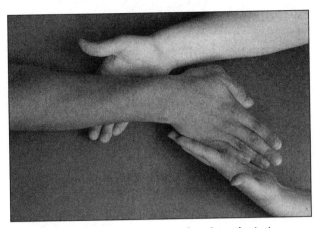

Figure 8-15 Proper positioning for ulnar deviation grades 5–3. Source: Delmar/Cengage Learning

Testing for Ulnar Deviation
Grades 5, 4, 3 (Normal, Good, Fair)
Gravity Resisted

POSITION OF PATIENT: Short sitting with hand resting on table forearm pronated.

POSITION OF THERAPIST: Standing in front of patient with supporting hand on forearm and resistance hand against the ulnar surface of the hand (see Figure 8-15).

TEST: Patient is instructed to move hand into ulnar deviation and hold against resistance.

DIRECTIONS: Say to the patient, "Leading with your little finger, bend your wrist and hold the position. Don't let me straighten it."

GRADING:

- **Grade 5 (Normal):** Patient moves to position and holds against maximum resistance.
- **Grade 4 (Good):** Patient moves to position and holds against strong (but not full) resistance.
- **Grade 3 (Fair):** Patient moves to position but tolerates no resistance.

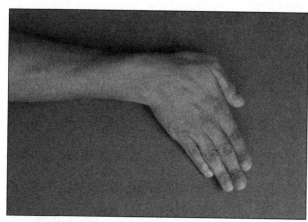

Figure 8-16 Proper positioning for ulnar deviation grades 2–0. Source: Delmar/Cengage Learning

Testing for Ulnar Deviation Grades 2, 1, 0 (Poor, Trace, None) Gravity Minimal

POSITION OF PATIENT: Short sitting with hand resting on table, forearm pronated.

POSITION OF THERAPIST: Standing in front of patient with one hand on distal forearm ulnar surface to palpate as necessary (see Figure 8-16).

TEST: Patient is instructed to move hand into ulnar deviation.

DIRECTIONS: Say to the patient, "Leading with your little finger, bend your wrist."

GRADING:

- **Grade 2 (Poor):** Patient moves through partial range.
- **Grade 1 (Trace):** Therapist notes contraction but no actual motion.
- **Grade 0 (None):** No contraction noted.

Substitutions

There is one primary substitution to watch for during MMT of the wrist:

- The most common substitution with wrist extension occurs when the fingers' extensors activate and assist with the motion. The best way to combat this is to make sure the fingers stay relaxed during the test.

RANGE OF MOTION

The following section discusses proper technique for measuring ROM for the wrist. The four wrist motions are flexion, extension, radial deviation, and ulnar deviation.

Wrist Flexion

Wrist flexion occurs in the sagittal plane around a medial/lateral or frontal axis. Normal AROM is 0°–80°, according to the American Academy of Orthopaedic Surgeons (1965). The end-feel is firm due to the tension placed on the soft tissue structures in the area as the motion is made.

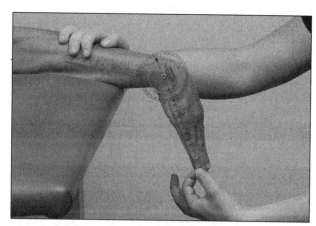

Figure 8-17 Proper positioning for wrist flexion.

Source: Delmar/Cengage Learning

POSITION OF PATIENT: Short sitting with forearm pronated and supported by the table and wrist over edge of table. From this position patient will allow wrist to drop into flexion.

POSITION OF THERAPIST: Standing or sitting to the test side of patient to provide support as patient moves and to position the goniometer. Therapist will need to stabilize the distal forearm.

POSITION OF GONIOMETER:

- **Fulcrum:** Over the triquetrum on the lateral surface of the wrist (see Figure 8-17)
- **Stationary arm:** Aligned with the midline of the lateral ulna
- **Movable arm:** Aligned with the lateral midline of the fifth metacarpal

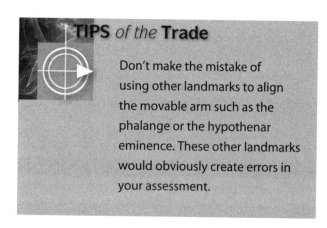

TIPS *of the* **Trade**

Don't make the mistake of using other landmarks to align the movable arm such as the phalange or the hypothenar eminence. These other landmarks would obviously create errors in your assessment.

Wrist Extension

Wrist extension occurs in the sagittal plane around a medial/lateral or frontal axis. Normal AROM is 0°–70°, according to the American Academy of Orthopaedic Surgeons (1965). The end-feel for wrist extension is firm due to the tension placed on the soft tissue structures in the area as the motion is made.

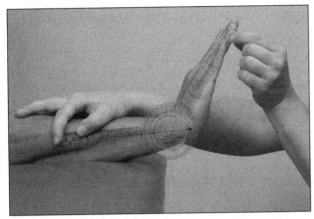

Figure 8-18 Proper positioning for wrist extension.

Source: Delmar/Cengage Learning

POSITION OF PATIENT: Short sitting with forearm pronated and supported by the table and wrist over edge of table. From this position patient will lift the wrist into extension.

POSITION OF THERAPIST: Standing or sitting to the test side of patient to provide support as patient moves and to position the goniometer. Therapist will need to stabilize the distal forearm.

POSITION OF GONIOMETER:

- **Fulcrum:** Over the triquetrum on the lateral surface of the wrist (see Figure 8-18)
- **Stationary arm:** Aligned with the midline of the lateral ulna
- **Movable arm:** Aligned with the lateral midline of the fifth metacarpal

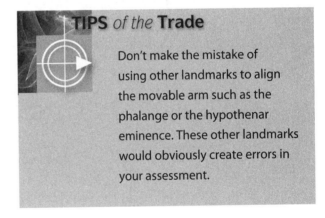

TIPS *of the* **Trade**

Don't make the mistake of using other landmarks to align the movable arm such as the phalange or the hypothenar eminence. These other landmarks would obviously create errors in your assessment.

Radial Deviation

Wrist radial deviation occurs in the frontal plane around an anterior/posterior or sagittal axis. Normal AROM is 0°–20°, according to the American Academy of Orthopaedic Surgeons (1965). The normal end-feel is hard due to the contact that is encountered between the radial styloid process and the scaphoid at end range.

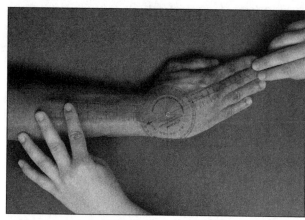

Figure 8-19 Proper positioning for radial deviation.

Source: Delmar/Cengage Learning

POSITION OF PATIENT: Short sitting with forearm pronated and supported on a table. From this position, patient will slide hand toward the thumb side into radial deviation.

POSITION OF THERAPIST: Standing or sitting on test side of patient to provide support as patient moves and to position the goniometer.

POSITION OF GONIOMETER:

- **Fulcrum:** Centered on the dorsal aspect of the wrist over the capitate (see Figure 8-19)
- **Stationary arm:** Aligned with the dorsal midline of the forearm
- **Movable arm:** Aligned with the third metacarpal

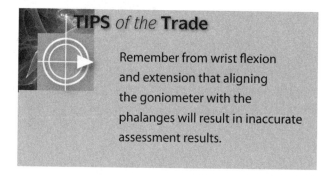

TIPS *of the* **Trade**

Remember from wrist flexion and extension that aligning the goniometer with the phalanges will result in inaccurate assessment results.

Ulnar Deviation

Wrist ulnar deviation occurs in the frontal plane around an anterior/posterior or sagittal axis. Normal AROM is 0°–30°, according to the American Academy of Orthopaedic Surgeons (1965). The normal end-feel is firm due to the tension placed on the soft tissue structures in the area as the motion is made.

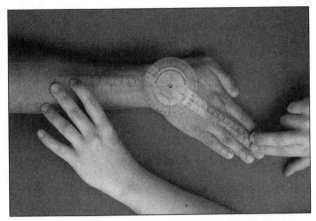

Figure 8-20 Proper positioning for ulnar deviation.

Source: Delmar/Cengage Learning

POSITION OF PATIENT: Short sitting with forearm pronated and supported on a table. From this position, patient will slide hand toward the little finger into ulnar deviation.

POSITION OF THERAPIST: Standing or sitting on test side of patient to provide support as patient moves and to position the goniometer.

POSITION OF GONIOMETER:

- **Fulcrum:** Centered on the dorsal aspect of the wrist over the capitate (see Figure 8-20)
- **Stationary arm:** Aligned with the dorsal midline of the forearm
- **Movable arm:** Aligned with the third metacarpal

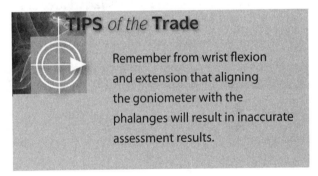

TIPS *of the* **Trade**

Remember from wrist flexion and extension that aligning the goniometer with the phalanges will result in inaccurate assessment results.

FUNCTIONAL APPLICATION

A review of common hand placements will show that most ADLs require more wrist extension than flexion and more ulnar deviation than radial deviation. More complex activities like turning a steering wheel, opening a jar, or turning a door knob require the greatest overall amounts of wrist ROM. Ryu and associates (1991) researched 31 tasks involving personal care, food preparation, and other miscellaneous ADLs and determined that all could be performed with 54° of flexion, 60° of extension, 17° of radial deviation, and 40° of ulnar deviation. Keeping in mind that assessment of function is key to rehabilitation, using those numbers as a quick screen for pathologies involving the wrist would be a timesaver.

LEARNER CHALLENGE

1. List wrist joint motions. Then identify the plane and axis in which they occur.
2. Palpate the following wrist landmarks: triquetrum, capitate, metacarpals 1–5, thenar eminence, and hypothenar eminence.
3. On a lab partner, use a china marker to shade in the flexor carpi ulnaris, the flexor carpi radialis, the extensor carpi radialis longus and brevis, and the extensor carpi ulnaris on one arm. Instruct lab partner to perform wrist flexion and extension and observe/palpate the movement under your shaded areas. Then have your lab partner perform ulnar and radial deviation and observe/palpate the movement under your shaded areas.
4. Fill in the following tables summarizing MMT and ROM measurements of the wrist.

A) Manual Muscle Testing for Grades 5, 4, 3 Gravity Resisted			
MOTION	TESTING POSITION	STABILIZING HAND	RESISTANCE HAND
Wrist Flexion			
Wrist Extension			
Radial Deviation			
Ulnar Deviation			

B) Manual Muscle Testing for Grades 2, 1, 0 Gravity Minimal

MOTION	TESTING POSITION	STABILIZING HAND	RESISTANCE HAND	PALPATION
Wrist Flexion				
Wrist Extension				
Radial Deviation				
Ulnar Deviation				

C) Range of Motion

MOTION	MOVABLE ARM	STATIONARY ARM	FULCRUM	NORMAL ROM
Wrist Flexion				
Wrist Extension				
Radial Deviation				
Ulnar Deviation				

NOTES

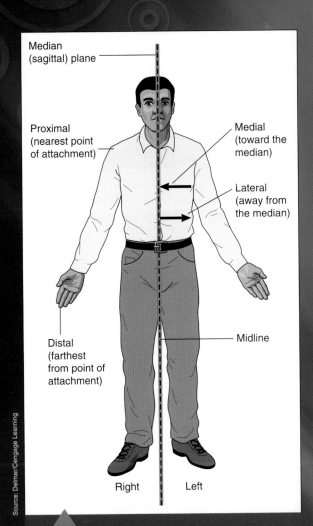

Median (sagittal) plane

Proximal (nearest point of attachment)

Medial (toward the median)

Lateral (away from the median)

Distal (farthest from point of attachment)

Midline

Right   Left

CP 1-1 Directional terms, body in anatomical position

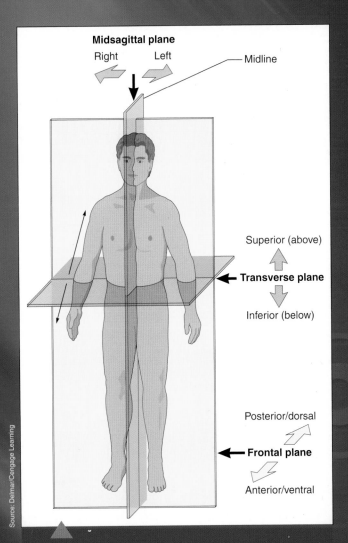

Midsagittal plane

Right   Left

Midline

Superior (above)

Transverse plane

Inferior (below)

Posterior/dorsal

Frontal plane

Anterior/ventral

CP 1-2 Planes of movement, body in fundamental position

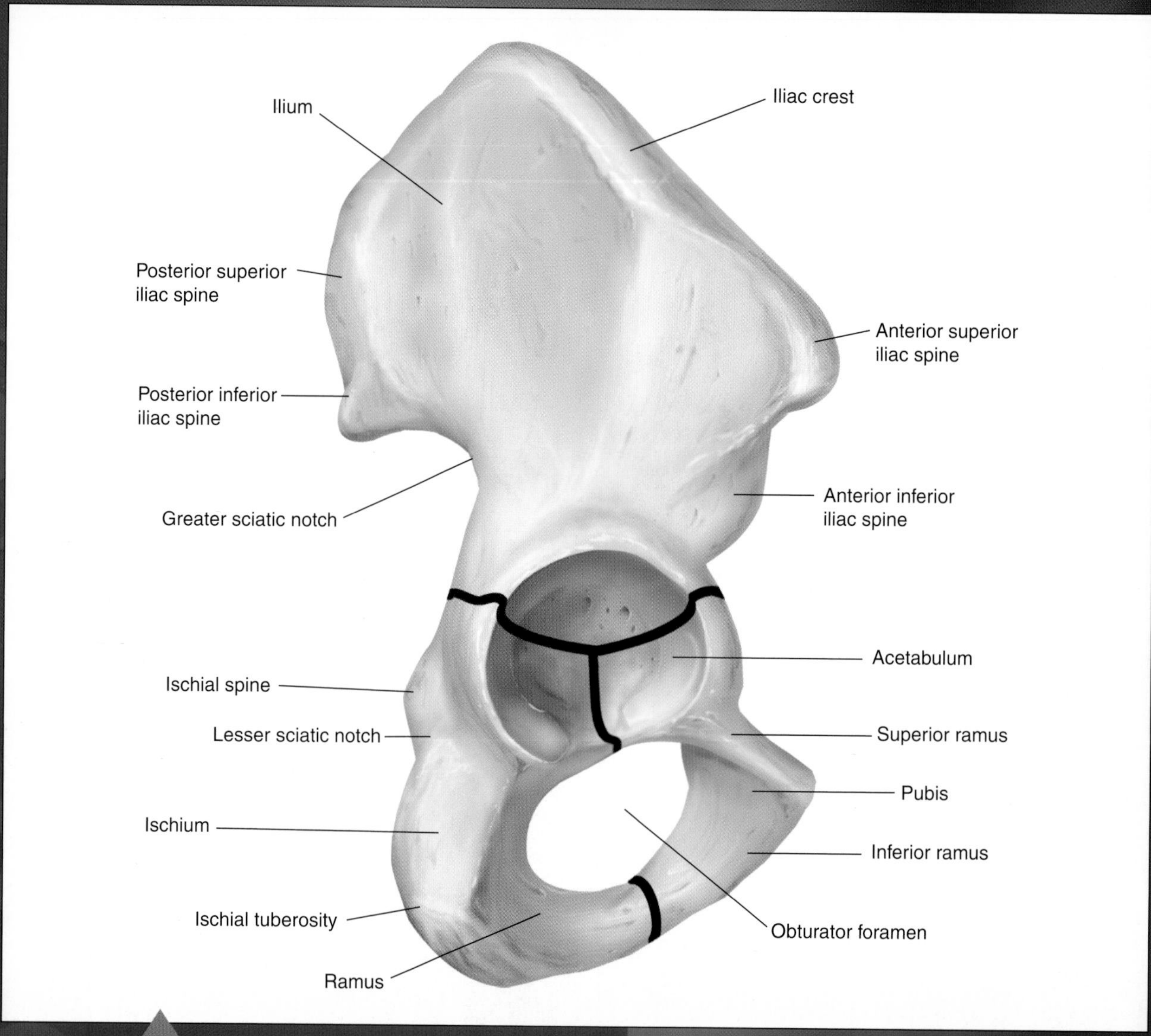

Ilium
Iliac crest
Posterior superior iliac spine
Anterior superior iliac spine
Posterior inferior iliac spine
Anterior inferior iliac spine
Greater sciatic notch
Acetabulum
Ischial spine
Lesser sciatic notch
Superior ramus
Pubis
Ischium
Inferior ramus
Ischial tuberosity
Obturator foramen
Ramus
Source: Delmar/Cengage Learning

CP 2-3 Right hip bone lateral view

CP 2-4 Femur

Head

Greater trochanter

Neck

Greater trochanter

Lesser trochanter

Pectineal line

Body

Linea aspera

Medial epicondyle

Lateral epicondyle

Lateral epicondyle

Lateral condyle

Adductor tubercle

Lateral condyle

Patellar surface

Medial condyle

Intercondyloid notch

Anterior View

Posterior View

Source: Delmar/Cengage Learning

CP 2-6 Ligamentum terres

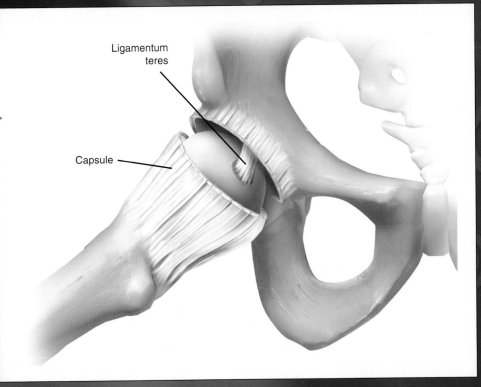

Ligamentum teres

Capsule

Source: Delmar/Cengage Learning

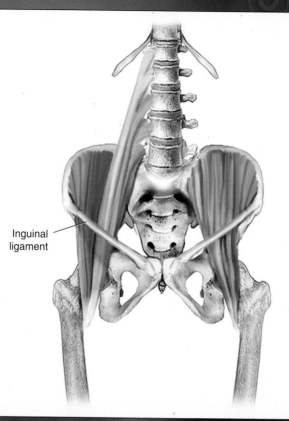

Inguinal
ligament

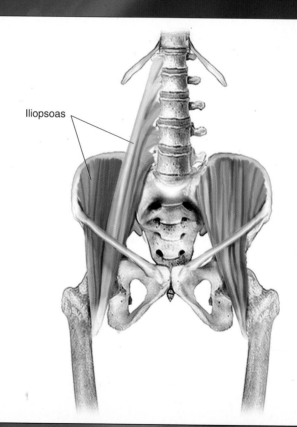

Iliopsoas

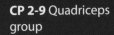

CP 2-9 Quadriceps group ▶

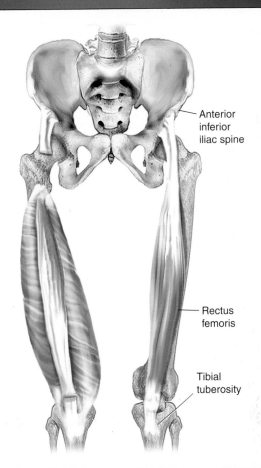

Anterior inferior iliac spine

Rectus femoris

Tibial tuberosity

CP 2-13 Hamstring muscles: semitendinosus, biceps fermoris, and semimembranosus ▶

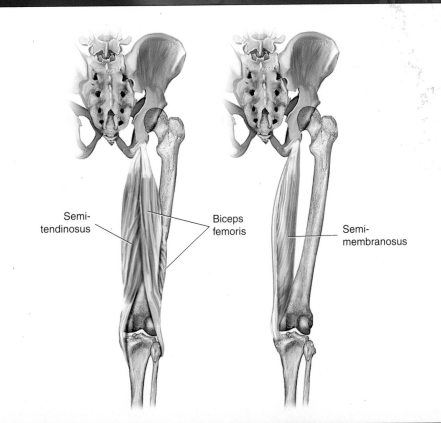

Semi-tendinosus

Biceps femoris

Semi-membranosus

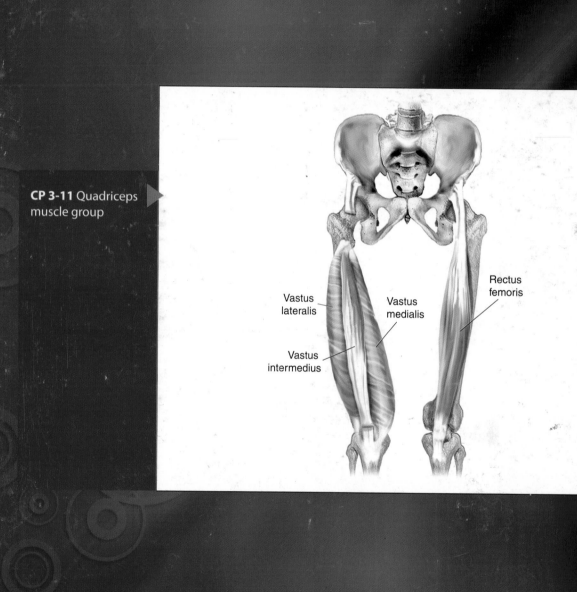

Vastus
lateralis

Vastus
medialis

Rectus
femoris

Vastus
intermedius

CP 4-1 Ankle and foot motions

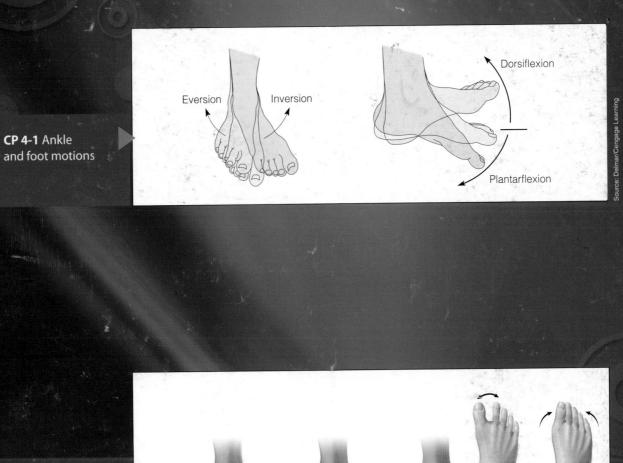

Eversion

Inversion

Dorsiflexion

Plantarflexion

CP 4-3 Motions of toes

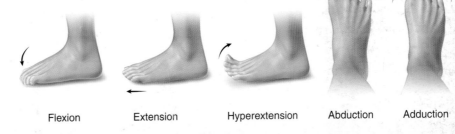

Flexion

Extension

Hyperextension

Abduction

Adduction

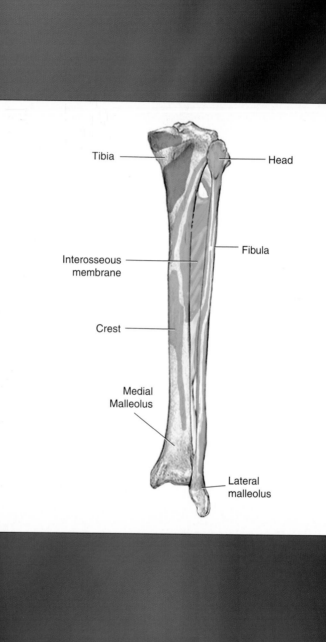

Tibia

Head

Fibula

Interosseous membrane

Crest

Medial Malleolus

Lateral malleolus

CP 4-8 Lateral ligaments

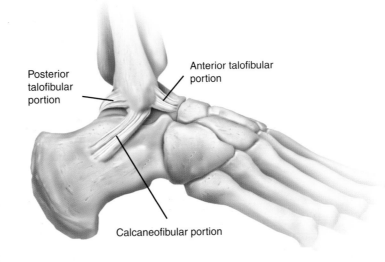

Posterior talofibular portion

Anterior talofibular portion

Calcaneofibular portion

CP 4-9 Tarsal ligaments

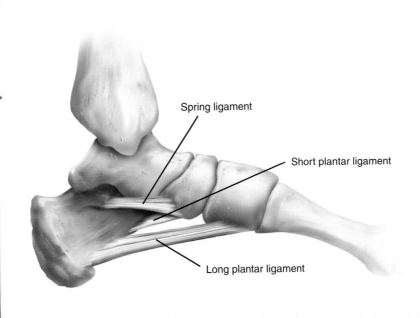

Spring ligament

Short plantar ligament

Long plantar ligament

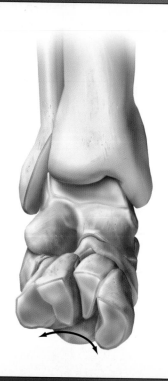

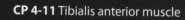

CP 4-10B Transverse arch of the foot

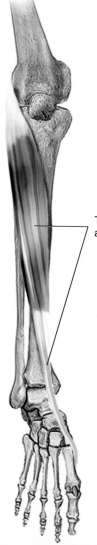

Tibialis anterior

CP 4-11 Tibialis anterior muscle

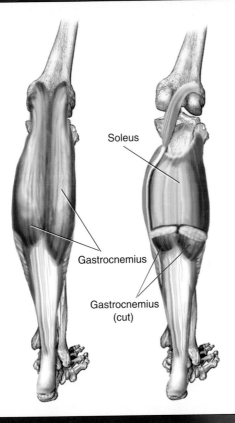

Soleus

Gastrocnemius

Gastrocnemius
(cut)

CP 4-14 Gastrocnemius and soleus muscles

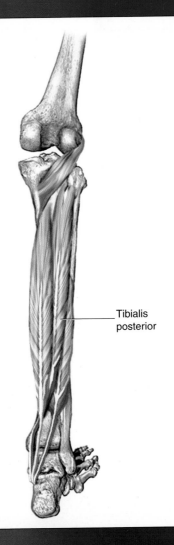

Tibialis
posterior

CP 4-20 Tibialis posterior muscle

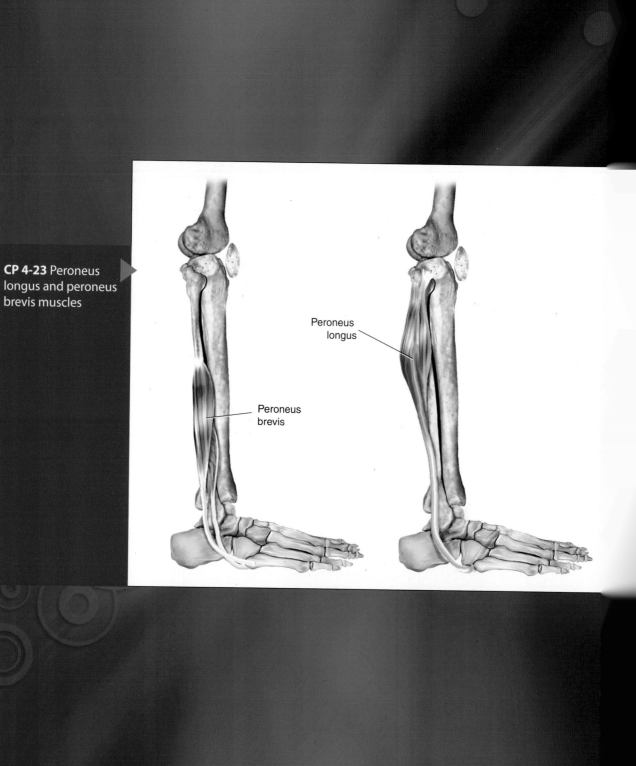

CP 4-23 Peroneus longus and peroneus brevis muscles

Peroneus longus

Peroneus brevis

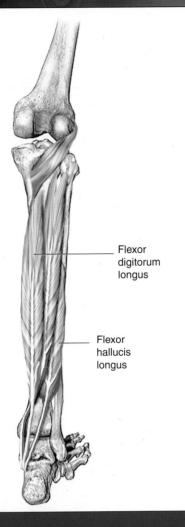

CP 4-26 Flexor hallucis longus and flexor digitorum longus muscles

Flexor digitorum longus

Flexor hallucis longus

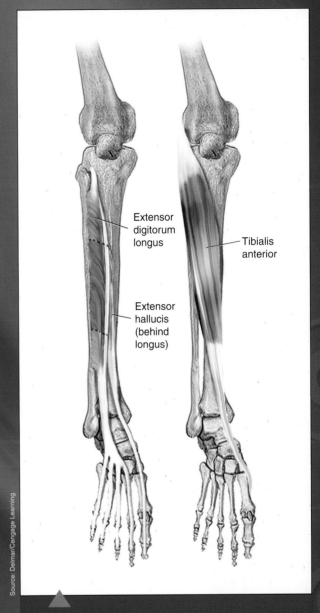

Extensor digitorum longus

Extensor hallucis (behind longus)

Tibialis anterior

CP 4-29 Extensor hallucis longus and extensor digitorum longus muscles

Source: Delmar/Cengage Learning

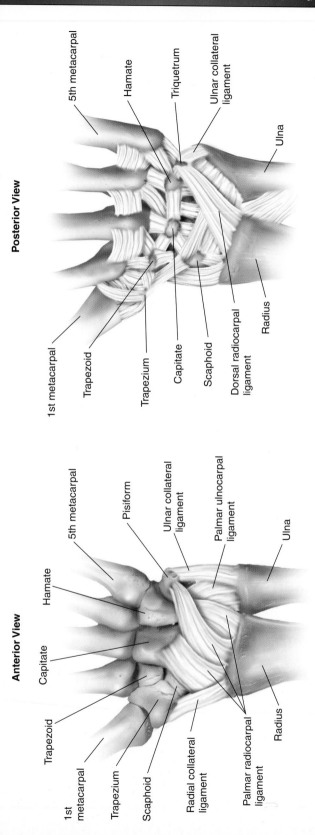

Posterior View

5th metacarpal

Hamate

Triquetrum

Ulnar collateral
ligament

Ulna

1st metacarpal

Trapezoid

Trapezium

Capitate

Scaphoid

Dorsal radiocarpal
ligament

Radius

Anterior View

Hamate

Capitate

5th metacarpal

Pisiform

Ulnar collateral
ligament

Palmar ulnocarpal
ligament

Ulna

Trapezoid

1st
metacarpal

Trapezium

Scaphoid

Radial collateral
ligament

Palmar radiocarpal
ligament

Radius

CP 8-3 (A) Ligaments of the wrist anterior (B) Ligaments of the wrist posterior

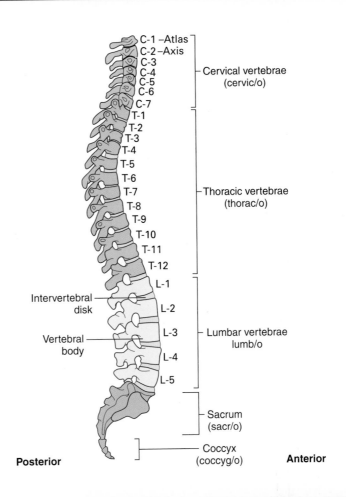

Source: Delmar/Cengage Learning

CP 10-2 Anterior/ posterior curves of vertebral column

C-1 –Atlas
C-2 –Axis
C-3
C-4
C-5
C-6
C-7

Cervical vertebrae (cervic/o)

T-1
T-2
T-3
T-4
T-5
T-6
T-7
T-8
T-9
T-10
T-11
T-12

Thoracic vertebrae (thorac/o)

Intervertebral disk

L-1
L-2
L-3
L-4
L-5

Lumbar vertebrae lumb/o

Vertebral body

Sacrum (sacr/o)

Coccyx (coccyg/o)

Posterior

Anterior

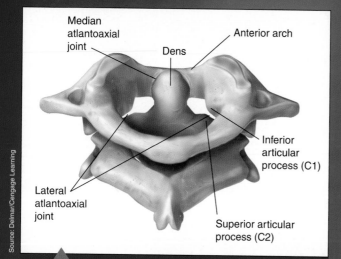

Median atlantoaxial joint

Anterior arch

Dens

Inferior articular process (C1)

Lateral atlantoaxial joint

Superior articular process (C2)

CP 10-3 Atlanto-occipital joint

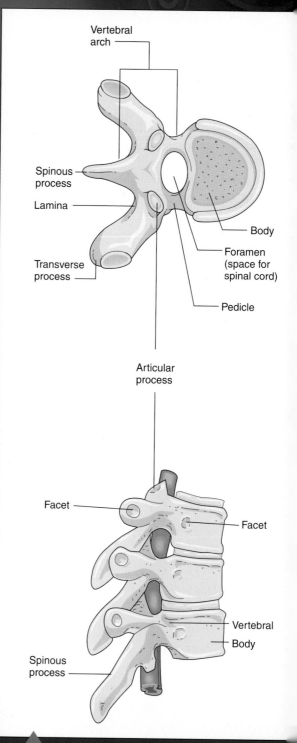

Vertebral arch

Spinous process

Lamina

Transverse process

Body

Foramen (space for spinal cord)

Pedicle

Articular process

Facet

Facet

Vertebral Body

Spinous process

CP 10-4 Superior and lateral view of vertebrae with facet joint

CP 10-8 Posterior suboccipital muscles

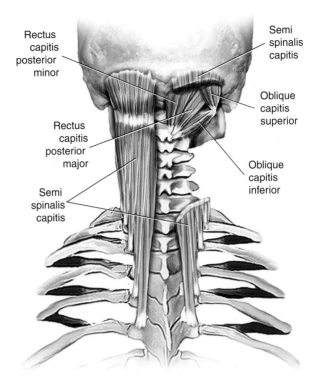

Rectus capitis posterior minor

Semi spinalis capitis

Oblique capitis superior

Rectus capitis posterior major

Oblique capitis inferior

Semi spinalis capitis

CP 10-11 Anterior suboccipital muscles

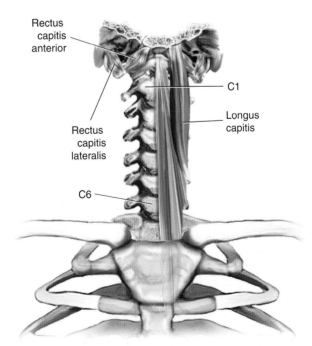

Rectus capitis anterior

C1

Longus capitis

Rectus capitis lateralis

C6

CP 10-13 Posterior cervical muscles

Upper trapezius
C1
C2
Splenius cervicis
Spinalis cervicis (often absent)
C5
C7
T1
Semispinalis cervicis
Longissimus cervicis
Iliocostalis cervicis
Rib 5
T5
Rib 6

CP 10-16 Anterior cervical muscles

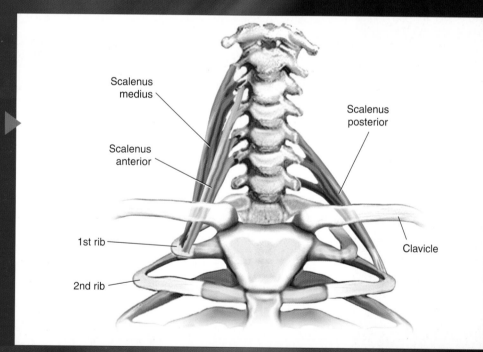

Scalenus medius
Scalenus posterior
Scalenus anterior
Clavicle
1st rib
2nd rib

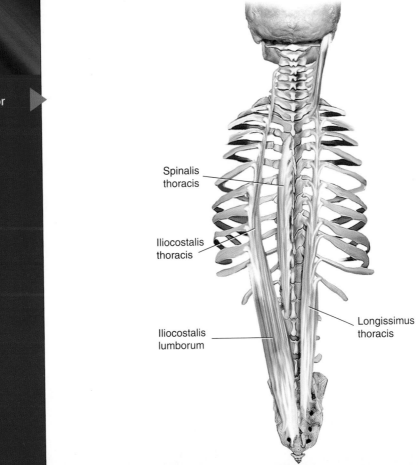

CP 10-18 Erector spinae muscle group

Spinalis
thoracis

Iliocostalis
thoracis

Longissimus
thoracis

Iliocostalis
lumborum

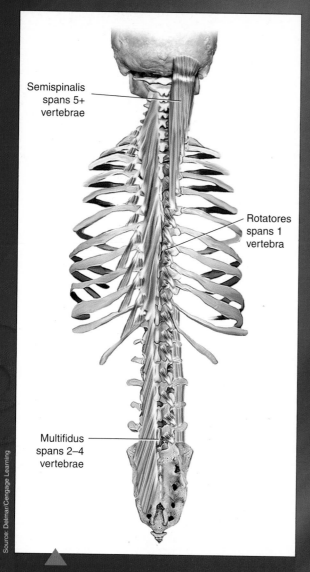

Semispinalis spans 5+ vertebrae

Rotatores spans 1 vertebra

Multifidus spans 2–4 vertebrae

CP 10-19 Transversospinalis muscle group

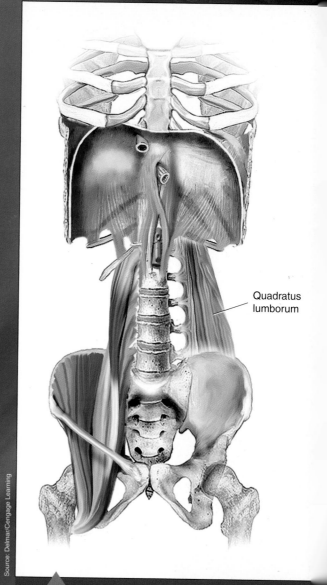

Quadratus lumborum

CP 10-20 Quadratus lumborum

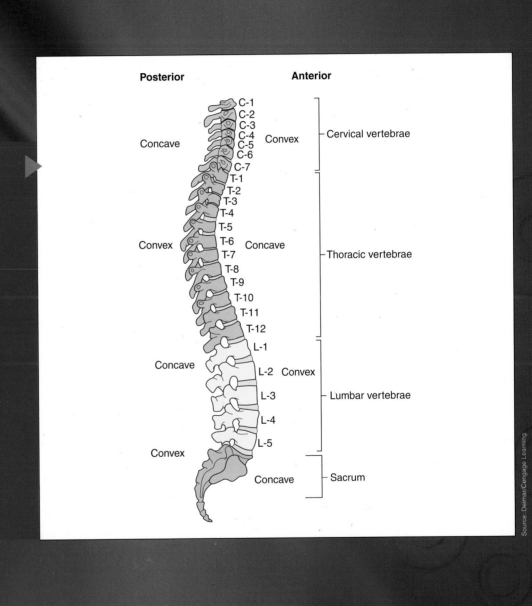

CP 11-1 Spinal column curves

Posterior   Anterior

Concave   Convex   — Cervical vertebrae

C-1
C-2
C-3
C-4
C-5
C-6
C-7

Convex   Concave   — Thoracic vertebrae

T-1
T-2
T-3
T-4
T-5
T-6
T-7
T-8
T-9
T-10
T-11
T-12

Concave   Convex   — Lumbar vertebrae

L-1
L-2
L-3
L-4
L-5

Convex   Concave   — Sacrum

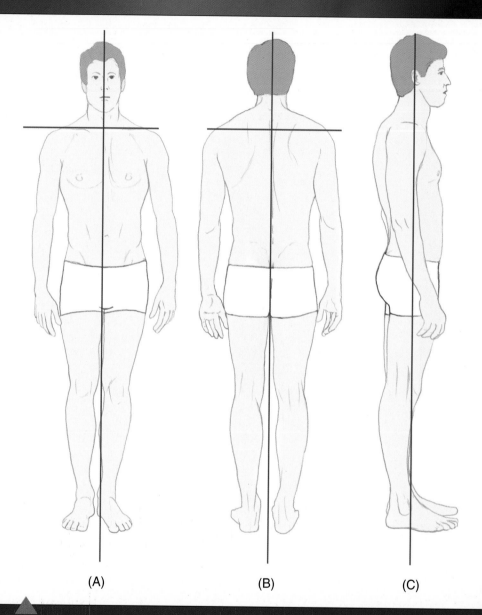

Source: Delmar/Cengage Learning

CP 11-2 (A) Anterior view of posture (B) Posterior view of posture (C) Lateral view of posture

GENERAL ANATOMY

These images provide general points of reference for the various parts of the body discussed throughout this worktext.

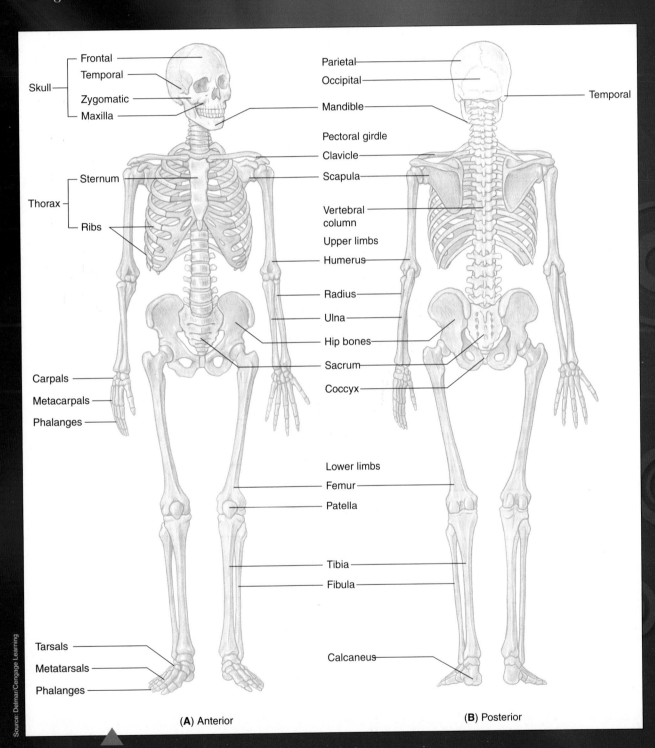

CP-1 The human skeletal system (A) Anterior view (B) Posterior view

Source: Delmar/Cengage Learning

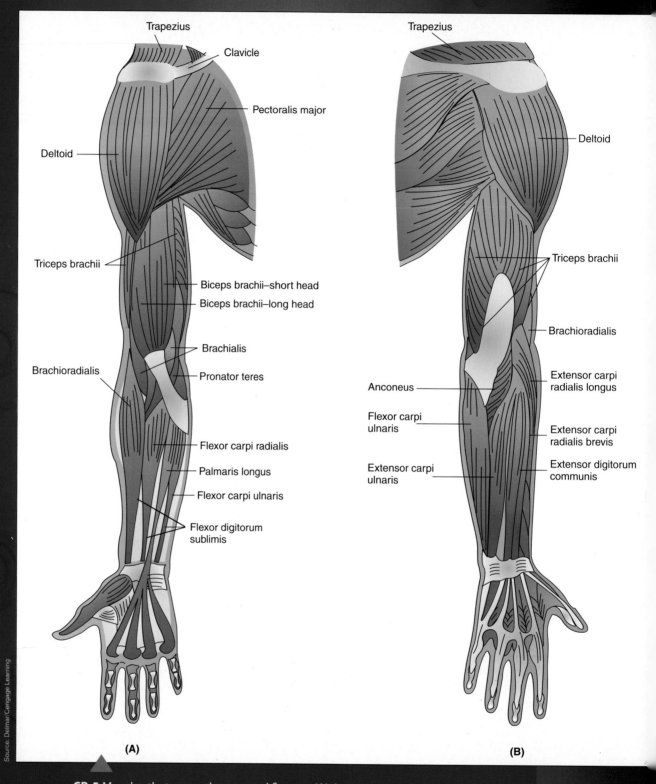

Trapezius

Clavicle

Pectoralis major

Deltoid

Triceps brachii

Biceps brachii–short head

Biceps brachii–long head

Brachialis

Brachioradialis

Pronator teres

Flexor carpi radialis

Palmaris longus

Flexor carpi ulnaris

Flexor digitorum
sublimis

(A)

Trapezius

Deltoid

Triceps brachii

Brachioradialis

Extensor carpi
radialis longus

Anconeus

Flexor carpi
ulnaris

Extensor carpi
radialis brevis

Extensor carpi
ulnaris

Extensor digitorum
communis

(B)

CP-5 Muscles that move the arm and fingers: (A) Anterior view (B) Posterior view

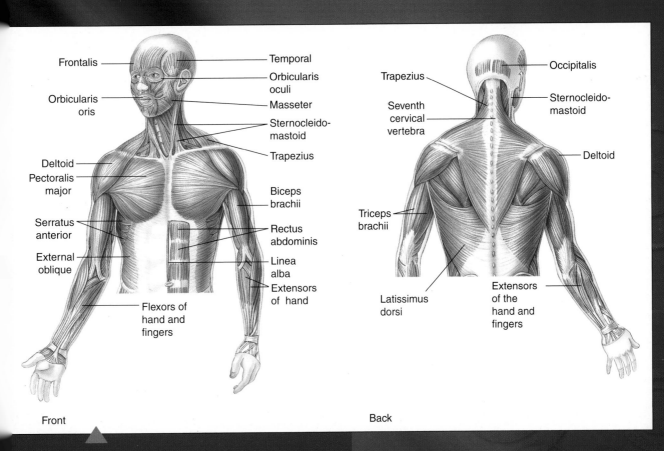

Front

Back

Frontalis

Temporal

Orbicularis
oculi

Orbicularis
oris

Masseter

Sternocleido-
mastoid

Trapezius

Deltoid

Pectoralis
major

Biceps
brachii

Serratus
anterior

Rectus
abdominis

External
oblique

Linea
alba

Extensors
of hand

Flexors of
hand and
fingers

Trapezius

Occipitalis

Seventh
cervical
vertebra

Sternocleido-
mastoid

Deltoid

Triceps
brachii

Latissimus
dorsi

Extensors
of the
hand and
fingers

CP-6 Muscles of the upper extremities

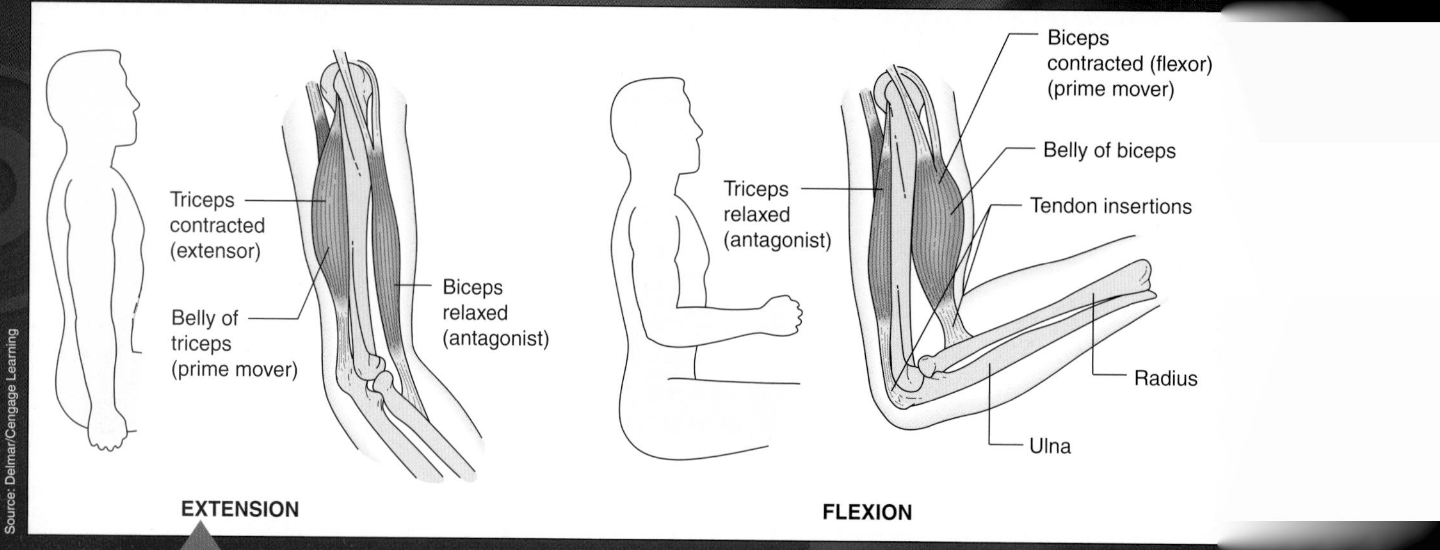

Triceps contracted (extensor)
Belly of triceps (prime mover)
Biceps relaxed (antagonist)
EXTENSION
Biceps contracted (flexor) (prime mover)
Belly of biceps
Tendon insertions
Triceps relaxed (antagonist)
Radius
Ulna
FLEXION
Source: Delmar/Cengage Learning

CP-7 Extension and flexion of the upper extremities

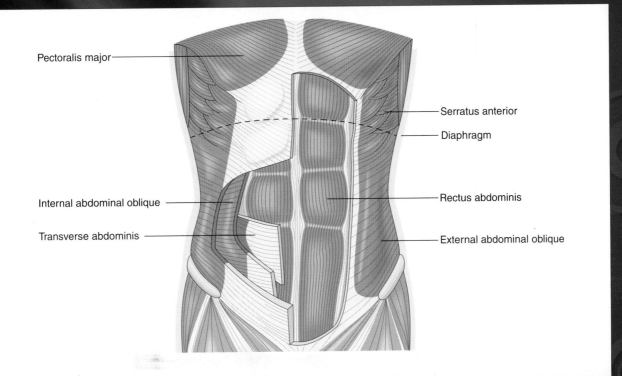

Pectoralis major

Serratus anterior

Diaphragm

Internal abdominal oblique

Transverse abdominis

Rectus abdominis

External abdominal oblique

CP-8 Muscles of the trunk

CP-9 Divisions of a vertebral column

Cervical vertebrae region:
1
2
3
4
5
6
7

(1) Cervical vertebrae
(7)
$C_1 - C_7$

Thoracic vertebrae region:
1
2
3
4
5
6
7
8
9
10
11
12

(2) Thoracic vertebrae
(12)
$T_1 - T_{12}$

Intervertebral disk

Vertebral body

Lumbar vertebrae region:
1
2
3
4
5

(3) Lumbar vertebrae
(5)
$L_1 - L_5$

(4) Sacrum

(5) Coccyx

Source: Delmar/Cengage Learning

THE HAND

OBJECTIVES

Upon completion of this chapter, the reader will be able to:

- Describe the joints of the hand.

- Identify the bony landmarks significant to the joints of the hand.

- Name the major ligaments and their purpose.

- Describe any supporting structures important to the joints of the hand.

- Describe the major motions of the joints of the hand and name the muscles that perform them.

- Identify the origins, insertions, and innervations of the muscles of the joints of the hand.

- Perform proper manual muscle testing on the major muscles of the joints of the hand grades 5–0.

- Be aware of possible substitutions during manual muscle testing on the joints of the hand.

- Accurately perform range of motion testing using the goniometer on the joints of the hand.

MUSCULOSKELETAL OVERVIEW

What a profoundly versatile structure the human hand is! It is made up of the thumb and four fingers. These structures can be further broken down into the metacarpal bones and phalanges for all five digits. The hand is the terminal point for the upper extremity. As we have worked our way down the upper extremity in previous chapters, this concept has been reiterated several times. The primary function of all the other upper extremity joints is to provide perfect placement for the hand to accomplish whatever task is set before it. This rather fragile-looking structure is capable of intricate movements such as needlework as well as gross motions such as grasping a jar to twist off the lid. The hand possesses the capability and coordination for each digit to work independently of the others in activities such as playing musical instruments, keyboarding, or performing sign language. The digits can also work together to grip the handle of a gardening tool or grasp a bag of garbage to haul to the curb.

Joints

The hand is made up of numerous joints (see Figure 9-1). The *carpometacarpal (CMC) joint* refers to the articulation between the distal row of carpal bones and the proximal end of the metacarpals. While these nonaxial joints provide stability rather than mobility, the fact that each digit begins individually at this joint provides some "give" during actions such as **opposition** of the first and fifth digits. All four fingers as well as the thumb have a CMC joint. The metacarpophalangeal (MCP) joint is located at what we often refer to as the knuckle of the hand. This joint encompasses the distal end of the metacarpal joint and the proximal end of the proximal phalanx. Again all four fingers and the thumb have an MCP joint. As we move on down the hand, we encounter the proximal interphalangeal (PIP) joint, which is made up of the distal end of the proximal phalanx and the proximal end of the middle phalanx. The final, most distal, joint of the hand is the distal interphalangeal (DIP), comprised of the

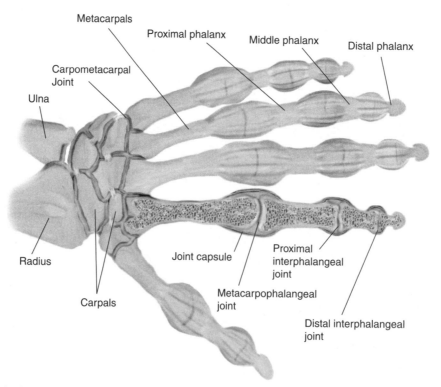

Figure 9-1 Joints of the hand. Source: Delmar/Cengage Learning

distal end of the middle phalanx and the proximal end of the distal phalanx. In these final two joints, the thumb differs from the fingers. While the fingers have two interphalangeal joints, the thumb has only one. Thus, this joint in the thumb is referred to as simply the *interphalangeal (IP) joint*. Some significant differences regarding the movement of the thumb will be discussed later in this chapter.

Motions available to digits 2–5 are flexion/extension and abduction/adduction at the MCP joints and also flexion/extension of the PIP and DIP joints. The thumb has the ability to flex/extend, abduct/adduct, and oppose/repose. As we work through muscle testing, we will examine finger actions separately from the actions of the thumb.

Bones

Landmarks of the hand involve many different bony structures (see Figure 9-2). The carpal bones (discussed previously in Chapter 8) include the scaphoid, lunate, triquetrum, pisiform, trapezoid, trapezium, capitate, and hamate. They form two rows at the base of the hand. Each digit has a long

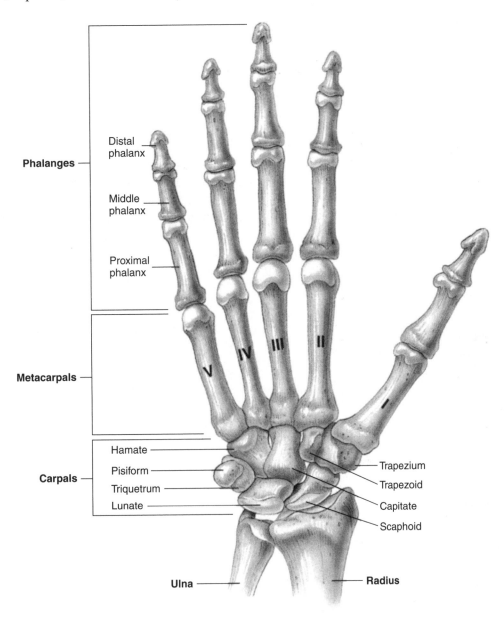

Figure 9-2 Bones of the hand. Source: Delmar/Cengage Learning

metacarpal bone that extends through the hand itself and connects to the bones of each digit. These are numbered, not named, to coincide with the digit. Numbering begins with the thumb as 1 and ending with the little finger as 5. The same numbering system holds true for the phalanges as a whole, although we often refer to them by other terms used in everyday life such as the thumb, index finger, middle finger, ring finger, and little finger.

> **TIPS** *of the* **Trade**
>
> It is easy to make an error when recording information about the digits using the number system. Remember, the thumb is counted as digit or phalange 1.

The makeup of each phalange is as follows: the fingers have three bones named for their location: the proximal phalanx, middle phalanx, and distal phalanx. The thumb has two bones, the proximal and distal phalanx.

Ligaments

The hand is most remarkable for the amount of available flexibility, but of course, a significant degree of stability is required as well. Two primary structures provide stability to the hand. The first is the flexor retinaculum (see Figure 9-3). This dense band of tissue crosses the wrist and hand on the palmar or anterior surface. It is made up of two ligaments. The palmar carpal ligament is more superficially located and functions to hold the finger flexor tendons close to the wrist, especially as the wrist flexes. The transverse carpal ligament, as the name indicates, runs transversely or medial/lateral across the carpal bones. It has medial attachments on the pisiform and the hook of the hamate and lateral attachments on the scaphoid and trapezium. As this ligament arches over the carpal bones, it creates a tunnel through which run the long finger flexor tendons and the median nerve. This ligament is the one often cut to relieve symptoms of carpal tunnel syndrome.

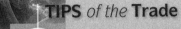
The second primary structure is the extensor retinaculum (see Figure 9-4). This band of connective tissue crosses the wrist on the extensor surface and provides a similar function as its counterpart in that it holds the extensor finger tendons close to the bones during wrist extension.

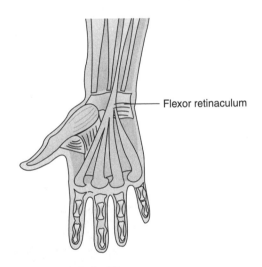

Anterior View

Figure 9-3 Flexor retinaculum. Source: Delmar/Cengage Learning

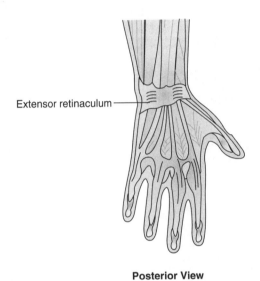

Posterior View

Figure 9-4 Extensor retinaculum. Source: Delmar/Cengage Learning

MUSCLE TESTING OF THE HAND

Because it is important to review the muscles associated with each movement, the individual sections begin with a table of the muscles responsible for the movement being tested, followed by a depiction of the primary muscles.

MCP Flexion

Table 9-1 lists the primary and accessory muscles responsible for MCP flexion. The lumbricals (see Figure 9-5), dorsal interossei (see Figure 9-6), and palmar interossei (see Figure 9-7) muscles are the primary movers for this motion.

TABLE 9-1	MUSCLES RESPONSIBLE FOR MCP FLEXION		
PRIMARY MUSCLES	**ORIGIN**	**INSERTION**	**INNERVATION**
First lumbricalis	Tendons of the flexor digitorum profundus, index finger radial side	Tendon of the extensor digitorum, index finger radial side	Median
Second lumbricalis	Tendons of the flexor digitorum profundus, middle finger radial side	Tendon of the extensor digitorum, middle finger radial side	Median
Third lumbricalis	Tendons of the flexor digitorum profundus, middle and ring finger radial side	Tendon of the extensor digitorum, ring finger radial side	Ulnar
Fourth lumbricalis	Tendons of the flexor digitorum profundus, ring and little finger radial side	Tendon of the extensor digitorum, little finger radial side	Ulnar
Dorsal interossei	Between respective metacarpal bones (i.e., first dorsal between thumb and index finger)	Base of respective proximal phalanx	Ulnar
Palmar interossei	Metacarpal bones 2, 4, 5 (none on the middle finger)	Base of respective proximal phalanx	Ulnar
ACCESSORY MUSCLES	**ORIGIN**	**INSERTION**	**INNERVATION**
Flexor digitorum superficialis	Common flexor tendon, coronoid process, and radius	Sides of middle phalanx of the four fingers	Median
Flexor digitorum profundus	Upper 3/4 of the ulna	Distal phalanx of the four fingers	Median and ulnar
Flexor digiti minimi	Hamate and flexor retinaculum	Base of proximal phalanx of the fifth finger	Ulnar nerve
Opponens digiti minimi	Hamate and flexor retinaculum	Fifth metacarpal	Ulnar

Anterior View

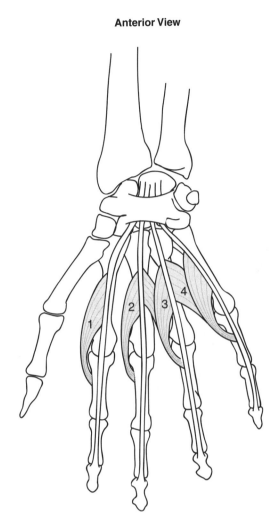

Figure 9-5 Lumbricales. Source: Delmar/Cengage Learning

Posterior View

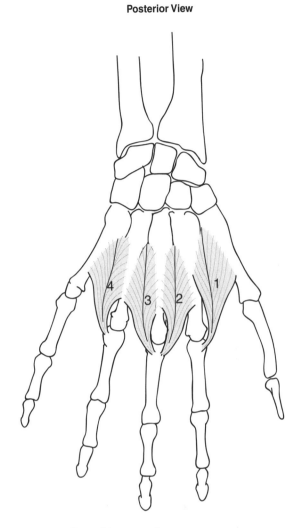

Figure 9-6 Dorsal interossei. Source: Delmar/Cengage Learning

Anterior View

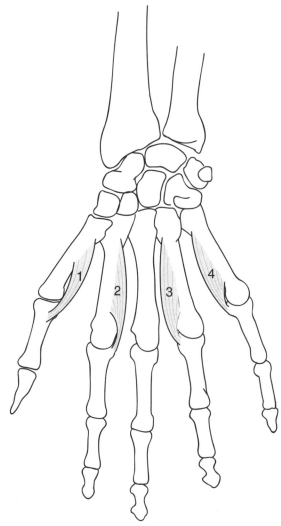

Figure 9-7 Palmar interossei. Source: Delmar/Cengage Learning

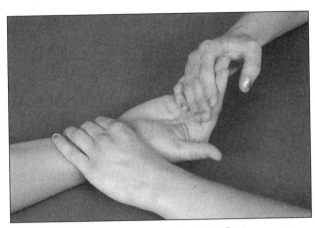

Figure 9-8 Proper positioning for MCP flexion grades 5–3. Source: Delmar/Cengage Learning

Testing for MCP Flexion Grades 5, 4, 3 (Normal, Good, Fair) Gravity Resisted

POSITION OF PATIENT: Forearm supinated, wrist neutral with metacarpophalangeal joints fully extended and all interphalangeal joints flexed (see Figure 9-8).

POSITION OF THERAPIST: One hand provides stabilization of the metacarpals proximally while the other hand provides resistance on the palmar surface of the proximal phalanges.

TEST: Patient instructed to flex MP joint while extending IP joints and hold against resistance. Each finger may be tested individually or as a unit.

DIRECTIONS: Say to the patient, "Bend your fingers at the knuckles and hold them there. Don't let me straighten them."

GRADING:

- **Grade 5 (Normal):** Patient achieves position and holds against maximum resistance.
- **Grade 4 (Good):** Patient achieves position and holds against strong (but not full) resistance.
- **Grade 3 (Fair):** Patient achieves position but tolerates no resistance.

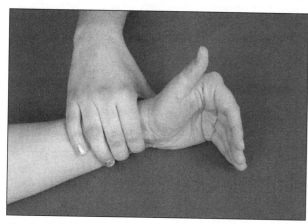

Figure 9-9 Proper positioning for MCP flexion grades 2–0. Source: Delmar/Cengage Learning

Testing for Grades 2, 1, 0 (Poor, Trace, None) Gravity Minimized

POSITION OF PATIENT: Forearm and wrist in neutral position to reduce gravitational influences; MP joints are flexed, IP joints extended (see Figure 9-9).

POSITION OF THERAPIST: Stabilize metacarpals.

TEST: Patient attempts motion.

DIRECTIONS: Say to the patient, "Try to bend your fingers at the knuckles."

GRADING:

- **Grade 2 (Poor):** Patient moves through partial range.
- **Grade 1 (Trace):** Patient shows slight motion.
- **Grade 0 (None):** No movement noted.

Finger PIP and DIP Flexion

Table 9-2 presents the primary and accessory muscles responsible for finger PIP and DIP flexion. The flexor digitorum superficialis (see Figure 9-10) and flexor digitorum profundus (see Figure 9-11) muscles are the primary movers for these motions.

TABLE 9-2	MUSCLES RESPONSIBLE FOR FINGER PIP AND DIP FLEXION		
PRIMARY MUSCLES	**ORIGIN**	**INSERTION**	**INNERVATION**
Flexor digitorum superficialis	Common flexor tendon, coronoid process, and radius	Sides of middle phalanx of the four fingers	Median
Flexor digitorum profundus	Upper 3/4 of the ulna	Distal phalanx of the four fingers	Median and ulnar
ACCESSORY MUSCLES	**ORIGIN**	**INSERTION**	**INNERVATION**
Flexor digitorum profundus	Upper 3/4 of the ulna	Distal phalanx of the four fingers	Median and ulnar

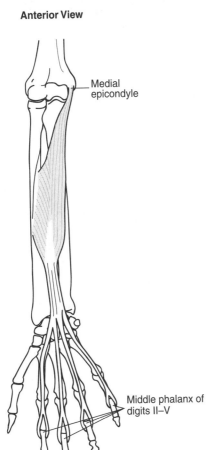

Anterior View

Medial epicondyle

Middle phalanx of digits II–V

Figure 9-10 Flexor digitorum superficialis.

Source: Delmar/Cengage Learning

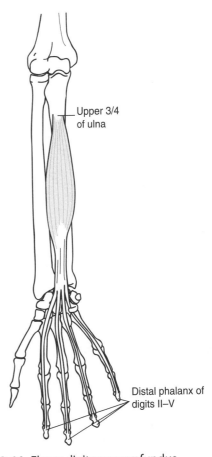

Anterior View

Upper 3/4 of ulna

Distal phalanx of digits II–V

Figure 9-11 Flexor digitorum profundus.

Source: Delmar/Cengage Learning

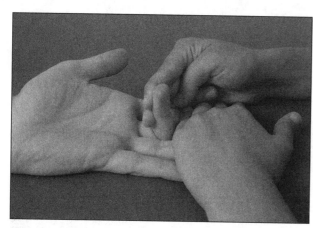

Figure 9-12 Proper positioning for PIP grades 5–3.

Source: Delmar/Cengage Learning

Testing for PIP Flexion Grades 5, 4, 3 (Normal, Good, Fair) Gravity Resisted

POSITION OF PATIENT: Forearm supinated with wrist neutral and finger to be tested slightly flexed (see Figure 9-12).

POSITION OF THERAPIST: Isolate finger to be tested by stabilizing all other fingers in full extension leaving test finger slightly flexed. Other hand provides resistance at the PIPs.

TEST: Patient flexes PIP joint only leaving DIP extended and holds against resistance.

DIRECTIONS: Say to the patient, "Bend the middle joint of this finger and hold it there. Don't let me straighten it."

GRADING:

- **Grade 5 (Normal):** Patient achieves position and holds against maximum resistance.
- **Grade 4 (Good):** Patient achieves position and holds against strong (but not full) resistance.
- **Grade 3 (Fair):** Patient achieves position but tolerates no resistance.

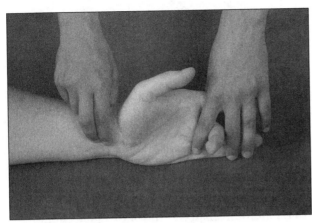

Figure 9-13 Proper positioning for PIP grades 2–0.

Source: Delmar/Cengage Learning

Testing for PIP Flexion Grades 2, 1, 0 (Poor, Trace, None) Gravity Minimized

POSITION OF PATIENT: Forearm neutral with wrist neutral and finger to be tested slightly flexed (see Figure 9-13).

POSITION OF THERAPIST: Isolate finger to be tested by stabilizing all other fingers in full extension, leaving test finger slightly flexed. Other hand rests on wrist to palpate depending on patient response.

TEST: Patient flexes PIP joint, leaving only DIP extended.

DIRECTIONS: Say to the patient, "Attempt to bend the middle joint of this finger."

GRADING:

- **Grade 2 (Poor):** Patient moves through partial range.
- **Grade 1 (Trace):** Patient shows slight motion or contraction is palpable.
- **Grade 0 (None):** No activity noted.

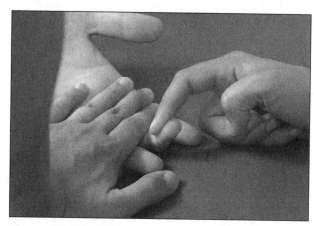

Figure 9-14 Proper positioning for DIP grades 5–3.

Source: Delmar/Cengage Learning

Testing for DIP Flexion Grades 5, 4, 3 (Normal, Good, Fair) Gravity Resisted

POSITION OF PATIENT: Forearm supinated, with wrist neutral and PIP joint extended (see Figure 9-14).

POSITION OF THERAPIST: Stabilize the middle phalanx in extension with fingers of one hand while providing resistance to the distal phalanx into extension or palpating for contraction as needed.

TEST: Patient instructed to flex distal phalanx and hold against resistance.

DIRECTIONS: Say to the patient, "Bend the tip of your finger and hold it. Don't let me straighten it."

GRADING:

- **Grade 5 (Normal):** Patient achieves position and holds against maximum resistance.
- **Grade 4 (Good):** Patient achieves position and holds against strong (but not full) resistance.
- **Grade 3 (Fair):** Patient achieves position but tolerates no resistance.

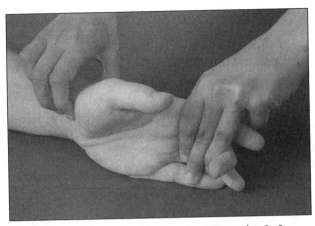

Figure 9-15 Proper positioning for DIP grades 2–0.

Source: Delmar/Cengage Learning

Testing for DIP Flexion Grades 2, 1, 0 (Poor, Trace, None) Gravity Minimized

POSITION OF PATIENT: Forearm neutral, wrist neutral, and PIP joint extended (see Figure 9-15).

POSITION OF THERAPIST: Stabilize the middle phalanx in extension with fingers of one hand while palpating at wrist for contraction as needed.

TEST: Patient instructed to flex distal phalanx.

DIRECTIONS: Say to the patient, "Bend the tip of your finger."

GRADING:

- **Grade 2 (Poor):** Patient moves through partial range.
- **Grade 1 (Trace):** Patient shows slight motion or contraction is palpable.
- **Grade 0 (None):** No activity noted.

Finger MP Extension

The primary muscles responsible for finger MP extension are listed in Table 9-3. The extensor digitorum (see Figure 9-16), extensor indicis (see Figure 9-17), and extensor digiti minimi (see Figure 9-18) muscles are the primary movers for this motion.

TABLE 9-3	MUSCLES RESPONSIBLE FOR FINGER MP EXTENSION		
PRIMARY MUSCLES	**ORIGIN**	**INSERTION**	**INNERVATION**
Extensor digitorum	Lateral epicondyle of humerus	Base of distal phalanx digits 2–5	Radial
Extensor indicis	Distal ulna	Base of distal phalanx of second digit	Radial
Extensor digiti minimi	Lateral epicondyle of humerus	Base of fifth distal phalanx	Radial

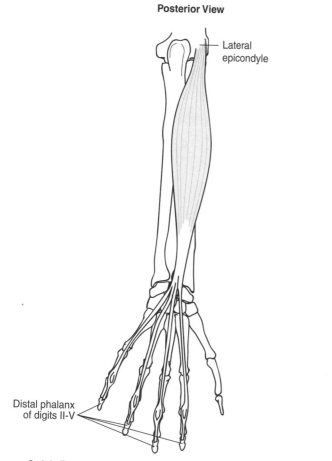

Figure 9-16 Extensor digitorum. Source: Delmar/Cengage Learning

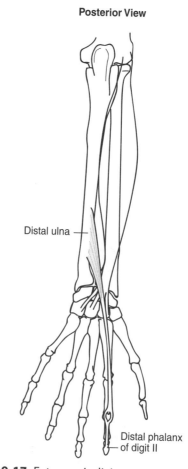

Figure 9-17 Extensor indicis. Source: Delmar/Cengage Learning

Posterior View

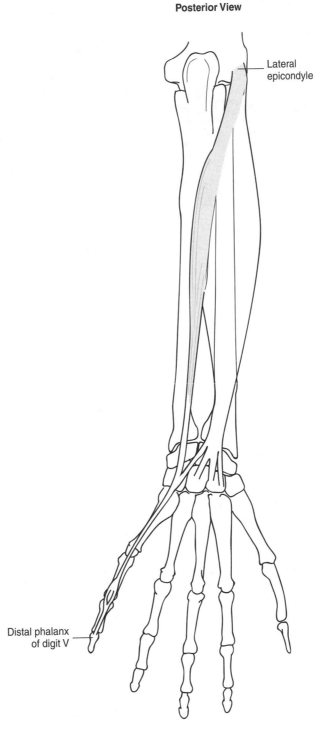

Lateral epicondyle

Distal phalanx of digit V

Figure 9-18 Extensor digiti minimi. Source: Delmar/Cengage Learning

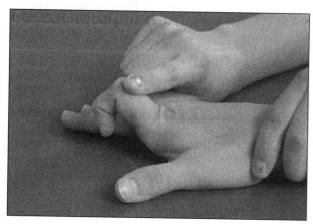

Figure 9-19 Proper positioning for finger MP extension grades 5–3. Source: Delmar/Cengage Learning

Testing for Finger MP Extension Grades 5, 4, 3 (Normal, Good, Fair) Gravity Resisted

POSITION OF PATIENT: Forearm pronated, wrist neutral, and all MP and IP joints in neutral (see Figure 9-19).

POSITION OF THERAPIST: Stabilize under the distal forearm. Apply digital resistance across the center of proximal phalanges 2–5.

TEST: Patient instructed to extend MP joints only and hold against resistance. IP joints should stay slightly flexed.

DIRECTIONS: Say to the patient, "Straighten your knuckle and hold it. Don't let me bend it."

GRADING:

- **Grade 5 (Normal):** Patient achieves position and holds against maximum resistance.
- **Grade 4 (Good):** Patient achieves position and holds against strong (but not full) resistance.
- **Grade 3 (Fair):** Patient achieves position but tolerates no resistance.

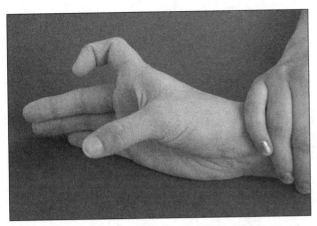

Figure 9-20 Proper positioning for finger MP extension grades 2–0. Source: Delmar/Cengage Learning

Testing for Finger MP Extension Grades 2, 1, 0 (Poor, Trace, None) Gravity Minimized

POSITION OF PATIENT: Forearm neutral, wrist neutral, and all MP and IP joints in neutral (see Figure 9-20).

POSITION OF THERAPIST: Stabilize under the distal forearm. Palpate tendons as needed.

TEST: Patient instructed to extend MP joints only. IP joints should stay slightly flexed.

DIRECTIONS: Say to the patient, "Straighten your knuckles."

GRADING:

- **Grade 2 (Poor):** Patient moves through partial range.
- **Grade 1 (Trace):** Patient shows slight motion.
- **Grade 0 (None):** No movement noted.

Finger Abduction

The primary and accessory muscles responsible for finger abduction are listed in Table 9-4. The dorsal interossei (refer to Figure 9-6) and abductor digiti minimi (see Figure 9-21) muscles are the primary movers for this motion.

TABLE 9-4	MUSCLES RESPONSIBLE FOR FINGER ABDUCTION		
PRIMARY MUSCLES	**ORIGIN**	**INSERTION**	**INNERVATION**
Dorsal interossei	Between respective metacarpal bones (i.e., first dorsal between thumb and index finger)	Base of respective proximal phalanx	Ulnar
Abductor digiti minimi	Pisiform and tendon of the flexor carpi ulnaris	Proximal phalanx of the fifth digit	Ulnar
ACCESSORY MUSCLES	**ORIGIN**	**INSERTION**	**INNERVATION**
Extensor digitorum	Lateral epicondyle of the humerus	Base of distal phalanx of fingers 2–5	Radial nerve
Extensor digiti minimi	Lateral epicondyle of the humerus	Base of distal phalanx of fifth finger	Radial nerve

Anterior View

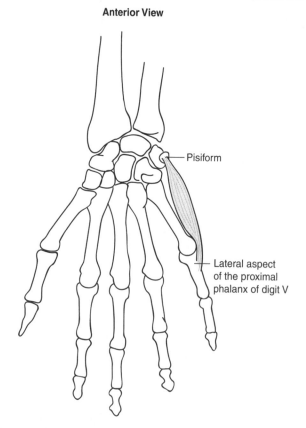

Pisiform

Lateral aspect of the proximal phalanx of digit V

Figure 9-21 Abductor digiti minimi. Source: Delmar/Cengage Learning

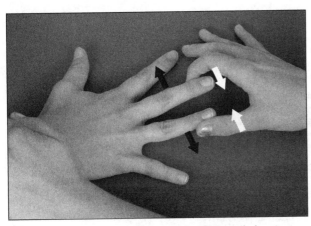

Figure 9-22 Proper positioning for finger abduction all grades. Source: Delmar/Cengage Learning

Testing for Finger Abduction Grades 5–0 (Normal to None)

POSITION OF PATIENT: Forearm pronated, wrist neutral, fingers splayed in extension and adduction (see Figure 9-22).

POSITION OF THERAPIST: One hand supports wrist while the other hand applies resistance on the lateral side of one finger and the medial side of the adjacent finger.

TEST: Patient is instructed to abduct fingers and hold against resistance, while each pair of fingers is tested separately by trying to adduct the adjacent fingers.

DIRECTIONS: Say to the patient, "Spread your fingers apart and hold them there. Don't let me bring them together."

GRADING:

- **Grades 5, 4 (Normal, Good):** Very much a judgment call as compared with other fingers and with the tests done on the uninvolved hand as these muscles do not tolerate much resistance.
- **Grade 3 (Fair):** Patient achieves position with any given pair of fingers but tolerates no resistance.
- **Grade 2 (Poor):** Patient moves through partial range.
- **Grade 1 (Trace):** Patient shows slight motion.
- **Grade 0 (None):** No movement noted.

Finger Adduction

Table 9-5 shows the primary and accessory muscles responsible for finger adduction. The palmar interossei muscle is the primary mover for this motion (refer to Figure 9-7).

TABLE 9-5	MUSCLES RESPONSIBLE FOR FINGER ADDUCTION		
PRIMARY MUSCLES	**ORIGIN**	**INSERTION**	**INNERVATION**
Palmar interossei	Metacarpal bones 2, 4, 5 (none on the middle finger)	Base of respective proximal phalanx	Ulnar
ACCESSORY MUSCLES	**ORIGIN**	**INSERTION**	**INNERVATION**
Extensor indicis	Distal ulna	Base of distal phalanx of the second finger	Radial

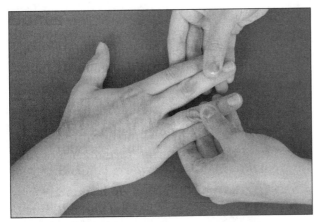

Figure 9-23 Proper positioning for finger adduction grades 5–3. Source: Delmar/Cengage Learning

Testing for Finger Adduction Grades 5, 4, 3 (Normal, Good, Fair)

POSITION OF PATIENT: Forearm pronated, wrist neutral, fingers extended and adducted (see Figure 9-23).

POSITION OF THERAPIST: Careful to grasp the middle phalanx only, the therapist grasps two adjoining fingers, applying resistance in the direction of abduction trying to separate the fingers. Each finger is done separately.

TEST: Patient is instructed to adduct fingers and hold against resistance.

DIRECTIONS: Say to the patient, "Hold your fingers tight against each other. Don't let me spread them apart."

GRADING:

- **Grades 5, 4 (Normal, Good):** Very much a judgment call as compared with other fingers and with the tests done on the uninvolved hand as these muscles do not tolerate much resistance.
- **Grade 3 (Fair):** Patient achieves position with any given pair of fingers but tolerates no resistance.

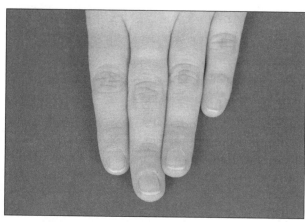

Figure 9-24 Proper positioning for finger adduction grades 2–0. Source: Delmar/Cengage Learning

Testing for Finger Adduction Grades 2, 1, 0 (Poor, Trace, None)

POSITION OF PATIENT: Forearm pronated, wrist neutral, fingers extended and abducted initially.

POSITION OF THERAPIST: Fingers placed on the side of the moving finger to note any movement.

TEST: Patient attempts to adduct fingers (see Figure 9-24).

DIRECTIONS: Say to the patient, "Move this finger closer to the one next to it."

GRADING:

- **Grade 2 (Poor):** Patient moves through partial range.
- **Grade 1 (Trace):** Patient shows slight motion.
- **Grade 0 (None):** No movement noted.

Thumb MP and IP Flexion

Table 9-6 presents the primary muscles responsible for thumb MP and IP flexion. The flexor pollicis brevis (see Figure 9-25) and flexor pollicis longus (see Figure 9-26) muscles are the primary movers for MP flexion and IP flexion respectively.

TABLE 9-6	MUSCLES RESPONSIBLE FOR THUMB MP AND IP FLEXION		
PRIMARY MUSCLES	**ORIGIN**	**INSERTION**	**INNERVATION**
MP Flexion: flexor pollicis brevis	Trapezium and flexor retinaculum	Proximal phalanx of thumb	Median
IP Flexion: flexor pollicis longus	Anterior surface of radius	Distal phalanx of thumb	Median nerve

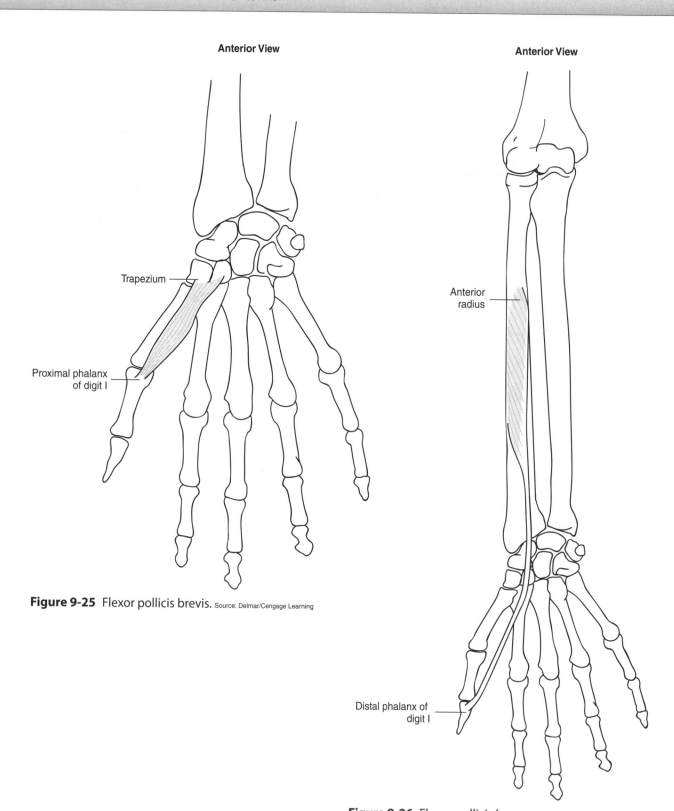

Anterior View

Trapezium

Proximal phalanx
of digit I

Figure 9-25 Flexor pollicis brevis. Source: Delmar/Cengage Learning

Anterior View

Anterior
radius

Distal phalanx of
digit I

Figure 9-26 Flexor pollicis longus. Source: Delmar/Cengage Learning

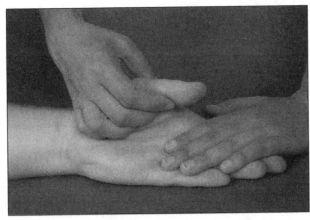

Figure 9-27 Proper positioning for thumb MP flexion all grades. Source: Delmar/Cengage Learning

Testing for MP Flexion Grades 5–0 (Normal to None)

POSITION OF PATIENT: Forearm supinated, wrist, CMC, and IP joints neutral. Thumb lies relaxed along the second metacarpal (see Figure 9-27).

POSITION OF THERAPIST: One hand stabilizes first metacarpal to avoid substitution. Resistance hand gives digital resistance on the proximal phalanx.

TEST: Patient is instructed to move thumb into MP flexion and hold against resistance.

DIRECTIONS: Say to the patient, "Bend the knuckle of your thumb and hold it. Don't let me straighten it."

GRADING:

- **Grade 5 (Normal):** Patient achieves position and holds against maximum resistance.
- **Grade 4 (Good):** Patient achieves position and holds against strong (but not full) resistance.
- **Grade 3 (Fair):** Patient achieves position and holds against just a slight amount of resistance because positioning is gravity decreased.
- **Grade 2 (Poor):** Patient achieves position.
- **Grade 1 (Trace):** Muscle is palpable just lateral to the flexor pollicis longus tendon in the thenar eminence.
- **Grade 0 (None):** No activity is noted or palpated.

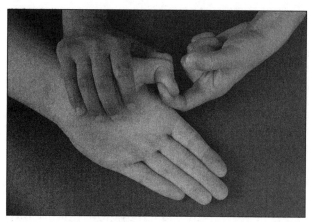

Figure 9-28 Proper positioning for thumb IP flexion all grades. Source: Delmar/Cengage Learning

Testing for IP Flexion Grades 5–0 (Normal to None)

POSITION OF PATIENT: Forearm supinated, wrist neutral, and MP joint in extension (see Figure 9-28).

POSITION OF THERAPIST: One hand stabilizes at the MP joint. Other hand applies digital resistance against the palmar surface of the distal phalanx.

TEST: Patient instructed to move IP joint into flexion and hold against resistance.

DIRECTIONS: Say to the patient, "Bend the tip of your thumb and hold it. Don't let me straighten it."

GRADING:

- **Grade 5 (Normal):** Patient achieves position and holds against maximum resistance.
- **Grade 4 (Good):** Patient achieves position and holds against strong (but not full) resistance.
- **Grade 3 (Fair):** Patient achieves position and holds against just a slight amount of resistance because positioning is gravity decreased.
- **Grade 2 (Poor):** Patient achieves position.
- **Grade 1 (Trace):** Activity is palpated. Tendon is palpable in the thenar eminence.
- **Grade 0 (None):** No activity noted or palpated.

Thumb MP and IP Extension

The primary muscles responsible for thumb MP and IP extension are listed in Table 9-7. The extensor pollicis brevis (see Figure 9-29) and extensor pollicis longus (see Figure 9-30) muscles are the primary movers for MP extension and IP extension respectively.

TABLE 9-7	MUSCLES RESPONSIBLE FOR THUMB MP AND IP EXTENSION		
PRIMARY MUSCLES	**ORIGIN**	**INSERTION**	**INNERVATION**
MP Extension: extensor pollicis brevis	Posterior surface of the distal radius	Base of the proximal phalanx	Radial
IP Extension: extensor pollicis longus	Mid-posterior surface of ulna, interosseous membrane	Base of distal phalanx	Radial

Posterior View

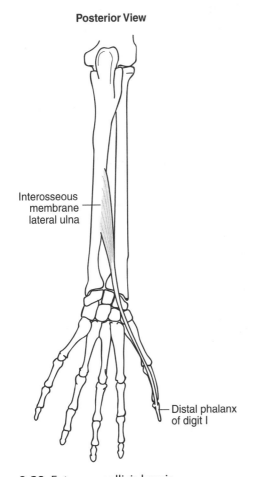

Interosseous membrane lateral ulna

Distal phalanx of digit I

Figure 9-29 Extensor pollicis brevis. Source: Delmar/Cengage Learning

Posterior View

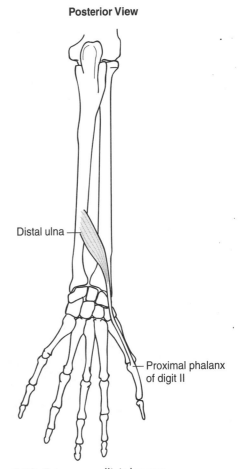

Distal ulna

Proximal phalanx of digit II

Figure 9-30 Extensor pollicis longus. Source: Delmar/Cengage Learning

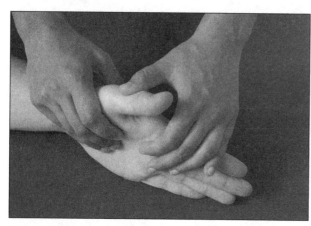

Figure 9-31 Proper positioning for thumb MP extension all grades. Source: Delmar/Cengage Learning

Testing for Thumb MP Extension Grades 5–0 (Normal to None)

POSITION OF PATIENT: Forearm and wrist in neutral; CMC and IP joints relaxed; MP joint abducted and flexed (see Figure 9-31).

POSITION OF THERAPIST: One hand stabilizes at the first metacarpal. The other hand applies digital resistance on the dorsal side of the proximal phalanx.

TEST: Patient is instructed to extend MP joint.

DIRECTIONS: Say to the patient, "Straighten the knuckle of your thumb. Don't let me bend it."

GRADING:

- **Grades 5 and 4 (Normal, Good):** Very much a judgment call as this is usually a weak muscle.
- **Grade 3 (Fair):** Patient achieves position and holds against a slight amount of resistance because positioning is gravity decreased.
- **Grade 2 (Poor):** Patient achieves position.
- **Grade 1 (Trace):** Activity is palpated. Tendon is palpable at the base of the first metacarpal between the abductor pollicis and the extensor pollicis longus tendons.
- **Grade 0 (None):** No activity noted.

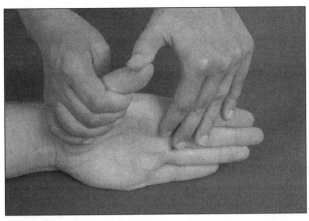

Figure 9-32 Proper positioning for thumb IP extension grades 5–3. Source: Delmar/Cengage Learning

Testing for Thumb IP Extension Grades 5, 4, 3 (Normal, Good, Fair)

POSITION OF PATIENT: Forearm and wrist neutral with ulnar border of the hand resting on the table and thumb relaxed (see Figure 9-32).

POSITION OF THERAPIST: One hand stabilizes at the proximal phalanx of the thumb. The other hand applies digital resistance to the dorsal surface of the distal phalanx.

TEST: Patient instructed to move distal phalanx of thumb into extension and hold against resistance.

DIRECTIONS: Say to the patient, "Straighten the tip of your thumb and hold it. Don't let me bend it."

GRADING:

- **Grades 5, 4 (Normal, Good):** Very much a judgment call as this is usually a weak muscle.
- **Grade 3 (Fair):** Patient achieves position.

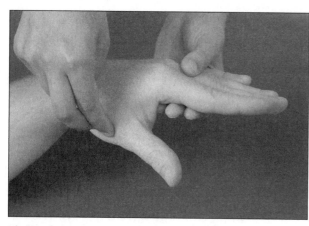

Figure 9-33 Proper positioning for thumb IP extension grades 2–0. Source: Delmar/Cengage Learning

Testing for Thumb IP Extension Grades 2, 1, 0 (Poor, Trace, None)

POSITION OF PATIENT: Forearm pronated, wrist neutral, and thumb relaxed (see Figure 9-33).

POSITION OF THERAPIST: One hand stabilizes on dorsal surface of the wrist. Other hand palpates as necessary.

TEST: Patient attempts to extend IP joint.

DIRECTIONS: Say to the patient, "Attempt to straighten the tip of your thumb."

GRADING:

- **Grade 2 (Poor):** Completes ROM in gravity decreased position.
- **Grade 1 (Trace):** Palpable muscle activity noted by palpating the extensor pollicis longus tendon along the dorsal surface of the proximal phalanx.
- **Grade 0 (None):** No activity noted.

Thumb Abduction

The primary and accessory muscles responsible for thumb abduction are presented in Table 9-8. The abductor pollicis longus (see Figure 9-34) and abductor pollicis brevis (see Figure 9-35) muscles are the primary movers for this motion.

TABLE 9-8	MUSCLES RESPONSIBLE FOR THUMB ABDUCTION		
PRIMARY MUSCLES	**ORIGIN**	**INSERTION**	**INNERVATION**
Abductor pollicis longus	Posterior surface of radius, interosseous membrane, and middle ulna	Base of the first metacarpal	Radial
Abductor pollicis brevis	Scaphoid, trapezium, and flexor retinaculum	Proximal phalanx of thumb	Median
ACCESSORY MUSCLES	**ORIGIN**	**INSERTION**	**INNERVATION**
Palmaris longus	Medial epicondyle of humerus	Palmar fascia	Median
Extensor pollicis brevis	Posterior distal radius	Base of proximal phalanx of thumb	Radial
Opponens pollicis	Trapezium and flexor retinaculum	First metacarpal	Median

Posterior View

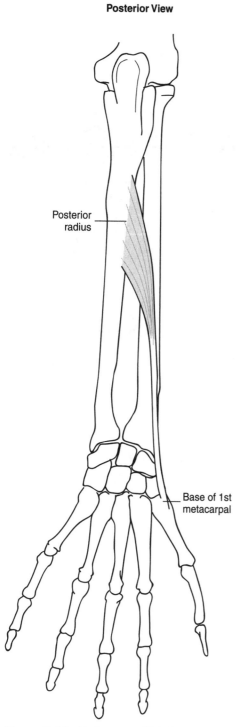

Posterior radius

Base of 1st metacarpal

Figure 9-34 Abductor pollicis longus.

Source: Delmar/Cengage Learning

Anterior View

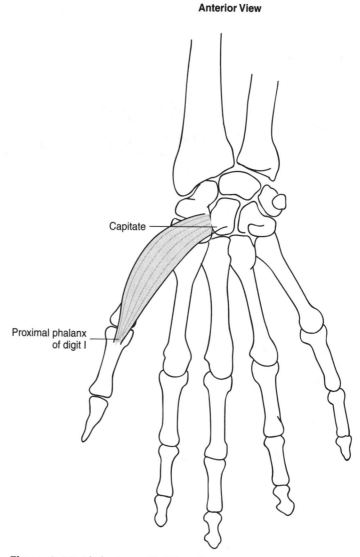

Capitate

Proximal phalanx of digit I

Figure 9-35 Abductor pollicis brevis. Source: Delmar/Cengage Learning

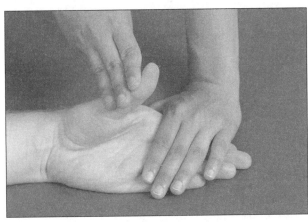

Figure 9-36 Proper positioning for abductor pollicis longus grades 5–0. Source: Delmar/Cengage Learning

Testing for Abductor Pollicis Longus Grades 5–0 (Normal to None)

POSITION OF PATIENT: Forearm supinated, wrist neutral, and thumb adducted (see Figure 9-36).

POSITION OF THERAPIST: One hand stabilizes metacarpals 2–5 and wrist. Other hand applies digital resistance on the distal end of the first metacarpal.

TEST: Patient instructed to abduct thumb and hold against resistance.

DIRECTIONS: Say to the patient, "Lift thumb away from fingers and hold it. Don't let me move it."

GRADING:

- **Grades 5, 4 (Normal, Good):** Completes ROM and holds against resistance; distinguishing between 5 and 4 may be difficult.

- **Grade 3 (Fair):** Completes ROM.

- **Grade 2 (Poor):** Completes some portion of ROM.

- **Grade 1 (Trace):** Palpable muscle activity noted by palpating the abductor pollicis longus tendon along the radial side of the base of the first metacarpal. It is the most lateral tendon on the wrist.

- **Grade 0 (None):** No activity noted.

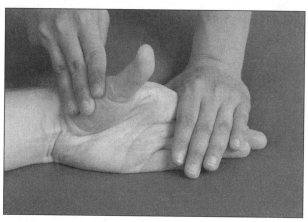

Figure 9-37 Proper positioning for abductor pollicis brevis grades 5–3. Source: Delmar/Cengage Learning

Testing for Abductor Pollicis Brevis Grades 5, 4, 3 (Normal, Good, Fair)

POSITION OF PATIENT: Forearm supinated, wrist neutral, and thumb adducted (see Figure 9-37).

POSITION OF THERAPIST: One hand stabilizes metacarpals 2–5 and wrist. Other hand applies digital resistance on the proximal phalanx of the thumb.

TEST: Patient instructed to abduct thumb and hold against resistance.

DIRECTIONS: Say to the patient, "Lift thumb away from fingers and hold it. Don't let me move it."

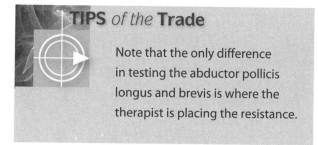

TIPS *of the* **Trade**

Note that the only difference in testing the abductor pollicis longus and brevis is where the therapist is placing the resistance.

GRADING:

- **Grade 5 (Normal):** Patient achieves position and holds against maximum resistance.
- **Grade 4 (Good):** Patient achieves position and holds against strong (but not full) resistance.
- **Grade 3 (Fair):** Patient achieves position and holds against just a slight amount of resistance because positioning is gravity decreased.

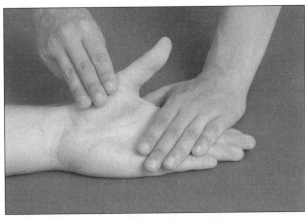

Figure 9-38 Proper positioning for abductor pollicis brevis grades 2–0. Source: Delmar/Cengage Learning

Testing for Abductor Pollicis Brevis Grades 2, 1, 0 (Poor, Trace, None)

POSITION OF PATIENT: Forearm and wrist in neutral, thumb relaxed (see Figure 9-38).

POSITION OF THERAPIST: One hand stabilizes wrist in neutral. Other hand prepares to palpate if necessary.

TEST: Patient attempts to abduct thumb.

DIRECTIONS: Say to the patient, "Move your thumb away from your fingers."

GRADING:

- **Grade 2 (Poor):** Completes partial range.
- **Grade 1 (Trace):** Activity is palpable. Muscle can be palpated in middle of the thenar eminence just medial to the opponens pollicis.
- **Grade 0 (None):** No activity noted.

Thumb Adduction

Table 9-9 lists the primary and accessory muscles responsible for thumb adduction. The adductor pollicis muscle is the primary mover for this motion (see Figure 9-39).

TABLE 9-9	MUSCLES RESPONSIBLE FOR THUMB ADDUCTION		
PRIMARY MUSCLES	**ORIGIN**	**INSERTION**	**INNERVATION**
Adductor pollicis	Capitate, base of the second metacarpal, palmar surface of the third metacarpal	Base of the proximal phalanx of thumb	Ulnar
ACCESSORY MUSCLES	**ORIGIN**	**INSERTION**	**INNERVATION**
First dorsal interosseus	Adjacent metacarpals	Base of proximal phalanx	Ulnar

Anterior View

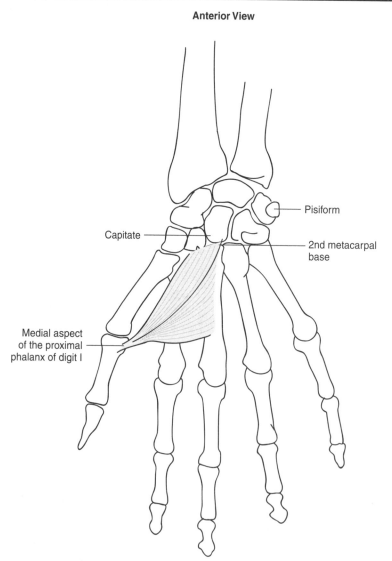

Figure 9-39 Adductor pollicis. Source: Delmar/Cengage Learning

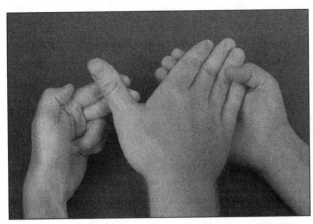

Figure 9-40 Proper positioning for thumb adduction grades 5–3. Source: Delmar/Cengage Learning

Testing for Thumb Adduction
Grades 5, 4, 3 (Normal, Good, Fair)

POSITION OF PATIENT: Forearm in pronation, wrist neutral, and thumb relaxed (see Figure 9-40).

POSITION OF THERAPIST: One hand stabilizes metacarpals 2–5. Other hand provides digital resistance along the medial surface of the proximal phalanx of the thumb.

TEST: Patient is instructed to adduct thumb and hold against resistance.

DIRECTIONS: Say to the patient, "Hold your thumb tightly to your fingers. Don't let me pull it away."

GRADING:

- **Grade 5 (Normal):** Patient achieves position and holds against maximum resistance.
- **Grade 4 (Good):** Patient achieves position and holds against strong (but not full) resistance.
- **Grade 3 (Fair):** Patient achieves position and holds against just a slight amount of resistance because positioning is gravity decreased.

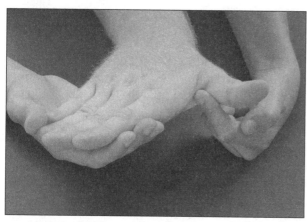

Figure 9-41 Proper positioning for thumb adduction grades 2–0. Source: Delmar/Cengage Learning

Testing for Thumb Adduction
Grades 2, 1, 0 (Poor, Trace, None)

POSITION OF PATIENT: Forearm and wrist in neutral and thumb abducted (see Figure 9-41).

POSITION OF THERAPIST: One hand stabilizes wrist. Other hand prepares to palpate if necessary.

TEST: Patient attempts to adduct thumb.

DIRECTIONS: Say to the patient, "Hold your thumb tightly against your fingers."

GRADING:

- **Grade 2 (Poor):** Completes full range.
- **Grade 1 (Trace):** Some activity noted or palpated. Muscle can be palpated on the palmar surface of the hand by "pinching" the web space between the thumb and first finger.
- **Grade 0 (Zero):** No activity noted.

Thumb Opposition

The primary and accessory muscles responsible for thumb opposition are shown in Table 9-10. The opponens pollicis (see Figure 9-42) and opponens digiti minimi (see Figure 9-43) muscles are the primary movers for this motion.

TABLE 9-10	MUSCLES RESPONSIBLE FOR THUMB OPPOSITION		
PRIMARY MUSCLES	**ORIGIN**	**INSERTION**	**INNERVATION**
Opponens pollicis	Trapezium and flexor retinaculum	First metacarpal	Median
Opponens digiti minimi	Hamate and flexor retinaculum	Fifth metacarpal	Ulnar
ACCESSORY MUSCLES	**ORIGIN**	**INSERTION**	**INNERVATION**
Abductor pollicis brevis	Scaphoid, trapezium, and flexor retinaculum	Proximal phalanx	Median
Flexor pollicis brevis	Trapezium and flexor retinaculum	Proximal phalanx	Median

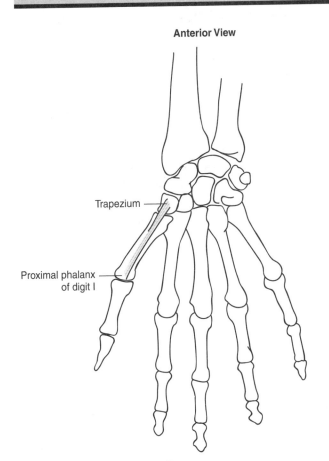

Figure 9-42 Opponens pollicis. Source: Delmar/Cengage Learning

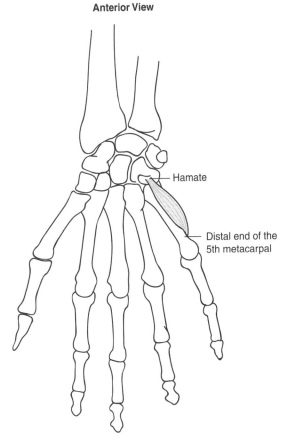

Figure 9-43 Opponens digiti minimi.
Source: Delmar/Cengage Learning

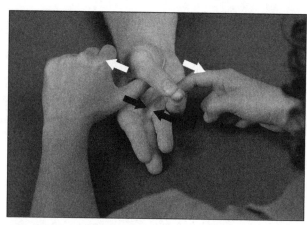

Figure 9-44 Proper positioning for thumb opposition grades 5–0. Source: Delmar/Cengage Learning

Testing for Thumb Opposition Grades 5–0 (Normal to None)

POSITION OF PATIENT: Forearm supinated, wrist neutral, thumb adducted, and MP and IP joints flexed (see Figure 9-44).

POSITION OF THERAPIST: One hand grasps the fifth metacarpal while the other hand grasps the first metacarpal. Resistance is applied to try to separate the thumb from the little finger.

TEST: Patient is instructed to touch the pad of the thumb to the pad of the little finger and hold against resistance.

DIRECTIONS: Say to the patient, "Touch the tip of your thumb to the tip of your little finger and hold it. Don't let me pull them apart."

GRADING:

- **Grade 5 (Normal):** Patient achieves position and holds against maximum resistance.
- **Grade 4 (Good):** Patient achieves position and holds against strong (but not full) resistance.
- **Grade 3 (Fair):** Patient achieves position but tolerates no resistance.
- **Grade 2 (Poor):** Patient moves through partial range.
- **Grade 1 (Trace):** Patient shows slight motion or contraction is palpable. The opponens pollicis can be palpated along the radial surface of the first metacarpal. The opponens digiti minimi can be palpated on the hypothenar eminence on the radial surface of the fifth metacarpal.
- **Grade 0 (None):** No activity noted.

Substitutions

Important substitutions to watch for during MMT of the hand are as follows:

- To avoid the long finger flexors substituting for the lumbricales during finger MP flexion, keep the IPs fully extended.
- If the DIP joint is allowed to flex during PIP flexion, that allows the flexor digitorum profundus to assist with motion.
- If the IP extensors relax during testing of flexors, it may cause passive IP flexion.
- Flexion of the wrist can produce IP extension. Keep the wrist in neutral for all testing of the digits.
- Fingers should be kept in a neutral flexion/extension position during finger adduction testing. Otherwise, the long finger flexors may contribute to the adduction motion.
- Substitution by the extensor pollicis longus can be noted in thumb MP extension if the motion occurs in conjunction with extension of the IP joint and CMC adduction.
- When testing the abductor pollicis longus, be aware that the extensor pollicis brevis may activate as well. This is noted if the line of pull is more toward the dorsal surface of the forearm.
- Make sure the thumb moves in a straight line when testing adduction. If the thumb angles down across the palm, the flexor pollicis longus and brevis have activated.
- Correct positioning for opposition is with the pads of the digits touching. If the thumb flexors (longus and brevis) are active, only the tips of the digits will touch.

RANGE OF MOTION

This section discusses proper techniques for measuring ROM for all joint motions of the fingers and thumb. The motions available at these joints include flexion, extension, abduction, and adduction.

MCP Flexion

The flexion motion of the metacarpophalangeal joint occurs in the sagittal plane around a medial-lateral or frontal axis. Normal AROM is 0°–90°, according to the American Academy of Orthopaedic Surgeons (1965). The end-feel is usually hard due to the contact of the proximal phalanx and the metacarpal.

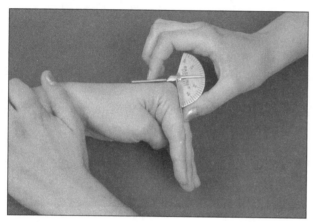

Figure 9-45 Proper positioning for MCP Flexion ROM.

Source: Delmar/Cengage Learning

POSITION OF PATIENT: Short sitting with forearm resting on a table. The forearm and wrist are in neutral with the fingers relaxed.

POSITION OF THERAPIST: One hand stabilizing the metacarpals and the goniometer while the other hand positions the goniometer and assists with proper positioning.

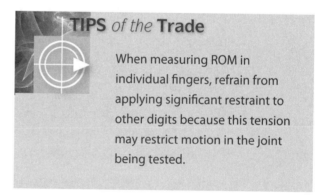

TIPS *of the* **Trade**

When measuring ROM in individual fingers, refrain from applying significant restraint to other digits because this tension may restrict motion in the joint being tested.

POSITION OF GONIOMETER:

- **Fulcrum:** Over the dorsal aspect of the MCP joint (see Figure 9-45)
- **Stationary arm:** Aligned with the dorsal midline of the metacarpal
- **Movable arm:** Aligned with the dorsal midline of the proximal phalanx

MCP Extension

Extension at the metacarpophalangeal joint occurs in the sagittal plane around a medial-lateral or frontal axis. Normal AROM in extension is 0°–45°. The end-feel is firm primarily due to the tension in the anterior joint capsule.

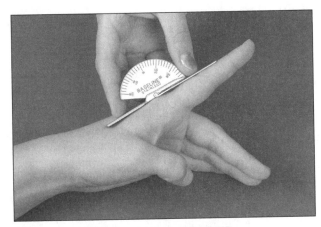

Figure 9-46 Proper positioning for MCP Extension ROM. Source: Delmar/Cengage Learning

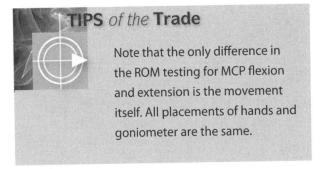

TIPS *of the* **Trade**

Note that the only difference in the ROM testing for MCP flexion and extension is the movement itself. All placements of hands and goniometer are the same.

POSITION OF PATIENT: Short sitting with forearm resting on a table. The forearm and wrist are in neutral with fingers relaxed.

POSITION OF THERAPIST: One hand stabilizing the metacarpals and the goniometer while the other hand positions the goniometer and assists with proper positioning.

POSITION OF GONIOMETER:

- **Fulcrum:** Over the dorsal aspect of the MCP joint (see Figure 9-46)
- **Stationary arm:** Aligned with the dorsal mid-line of the metacarpal
- **Movable arm:** Aligned with the dorsal mid-line of the proximal phalanx

MCP Abduction

Metacarpophalangeal abduction occurs in the frontal plane around an anterior-posterior or sagittal axis. Normal AROM is not listed in most sources. The end-feel is firm due to the tension that occurs in the soft tissue of the area.

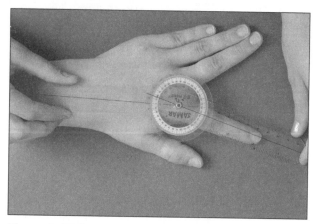

Figure 9-47 Proper positioning for MCP Abduction ROM. Source: Delmar/Cengage Learning

POSITION OF PATIENT: Short sitting with the forearm pronated and resting on the table. The wrist and MCP joints are in neutral.

POSITION OF THERAPIST: One hand positioned to stabilize the metacarpal. Both hands available to position the goniometer as needed.

POSITION OF GONIOMETER:

- **Fulcrum:** Over the dorsal aspect of the MCP joint (see Figure 9-47)
- **Stationary arm:** Aligned with the dorsal mid-line of the metacarpal
- **Movable arm:** Aligned with the dorsal mid-line of the proximal phalanx

MCP Adduction

While MCP adduction is muscle tested, it is not usually included in a ROM test as it is simply the return from MCP abduction (see Figure 9-48). No sources were found indicating normative ROM values for this motion.

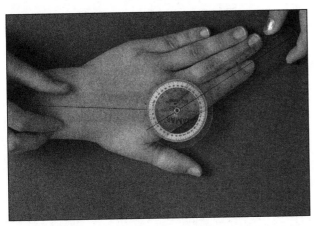

Figure 9-48 Proper positioning for MCP Adduction ROM. Source: Delmar/Cengage Learning

PIP Flexion

Proximal interphalangeal (PIP) flexion occurs in the sagittal plane around a medial-lateral or frontal axis. Normal AROM is 0°–100°, according to the American Academy of Orthopaedic Surgeons (1965). The end-feel may vary but is usually found to be hard due to bone-bone contact between the middle phalanx and the proximal phalanx.

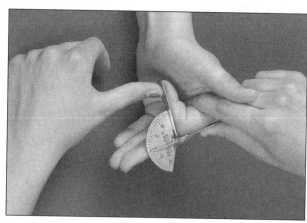

Figure 9-49 Proper positioning for PIP flexion ROM. Source: Delmar/Cengage Learning

POSITION OF PATIENT: Short sitting with forearm resting on a table. The forearm and wrist are in neutral with fingers relaxed.

POSITION OF THERAPIST: One hand stabilizing the proximal phalanx and the goniometer while the other hand positions the goniometer and assists with proper positioning.

POSITION OF GONIOMETER:

- **Fulcrum:** Over the dorsal aspect of the PIP joint (see Figure 9-49)

- **Stationary arm:** Aligned with the dorsal midline of the proximal phalanx

- **Movable arm:** Aligned with the dorsal midline of the middle phalanx

PIP Extension

Proximal interphalangeal (PIP) extension occurs in the sagittal plane around a medial-lateral or frontal axis. The normal AROM is 0°, according to the American Academy of Orthopaedic Surgeons (1965). The end-feel is firm due to the tension placed on the surrounding soft tissue.

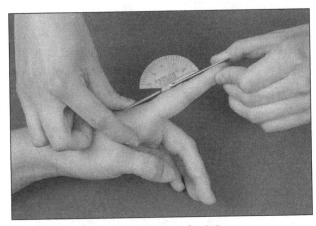

Figure 9-50 Proper positioning for PIP extension ROM. Source: Delmar/Cengage Learning

POSITION OF PATIENT: Short sitting with forearm resting on a table. The forearm and wrist are in neutral with the fingers relaxed.

POSITION OF THERAPIST: One hand stabilizing the proximal phalanx and the goniometer while the other hand positions the goniometer and assists with proper positioning.

POSITION OF GONIOMETER:

- **Fulcrum:** Over the dorsal aspect of the PIP joint (see Figure 9-50)
- **Stationary arm:** Aligned with the dorsal midline of the proximal phalanx
- **Movable arm:** Aligned with the dorsal midline of the middle phalanx

DIP Flexion

The flexion motion of the distal interphalangeal joint (DIP) occurs in the sagittal plane around a medial lateral or frontal axis. Normal AROM is 0°–90°, according to the American Academy of Orthopaedic Surgeons (1965). The end-feel is firm due to the tension placed on surrounding soft tissue during the motion.

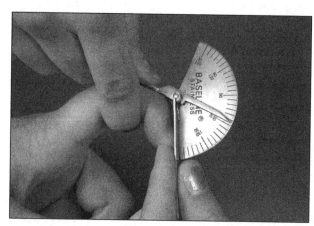

Figure 9-51 Proper positioning for DIP flexion ROM.

Source: Delmar/Cengage Learning

POSITION OF PATIENT: Short sitting with forearm resting on a table. The forearm and wrist are in neutral with the fingers relaxed.

POSITION OF THERAPIST: One hand stabilizing the middle phalanx and the goniometer while the other hand positions the goniometer and assists with proper positioning.

POSITION OF GONIOMETER:

- **Fulcrum:** Over the dorsal aspect of the DIP joint (see Figure 9-51)
- **Stationary arm:** Aligned with the dorsal midline of the middle phalanx
- **Movable arm:** Aligned with the dorsal midline of the distal phalanx

DIP Extension

The extension motion of the distal interphalangeal joint (DIP) occurs in the sagittal plane around a medial lateral or frontal axis. Normal AROM is 0°, according to the American Academy of Orthopaedic Surgeons (1965). The end-feel is firm due to the tension placed on surrounding soft tissue during the motion.

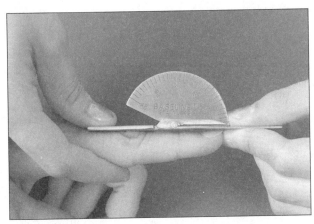

Figure 9-52 Proper positioning for DIP extension ROM.

Source: Delmar/Cengage Learning

POSITION OF PATIENT: Short sitting with forearm resting on a table. The forearm and wrist are in neutral with fingers relaxed.

POSITION OF THERAPIST: One hand stabilizing the middle phalanx and the goniometer while the other hand positions the goniometer and assists with proper positioning.

POSITION OF GONIOMETER:

- **Fulcrum:** Over the dorsal aspect of the DIP joint (see Figure 9-52)
- **Stationary arm:** Aligned with the dorsal midline of the middle phalanx
- **Movable arm:** Aligned with the dorsal midline of the distal phalanx

Thumb CMC Flexion

The thumb moves in different planes than the rest of the digits and therefore must be considered separately.

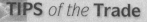

TIPS *of the* **Trade**

A wise anatomy and physiology instructor once shared this memory aid with me: To keep straight which is flexion/extension or abduction/adduction of the thumb, remember that when the thumb is flexing, all the joints of the thumb can perform the same action. When the thumb is abducting, the motion can only occur at the carpometacarpal (CMC) joint. Try it, and you'll see!

Thumb CMC flexion occurs in the frontal plane around an anterior-posterior or sagittal axis.

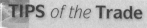

TIPS *of the* **Trade**

Remember to visualize the body in anatomical position when thinking about the thumb motions and positions.

The normal AROM is 0°–15°, according to the American Academy of Orthopaedic Surgeons (1965). The end-feel is often soft due to the muscle bulk of the thenar eminence coming in contact with the palm of the hand.

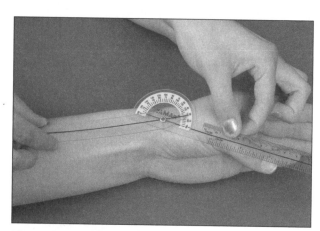

Figure 9-53 Proper positioning for thumb carpometacarpal flexion ROM. Source: Delmar/Cengage Learning

POSITION OF PATIENT: Short sitting with the forearm supinated, wrist in neutral, and the fingers relaxed. The arm is supported on a table.

POSITION OF THERAPIST: One hand stabilizing the wrist and carpals to inhibit movement while also stabilizing the stationary arm of the goniometer. The other hand guides the thumb into CMC flexion and aligns the movable arm of the goniometer.

POSITION OF GONIOMETER:

- **Fulcrum:** Over palmar aspect of the CMC joint (see Figure 9-53)
- **Stationary arm:** Aligned with the midline of the anterior surface of the radius
- **Movable arm:** Aligned with the midline of the anterior surface of the first metacarpal

Thumb CMC Extension

Thumb CMC extension occurs in the frontal plane around an anterior-posterior or sagittal axis. The normal AROM is 0°–20°, according to the American Academy of Orthopaedic Surgeons (1965). The end-feel is firm due to the tension in surrounding soft tissue during the motion.

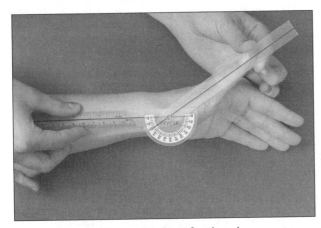

Figure 9-54 Proper positioning for thumb carpometacarpal extension ROM. Source: Delmar/Cengage Learning

POSITION OF PATIENT: Short sitting with the forearm supinated, wrist in neutral, and fingers relaxed. The arm is supported on a table.

POSITION OF THERAPIST: One hand stabilizing the wrist and carpals to inhibit movement while also stabilizing the stationary arm of the goniometer. The other hand guides the thumb into CMC extension and aligns the movable arm of the goniometer.

POSITION OF GONIOMETER:

- **Fulcrum:** Over palmar aspect of the CMC joint (see Figure 9-54)
- **Stationary arm:** Aligned with the midline of the anterior surface of the radius
- **Movable arm:** Aligned with the midline of the anterior surface of the first metacarpal

Thumb CMC Abduction

The motion of carpometacarpal (CMC) abduction occurs in a sagittal plane around a medial-later or frontal axis. The normal AROM is 0°–70°, according to the American Academy of Orthopaedic Surgeons (1965). The end-feel is firm due to the tension in surrounding soft tissue during the motion.

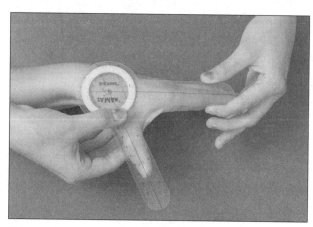

Figure 9-55 Proper positioning for thumb carpometacarpal abduction ROM. Source: Delmar/Cengage Learning

POSITION OF PATIENT: Short sitting with the arm resting on a table. The forearm, wrist, and thumb are in neutral.

POSITION OF THERAPIST: One hand stabilizes the carpal and the second metacarpal to avoid any wrist action while the other hand moves the first metacarpal away from the hand. Both hands also position the goniometer.

POSITION OF GONIOMETER:

- **Fulcrum:** Over the lateral aspect of the styloid process of the radius (see Figure 9-55)
- **Stationary arm:** Aligned with the lateral midline of the second metacarpal
- **Movable arm:** Aligned with the midline of the first metacarpal

Thumb CMC Opposition

CMC adduction is not usually measured as it is simply the return to the starting position for CMC abduction. Carpometacarpal opposition is actually a combination of movements occurring at the CMC joints of the thumb and the little finger. Therefore, it does not occur in a straight plane. The motion usually culminates in touching the tip of the thumb to either the tip or base of the fifth digit. The end-feel is soft due to the contact of the muscle bulk in the palm.

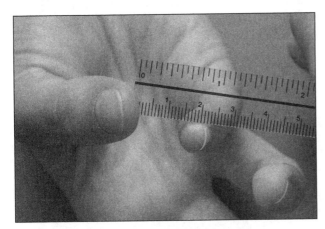

Figure 9-56 Proper positioning for thumb carpometacarpal opposition ROM. Source: Delmar/Cengage Learning

POSITION OF PATIENT: Short sitting with the forearm supinated and the wrist in neutral. All fingers and thumb are relaxed.

POSITION OF THERAPIST: One hand stabilizes the fifth metacarpal to prevent additional movements. The other hand guides the thumb in the motion and holds the goniometer if necessary.

POSITION OF GONIOMETER: The goniometer is not used in this case to measure an angle. Use the ruler located on the goniometer's arm to measure any gap between the thumb and fifth digit (see Figure 9-56). There is no need to take a measurement if the digits touch.

Thumb MCP Flexion

The thumb metacarpophalangeal (MCP) flexion motion occurs in the frontal plane around an anterior-posterior or sagittal axis. The normal AROM is 0°–50°, according to the American Academy of Orthopaedic Surgeons (1965). The end-feel is usually hard due to the bony contact of the proximal phalanx with the first metacarpal.

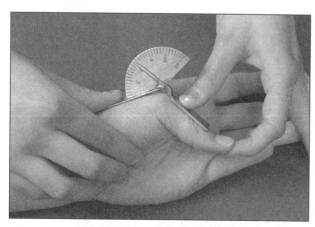

Figure 9-57 Proper positioning for thumb metacarpophalangeal flexion ROM. Source: Delmar/Cengage Learning

POSITION OF PATIENT: Short sitting with the forearm supinated and the wrist in neutral. All fingers and thumb are relaxed.

POSITION OF THERAPIST: One hand stabilizing the first metacarpal to inhibit movement while also stabilizing the stationary arm of the goniometer. The other hand guides the thumb into MCP flexion and aligns the movable arm of the goniometer.

POSITION OF GONIOMETER:

- **Fulcrum:** Over palmar aspect of the MCP joint (see Figure 9-57)
- **Stationary arm:** Aligned with the dorsal midline of the first metacarpal
- **Movable arm:** Aligned with the dorsal midline of the proximal phalange

Thumb MCP Extension

Thumb MCP extension occurs in the frontal plane around an anterior-posterior or sagittal axis. The normal AROM is 0°, according to the American Academy of Orthopaedic Surgeons (1965). The end-feel is firm due to the tension in surrounding soft tissue during the motion.

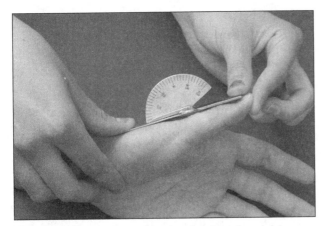

Figure 9-58 Proper positioning for thumb metacarpophalangeal extension ROM.

Source: Delmar/Cengage Learning

POSITION OF PATIENT: Short sitting with the forearm supinated, wrist in neutral, and fingers relaxed. The arm is supported on a table.

POSITION OF THERAPIST: One hand stabilizing the first metacarpal to inhibit movement while also stabilizing the stationary arm of the goniometer. The other hand guides the thumb into MCP extension and aligns the movable arm of the goniometer.

POSITION OF GONIOMETER:

- **Fulcrum:** Over dorsal aspect of the MCP joint (see Figure 9-58)
- **Stationary arm:** Aligned with the dorsal midline of the first metacarpal
- **Movable arm:** Aligned with the dorsal midline of the proximal phalanx

Thumb IP Flexion

The motion of thumb interphalangeal (IP) flexion occurs in a frontal plane around an anterior-posterior axis. The normal AROM is 0°–80°, according to the American Academy of Orthopaedic Surgeons (1965). The end-feel is firm due to the tension in surrounding soft tissue during the motion.

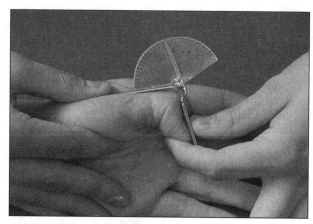

Figure 9-59 Proper positioning for thumb interphalangeal flexion ROM. Source: Delmar/Cengage Learning

POSITION OF PATIENT: Short sitting with the forearm supinated, wrist in neutral, and all fingers and thumb relaxed.

POSITION OF THERAPIST: One hand stabilizing the proximal phalanx to inhibit movement while also stabilizing the stationary arm of the goniometer. The other hand guides the thumb into IP flexion and aligns the movable arm of the goniometer.

POSITION OF GONIOMETER:

- **Fulcrum:** Over dorsal aspect of the IP joint (see Figure 9-59)
- **Stationary arm:** Aligned with the dorsal midline of the proximal phalanx
- **Movable arm:** Aligned with the dorsal midline of the distal phalanx

Thumb IP Extension

Thumb IP extension occurs in the frontal plane around an anterior-posterior or sagittal axis. The normal AROM is 0°–20°, according to the American Academy of Orthopaedic Surgeons (1965). The end-feel is firm due to the tension in surrounding soft tissue during the motion.

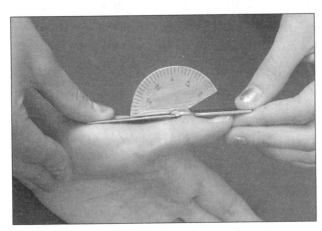

Figure 9-60 Proper positioning for thumb interphalangeal extension ROM. Source: Delmar/Cengage Learning

POSITION OF PATIENT: Short sitting with the forearm supinated, wrist in neutral, and fingers relaxed. The arm is supported on a table.

POSITION OF THERAPIST: One hand stabilizing the proximal phalanx to inhibit movement while also stabilizing the stationary arm of the goniometer. The other hand guides the thumb into IP extension and aligns the movable arm of the goniometer.

POSITION OF GONIOMETER:

- **Fulcrum:** Over dorsal aspect of the IP joint (see Figure 9-60)
- **Stationary arm:** Aligned with the dorsal midline of the proximal phalanx
- **Movable arm:** Aligned with the dorsal midline of the distal phalanx

FUNCTIONAL APPLICATION

As you reflect on all you have learned about the function of the upper extremity through the previous chapters, you can see that it is all about the hand. Upper extremity movement is primarily available to place the hand in an optimal position for various activities. Without normal functional capabilities of the hand, the human body would not be able to care for itself adequately. Studies abound regarding ROM needs at various joints of the hand; the summary of that varied research is that most mobility is required at the MCP joints. Although movement at the DIP is optimal, many activities could still be completed with little movement at this most distal joint if adequate motion is available at the MCP. Another conclusion is that interaction between the thumb and fingers is crucial. Many daily activities require opposition of thumb and fingers such as holding a glass, answering a telephone, or writing your name. Keep this functional information in mind as you assess patients.

LEARNER CHALLENGE

1. List all finger and thumb joint motions. Then identify the plane and axis in which they occur.

2. Palpate the following hand landmarks: metacarpals 1–5; thenar eminence; hypothenar eminence; proximal, middle, and distal phalanges for all fingers; and proximal and distal phalanges of the thumb.

3. On a lab partner, use a china marker to shade in the following extrinsic muscles on one arm/hand: flexor digitorum superficialis, extensor digitorum, and the extensor pollicis longus. On the other hand, use a china marker to shade in the following intrinsic muscles: flexor digiti minimi, dorsal interossei, and the abductor pollicis brevis. Instruct lab partner to perform finger flexion, extension, and abduction with the palm up, and observe/palpate the movement under your shaded areas. Then have your lab partner perform the same motions with the palm down and observe/palpate the movement under your shaded areas.

4. Fill in the following tables summarizing MMT and ROM measurements of the hand.

A) Manual Muscle Testing for Grades 5, 4, 3 Gravity Resisted			
MOTION	**TESTING POSITION**	**STABILIZING HAND**	**RESISTANCE HAND**
MCP Flexion			
Finger PIP Flexion			
Finger DIP Flexion			

continues

A) Manual Muscle Testing for Grades 5, 4, 3 Gravity Resisted *(continued)*

MOTION	TESTING POSITION	STABILIZING HAND	RESISTANCE HAND
Finger MP Extension			
Finger Abduction			
Finger Adduction			
Thumb MP Flexion			
Thumb IP Flexion			
Thumb MP Extension			
Thumb IP Extension			
Thumb Abduction			
Thumb Adduction			
Thumb Opposition			

B) Manual Muscle Testing for Grades 2, 1, 0 Gravity Minimal

MOTION	TESTING POSITION	STABILIZING HAND	RESISTANCE HAND	PALPATION
MCP Flexion				
Finger PIP Flexion				
Finger DIP Flexion				

continues

B)   Manual Muscle Testing for Grades 2, 1, 0 Gravity Minimal *(continued)*

MOTION	TESTING POSITION	STABILIZING HAND	RESISTANCE HAND	PALPATION
Finger MP Extension				
Finger Abduction				
Finger Adduction				
Thumb MP Flexion				
Thumb IP Flexion				
Thumb MP Extension				
Thumb IP Extension				
Thumb Abduction				
Thumb Adduction				
Thumb Opposition				

C)   Range of Motion

MOTION	MOVABLE ARM	STATIONARY ARM	FULCRUM	NORMAL ROM
MCP Flexion				
MCP Extension				

continues

C) Range of Motion *(continued)*

MOTION	MOVABLE ARM	STATIONARY ARM	FULCRUM	NORMAL ROM
MCP Abduction				
MCP Adduction				
PIP Flexion				
PIP Extension				
DIP Flexion				
DIP Extension				
Thumb CMC Flexion				
Thumb CMC Extension				
Thumb CMC Abduction				
Thumb CMC Opposition				
Thumb MCP Flexion				
Thumb MCP Extension				
Thumb IP Flexion				
Thumb IP Extension				

NOTES

THE TRUNK

OBJECTIVES

Upon completion of this chapter, the reader will be able to:

- Describe the structures of the spine.

- Identify the bony landmarks significant to the spine.

- Name the major ligaments and their purpose.

- Describe any supporting structures important to the spine.

- Describe the major motions of the trunk and name the muscles that perform them.

- Identify the origins, insertions, and innervations of the muscles of the trunk.

- Perform proper manual muscle testing on the major muscles of the trunk grades 5–0.

- Be aware of possible substitutions during manual muscle testing on the trunk.

- Accurately perform trunk range of motion testing using the goniometer or tape measure.

MUSCULOSKELETAL OVERVIEW

The simplest way to describe this complex structure is that it is a flexible rod. It is a major component of the axial skeleton and by design provides protection for the spinal cord and shock absorption for the whole body. This "flexible rod" is multi-jointed to provide available movement throughout. Perfectly balanced atop the spine is the skull, which provides protection for the brain.

The vertebral column or spinal column is made up of small irregular bones called *vertebrae*, which have many protrusions that allow for muscle and ligament attachments. The bones of the spinal column are divided into four sections (see Figure 10-1). The cervical area includes the first 7 bones; the next 12 are called the *thoracic vertebrae*; then come the 5 bones of the lumbar spine. At the base of the spine is the sacrum, which consists of 5 fused bones, and the coccyx, a small pointed structure made up of 4 fused bones.

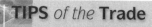

TIPS *of the* **Trade**

Remember, *vertebra* indicates the singular form, while *vertebrae* indicates the plural form of this medical term. These terms are often easily confused because their spelling is so similar.

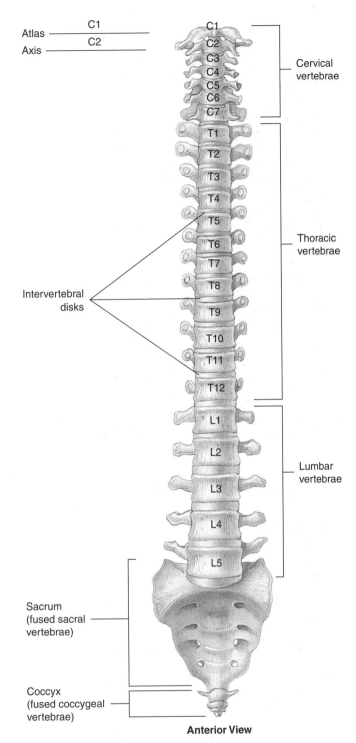

Atlas — C1
Axis — C2

C1
C2
C3
C4
C5
C6
C7

C1
C2
C3
C4
C5
C6
C7
} Cervical vertebrae

T1
T2
T3
T4
T5
T6
T7
T8
T9
T10
T11
T12
} Thoracic vertebrae

Intervertebral disks

L1
L2
L3
L4
L5
} Lumbar vertebrae

Sacrum (fused sacral vertebrae)

Coccyx (fused coccygeal vertebrae)

Anterior View

Figure 10-1 Vertebral column. Source: Delmar/Cengage Learning

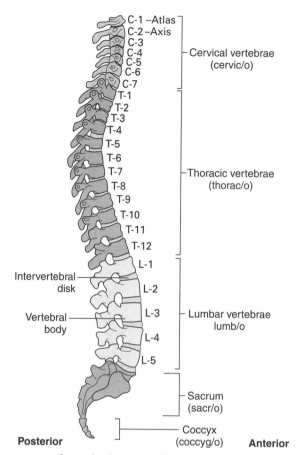

C-1 –Atlas
C-2 –Axis
C-3
C-4
C-5
C-6
C-7 — Cervical vertebrae (cervic/o)
T-1
T-2
T-3
T-4
T-5
T-6
T-7
T-8
T-9
T-10
T-11
T-12 — Thoracic vertebrae (thorac/o)
Intervertebral disk
Vertebral body
L-1
L-2
L-3
L-4
L-5 — Lumbar vertebrae lumb/o
Sacrum (sacr/o)
Coccyx (coccyg/o)
Posterior   **Anterior**

Figure 10-2 Anterior/posterior curves of vertebral column *(See color plate).* Source: Delmar/Cengage Learning

These vertebrae are situated on top of one another in an alternating anterior/posterior curved fashion (see Figure 10-2). These curves are referred to as a **lordotic curve,** which curves inward toward the center of the body (found in the lumbar and cervical regions), and a **kyphotic curve,** which curves outward away from the center of the body (found in the sacral and thoracic regions). These curves enhance the shock absorption capabilities of the spine.

The sacral area is nestled between the ilia of the pelvis, which gives it greater stability than found in other areas of the spine. The same is true in the thoracic area where the ribs are attached. Any area with more bony structure will be more stable. Because they have less bony structure, the cervical and lumbar regions are more flexible. The increased ROM also means that these areas are more prone to injury.

Joints

The spine has several joints, some of which connect it with surrounding structures and others that connect different parts of the spine itself. Superiorly the spine must connect with the skull. The atlanto-occipital joint is formed where the condyles of the occiput articulate with the superior articular processes of the atlas (see Figure 10-3). Cervical **rotation** occurs between the atlas (C1) and the axis (C2). The articulation at this juncture is vastly different than anywhere else along the spine. There are actually three joints located between the atlas and the axis. The median atlantoaxial joint occurs between the odontoid process of C2 and the anterior arch of C1. Two lateral atlantoaxial joints are located between the articular processes of the two vertebrae.

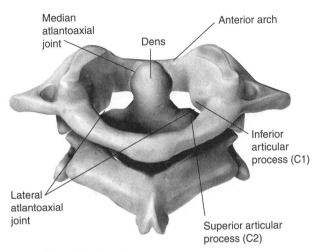

Figure 10-3 Atlanto-occipital joint (*See color plate*). Source: Delmar/Cengage Learning

Throughout the spine from C2 through S1, the articulations are essentially the same. Each vertebrae has two articulating surfaces (one on each side posteriorly). The superior articulating surface of the lower vertebra articulates with the inferior articulating surface of the adjacent upper vertebrae. These joints are called *facet joints* (see Figure 10-4). Each joint has its own joint capsule.

TIPS *of the* Trade

Remember each vertebra articulates with both the vertebrae above it and below it, and each vertebra has articulating surfaces on each side. That means each vertebra has four articulations or joints.

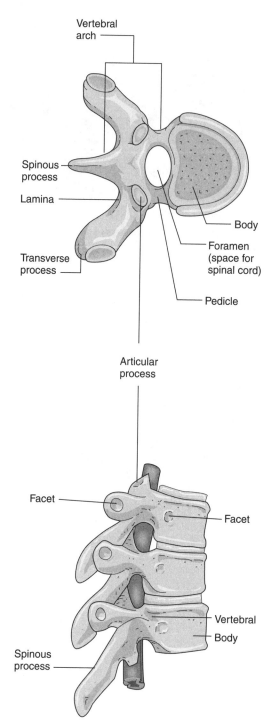

Figure 10-4 Superior and lateral view of vertebrae with facet joint (*See color plate*). Source: Delmar/Cengage Learning

Bones

Since many cervical muscles have attachments on the skull, the bony landmarks of the skull that are directly connected to spinal musculature will be discussed, along with those of the vertebral column (see Figures 10-5 and 10-6).

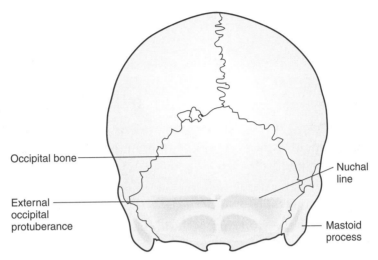

Occipital bone

Nuchal line

External occipital protuberance

Mastoid process

Figure 10-5 Bony landmarks of the skull. Source: Delmar/Cengage Learning

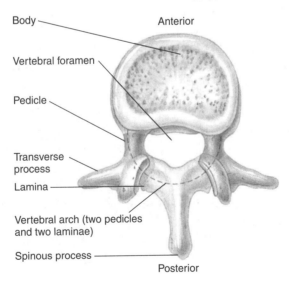

Body

Anterior

Vertebral foramen

Pedicle

Transverse process

Lamina

Vertebral arch (two pedicles and two laminae)

Spinous process

Posterior

Figure 10-6 Bony landmarks of the vertebrae. Source: Delmar/Cengage Learning

Skull

- **Mastoid process:** Bony prominence behind the ear
- **Occipital bone:** Posterior inferior portion of the skull
- **Occipital protuberance:** Prominence located in the center of the occiput
- **Nuchal line:** Ridge running in a horizontal direction from the occipital protuberance toward the mastoid process

Vertebrae

- **Body:** Anterior rounded portion of each vertebra (not present in C1, also called the *atlas*)
- **Neural or vertebral arch:** The posterior portion of the vertebra
- **Spinous process:** The center posterior projection of the vertebra; easily palpated
- **Transverse process:** Bilateral projections of the vertebra where the lamina meets the pedicle
- **Vertebral foramen:** Opening formed by the union of the body and the vertebral arch; the spinal cord passes through this structure
- **Intervertebral foramen:** The lateral opening between two vertebrae that allows for the passage of spinal nerves and vessels
- **Facet:** Projection on each transverse process with both a superior and inferior surface that allows for articulation with adjacent vertebra

Ligaments

The sheer numbers of vertebrae requiring support and stability would indicate this area of the body requires many ligaments to literally "hold things together" (see Figure 10-7). The anterior longitudinal ligament runs the length of the spinal column. Superiorly it is much thinner and becomes thicker inferiorly as it nears its attachment to the sacrum. The purpose of the anterior longitudinal ligament is to prevent excessive hyperextension. On the opposite side of the spine, we find the posterior longitudinal ligament. This ligament is located inside the vertebral foramen and serves the purpose of preventing excessive flexion. In terms of thickness you will find the reverse of the anterior longitudinal ligaments in that the posterior longitudinal ligament is thicker superiorly where it provides extra support for the skull. The posterior longitudinal ligament is much thinner inferiorly, which can predispose the lumbar area to instability and potential disk injury. In the cervical area the nuchal ligament (ligamentum nuchae) runs from the skull to C7. It is a strong but superficial ligament that actually serves two purposes. It provides stability to the cervical area and the skull and provides attachment points for muscles of the shoulder girdle and shoulder joint. The supraspinal ligament extends from C7 to the sacrum. It runs along the tips of the spinous processes. The interspinal ligaments connect adjacent spinous processes from C7 to the sacrum. The final ligament is also located on the posterior side of the spinal column and is named the *ligamentum flavum*. This ligament connects adjacent lamina on the anterior surface.

Sagittal Section View

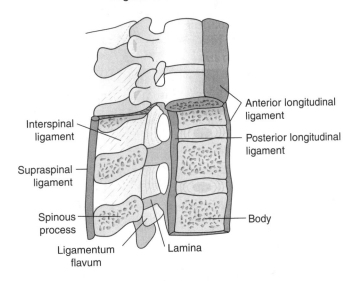

Interspinal ligament

Supraspinal ligament

Spinous process

Ligamentum flavum

Anterior longitudinal ligament

Posterior longitudinal ligament

Body

Lamina

Superior View

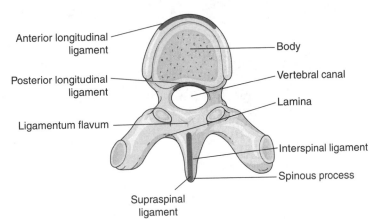

Anterior longitudinal ligament

Posterior longitudinal ligament

Ligamentum flavum

Supraspinal ligament

Body

Vertebral canal

Lamina

Interspinal ligament

Spinous process

Figure 10-7 Sagittal and superior view of ligaments. Source: Delmar/Cengage Learning

MUSCLE TESTING OF THE TRUNK

For the purpose of this worktext, the movements available in the spine are divided into cervical and thoraco-lumbar motions. The movements possible include flexion/extension, rotation, and **lateral flexion,** also called **side-bending.**

Capital Extension

Table 10-1 lists the primary and accessory muscles responsible for capital extension. The rectus capitis posterior major, rectus capitis posterior minor, longissimus capitis, obliquus capitis superior, obliquus capitis inferior, splenius capitis, and semispinalis capitis muscles are the primary movers for capital extension (see Figure 10-8).

TABLE 10-1	MUSCLES RESPONSIBLE FOR CAPITAL EXTENSION		
PRIMARY MUSCLES	**ORIGIN**	**INSERTION**	**INNERVATION**
Rectus capitis posterior major	Spinous process of the axis	Lateral inferior nuchal line of the occiput	C1
Rectus capitis posterior minor	Atlas (tubercle of posterior arch)	Lateral inferior nuchal line of the occiput	C1
Longissimus capitis	T1–T5 vertebrae transverse processes C4–C7 vertebrae articular processes	Posterior mastoid process	C1–C3
Obliquus capitis superior	Transverse process of atlas	Along nuchal line of occiput	C1
Obliquus capitis inferior	Lamina and spinous process of axis	Transverse process of atlas	C1
Splenius capitis	Lower half of nuchal ligament	Lateral occipital bone, mastoid process	C4–C8
Semispinalis capitis (also called *spinalis capitis*)	Transverse processes of C7–T6 and C4–C6 articular processes	Along nuchal line of occiput	Posterior primary division of spinal nerves
ACCESSORY MUSCLES	**ORIGIN**	**INSERTION**	**INNERVATION**
Upper trapezius	Occipital protuberance, middle third of nuchal line, spinous process of C7, and ligamentum nuchae	Lateral third of posterior clavicle	Accessory nerve (cranial nerve XI) C3–C4
Sternocleidomastoid	Sternum and clavicle	Mastoid process	Accessory nerve (cranial nerve XI) C2–C3

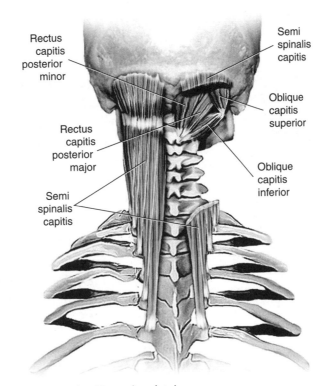

Figure 10-8 Posterior suboccipital muscles *(See color plate).* Source: Delmar/Cengage Learning

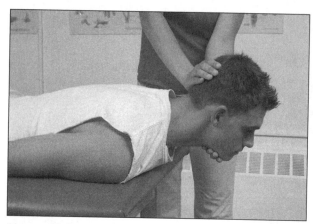

Figure 10-9 Proper positioning for capital extension grades 5–3. Source: Delmar/Cengage Learning

Testing for Capital Extension Grades 5, 4, 3 (Normal, Good, Fair) Gravity Resisted

POSITION OF PATIENT: Prone with head off the end of the treatment table (see Figure 10-9).

POSITION OF THERAPIST: Standing next to patient with one hand applying resistance at the occiput. The other hand below the head prepared to provide support in case the head gives way.

TEST: Resistance is applied as patient tilts upward chin only (no cervical movement allowed).

DIRECTIONS: Say to the patient, "Tip your head up and hold it. Don't let me push it down."

GRADING:

- **Grade 5 (Normal):** Patient achieves position and holds against maximum resistance.
- **Grade 4 (Good):** Patient achieves position and holds against strong (but not full) resistance.
- **Grade 3 (Fair):** Patient achieves position but tolerates no resistance.

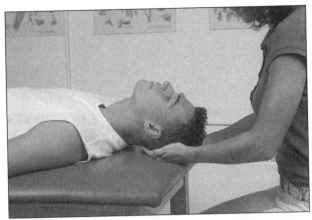

Figure 10-10 Proper positioning for capital extension grades 2–0. Source: Delmar/Cengage Learning

Testing for Capital Extension
Grades 2, 1, 0 (Poor, Trace, None)
Gravity Minimized

POSITION OF PATIENT: Supine with head supported on treatment table (see Figure 10-10).

POSITION OF THERAPIST: Standing at end of table facing patient with both hands supporting the head at the base of the occiput to allow palpation of muscles if needed.

TEST: Patient attempts to tilt chin upward.

DIRECTIONS: Say to the patient, "Tilt your chin upward."

GRADING:

- **Grade 2 (Poor):** Patient moves through partial range.
- **Grade 1 (Trace):** Patient shows slight motion or contraction is palpable.
- **Grade 0 (None):** No activity noted.

Capital Flexion

Table 10-2 presents the primary muscles responsible for capital flexion. The rectus capitis anterior, rectus capitis lateralis, and longus capitis muscles are the primary movers for capital flexion (see Figure 10-11).

TABLE 10-2	MUSCLES RESPONSIBLE FOR CAPITAL FLEXION		
PRIMARY MUSCLES	**ORIGIN**	**INSERTION**	**INNERVATION**
Rectus capitis anterior	Transverse process atlas	Basilar portion occiput	C1–C3
Rectus capitis lateralis	Transverse process atlas	Jugular process occiput	C1–C3
Longus capitis	C3–C6 transverse processes of vertebrae	Basilar portion occiput	C1–C3

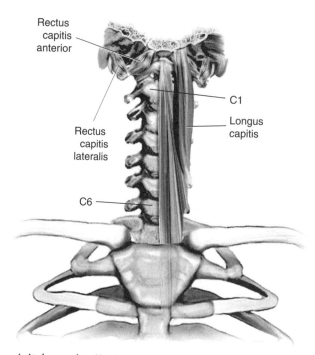

Figure 10-11 Anterior suboccipital muscles *(See color plate).* Source: Delmar/Cengage Learning

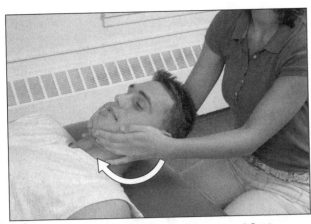

Figure 10-12 Proper positioning for capital flexion grades 5–0. Source: Delmar/Cengage Learning

Testing for Capital Flexion Grades 5–0 (Normal to None)

POSITION OF PATIENT: Supine with the head supported on the treatment table (see Figure 10-12).

POSITION OF THERAPIST: Standing at head of table with hands prepared to give resistance under the mandible by pulling upward and backward.

TEST: Resistance is applied as patient attempts to tuck chin toward the chest without raising the head from the table.

DIRECTIONS: Say to the patient, "Tip your chin toward your chest and hold it. Don't let me pull you back."

GRADING:

- **Grade 5 (Normal):** Patient achieves position and holds against maximum resistance.
- **Grade 4 (Good):** Patient achieves position and holds against strong (but not full) resistance.
- **Grade 3 (Fair):** Patient achieves position but tolerates no resistance.
- **Grade 2 (Poor):** Patient moves through partial range.
- **Grade 1 (Trace):** Patient shows slight motion or contraction is palpable.
- **Grade 0 (None):** No activity noted.

Cervical Extension

The primary and accessory muscles responsible for cervical extension are listed in Table 10-3. The longissimus cervicis, semispinalis cervicis, illiocostalis cervicis, splenius cervicis, upper trapezius, and spinalis cervicis muscles are the primary movers for cervical extension (see Figure 10-13).

TABLE 10-3	MUSCLES RESPONSIBLE FOR CERVICAL EXTENSION		
PRIMARY MUSCLES	**ORIGIN**	**INSERTION**	**INNERVATION**
Longissimus cervicis	Transverse processes T1–T5 vertebrae	Transverse processes C2–C6	C3–C8
Semispinalis cervicis	Transverse processes T1–T5	Spinous processes C2–C5	C2–C5
Iliocostalis cervicis	Ribs 3–6	Transverse processes C4–C6	C4–C8
Splenius cervicis	Spinous processes T3–T6	Transverse processes C1–C3	C3–C8
Upper trapezius	Occipital protuberance, middle third of nuchal line, spinous process of C7, and ligamentum nuchae	Lateral third of posterior clavicle	Accessory nerve (cranial nerve XI) 3–4 cervical
Spinalis cervicis	Spinous processes C7, ligamentum nuchae	Spinous process of C2–C3	C3–C8
ACCESSORY MUSCLES	**ORIGIN**	**INSERTION**	**INNERVATION**
Interspinales cervicis	Cervical spinous processes below	Cervical spinous processes above	C3–C8
Intertransversarii cervicis	Cervical transverse processes above	Cervical spinous processes below	C4–C8
Rotatores cervicis	Cervical transverse process below	Cervical base of spinous process above	C3–C8
Multifidi	Sacrum, aponeurosis of erector spinae, PSIS of ilium, L1–L5, transverse processes T1–T12, C4–C7	Spinous processes of higher vertebra	C2–C8
Levator scapulae	C1–C4 vertebrae (transverse process)	Scapula (vertebral border between superior angle and root of scapular spine)	C3–C4, dorsal scapular nerve (C5)

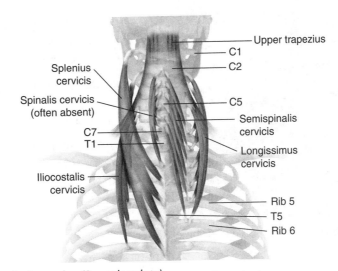

Figure 10-13 Posterior cervical muscles *(See color plate).* Source: Delmar/Cengage Learning

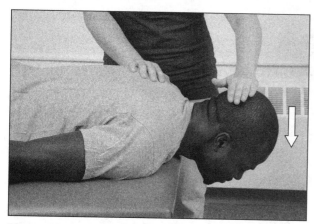

Figure 10-14 Proper positioning for cervical extension grades 5–3. Source: Delmar/Cengage Learning

Testing for Cervical Extension Grades 5, 4, 3 (Normal, Good, Fair) Gravity Resisted

POSITION OF PATIENT: Prone with head off the end of the treatment table (see Figure 10-14).

POSITION OF THERAPIST: Standing next to patient with one hand applying resistance at the occiput. The other hand may be placed below the head prepared to provide support in case the head gives way.

TEST: Resistance is applied as patient extends neck without tilting chin.

DIRECTIONS: Say to the patient, "Lift your head up and look toward the wall in front of you. Hold it. Don't let me push it down."

GRADING:

- **Grade 5 (Normal):** Patient achieves position and holds against maximum resistance.
- **Grade 4 (Good):** Patient achieves position and holds against strong (but not full) resistance.
- **Grade 3 (Fair):** Patient achieves position but tolerates no resistance.

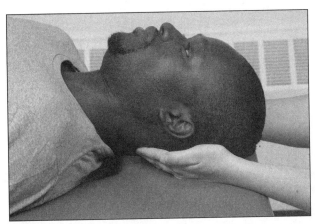

Figure 10-15 Proper positioning for cervical extension grades 2–0. Source: Delmar/Cengage Learning

Testing for Cervical Extension Grades 2, 1, 0 (Poor, Trace, None) Gravity Minimized

POSITION OF PATIENT: Supine with head supported on treatment table (see Figure 10-15).

POSITION OF THERAPIST: Standing at end of table facing patient with both hands supporting the head, with fingers placed distal to the base of the occiput to allow palpation of cervical muscles if needed.

TEST: Patient attempts to extend neck into the table.

DIRECTIONS: Say to the patient "Push your head and neck down into the table."

GRADING:

- **Grade 2 (Poor):** Patient moves through partial range.
- **Grade 1 (Trace):** Patient shows slight motion, or contraction is palpable.
- **Grade 0 (None):** No activity noted.

Cervical Flexion

The primary and accessory muscles responsible for cervical flexion are shown in Table 10-4. The sternocleidomastoid, longus colli, and scalenus anterior muscles are the primary movers for cervical flexion (see Figure 10-16).

TABLE 10-4	MUSCLES RESPONSIBLE FOR CERVICAL FLEXION		
PRIMARY MUSCLES	**ORIGIN**	**INSERTION**	**INNERVATION**
Sternocleidomastoid	Sternum and clavicle	Mastoid process	Accessory nerve (cranial XI) C2–C3
Longus colli: (1) superior oblique, (2) vertical intermediate, (3) scalenus anterior	(1) Transverse processes C3–C5, (2) T1–T3 and C5–C7 vertebrae, (3) transverse processes C3–C6	(1) atlas, (2) C2–C4, (3) transverse processes C5–C6	C2–C7
Scalenus anterior	Transverse processes C3–C6	First rib	C4–C6
ACCESSORY MUSCLES	**ORIGIN**	**INSERTION**	**INNERVATION**
Scalenus medius	Transverse processes C2–C7	First rib	C3–C8

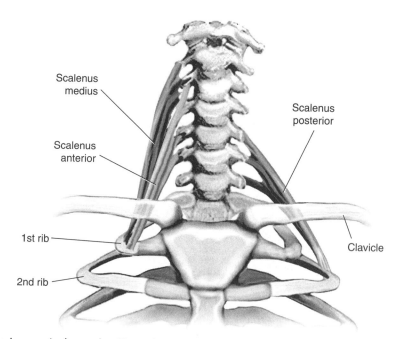

Figure 10-16 Anterior cervical muscles *(See color plate).* Source: Delmar/Cengage Learning

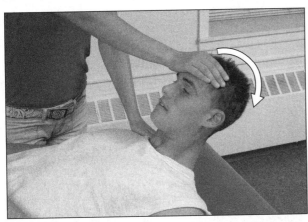

Figure 10-17 Proper positioning for cervical flexion grades 5–0. Source: Delmar/Cengage Learning

Testing for Cervical Flexion Grades 5–0 (Normal to None)

POSITION OF PATIENT: Supine with the head supported on the treatment table (see Figure 10-17).

POSITION OF THERAPIST: Standing at head of table prepared to give resistance with one hand against the forehead.

TEST: Resistance is applied as patient attempts to lift head straight up off the table.

DIRECTIONS: Say to the patient, "Lift your head and neck straight off the table and hold it. Don't let me push you back."

GRADING:

- **Grade 5 (Normal):** Patient achieves position and holds against maximum resistance.
- **Grade 4 (Good):** Patient achieves position and holds against strong (but not full) resistance.
- **Grade 3 (Fair):** Patient achieves position but tolerates no resistance.
- **Grade 2 (Poor):** Patient moves through partial range.
- **Grade 1 (Trace):** Patient shows slight motion, or contraction is palpable.
- **Grade 0 (None):** No activity noted.

Trunk Extension

Table 10-5 lists the primary and accessory muscles responsible for trunk extension. The iliocostalis thoracis, iliocostalis lumborum, longissimus thoracis, spinalis thoracis (see Figure 10-18), semispinalis thoracis, multifidi, rotatores thoracis and lumborum (see Figure 10-19), interspinales, and quadratus lumborum (see Figure 10-20) muscles are the primary movers for trunk extension.

TABLE 10-5	MUSCLES RESPONSIBLE FOR TRUNK EXTENSION		
PRIMARY MUSCLES	**ORIGIN**	**INSERTION**	**INNERVATION**
Iliocostalis thoracis	7–12 ribs	1–6 ribs, transverse process of C7	T1–T12 spinal
Iliocostalis lumborum	Erector spinae tendon, thoracolumbar fascia, iliac crest, sacrum	6–12 ribs	L1–L5 spinal
Longissimus thoracis	Erector spinae tendon, thoracolumbar fascia, transverse processes L1–L5	Transverse processes T1–T12, 2–12 ribs	T1–L1 spinal
Spinalis thoracis	Erector spinae tendon, T11–L2 spinous processes	T1–T4	T1–T12 spinal
Semispinalis thoracis	Transverse processes T6–T10	C6–T4 spinous processes	T1–T12 spinal
Multifidi	Sacrum, aponeurosis of erector spinae, PSIS of ilium, L1–L5, transverse processes T1–T12, C4–C7	Spinous processes of higher vertebra	C2–C8
Rotatores thoracis and lumborum	Transverse processes thoracic and lumbar	Next highest vertebra	T1–L5 spinal
Interspinales	Spinous process above	Spinous process below	T1–L4 spinal
Intertransversarii	Transverse process above	Transverse process below	Spinal (lumbar and sacral)
Quadratus lumborum	Iliac crest	Twelfth rib, transverse processes L1–L5	Twelfth thoracic and first lumbar
ACCESSORY MUSCLES	**ORIGIN**	**INSERTION**	**INNERVATION**
Gluteus maximus	Posterior sacrum and ilium	Posterior femur distal to greater trochanter, iliotibial band	Inferior gluteal (L5, S1, S2)

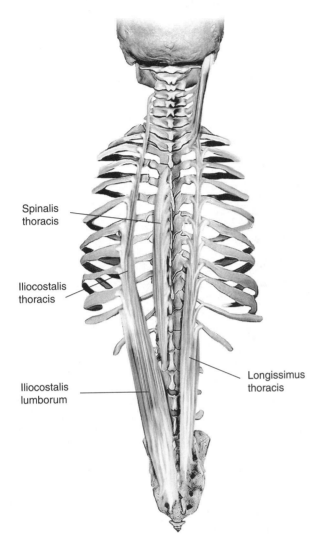

Spinalis
thoracis

Iliocostalis
thoracis

Iliocostalis
lumborum

Longissimus
thoracis

Figure 10-18 Erector spinae muscle group *(See color plate)*. Source: Delmar/Cengage Learning

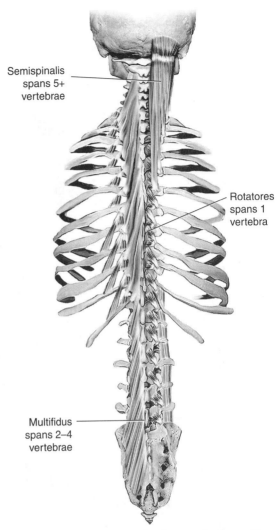

Semispinalis
spans 5+
vertebrae

Rotatores
spans 1
vertebra

Multifidus
spans 2–4
vertebrae

Figure 10-19 Transversospinalis muscle group *(See color plate)*. Source: Delmar/Cengage Learning

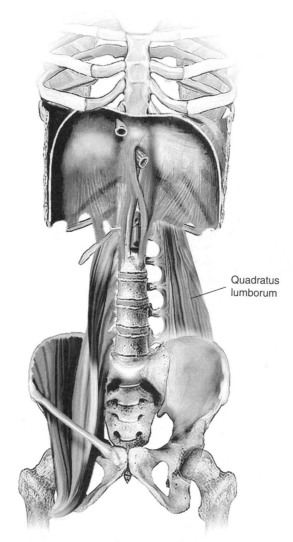

Figure 10-20 Quadratus lumborum *(See color plate).* Source: Delmar/Cengage Learning

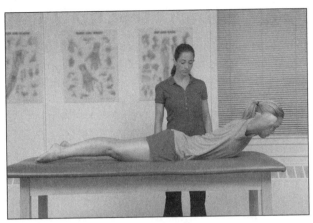

Figure 10-21 Proper positioning for lumbar spine extension grades 5, 4. Source: Delmar/Cengage Learning

Testing for Lumbar Spine Grades 5, 4 (Normal, Good)

POSITION OF PATIENT: Prone with hands clasped behind the head (see Figure 10-21).

POSITION OF THERAPIST: Standing to the side of patient to stabilize the lower body as needed.

TEST: Patient attempts to lift the chest off the table by extending the lumbar spine.

DIRECTIONS: Say to the patient, "Arch your back. Hold the position while I count to 5."

GRADING:

- **Grade 5 (Normal):** Patient achieves position and holds without signs of effort.
- **Grade 4 (Good):** Patient achieves position and holds but displays some wavering or sign of effort.

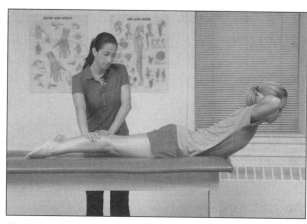

Figure 10-22 Proper positioning for thoracic spine extension grades 5, 4. Source: Delmar/Cengage Learning

Testing for Thoracic Spine Grades 5, 4 (Normal, Good)

POSITION OF PATIENT: Prone with upper body extending off the table to about mid sternum with hands clasped behind the head (see Figure 10-22).

POSITION OF THERAPIST: Standing to the side of patient to stabilize the lower body as needed.

TEST: Patient attempts to lift the upper body to horizontal position.

DIRECTIONS: Say to the patient, "Arch your back. Hold the position while I count to 5."

GRADING:

- **Grade 5 (Normal):** Patient achieves position and holds without signs of effort.
- **Grade 4 (Good):** Patient achieves position and holds but displays some wavering or sign of effort.

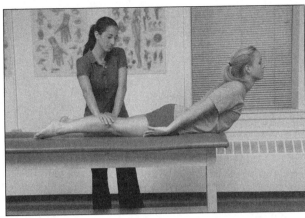

Figure 10-23 Proper positioning for thoraco-lumbar extension grade 3. Source: Delmar/Cengage Learning

Testing for Thoracic and Lumbar Spine Grade 3 (Fair)

POSITION OF PATIENT: Prone with upper body extending off the table to about mid sternum with arms at sides (see Figure 10-23).

POSITION OF THERAPIST: Standing to the side of patient to stabilize the lower body as needed.

TEST: Patient attempts to lift the upper body to horizontal position.

DIRECTIONS: Say to the patient, "Arch your back. Hold the position while I count to 5."

GRADING:

- **Grade 3 (Fair):** Patient achieves position.

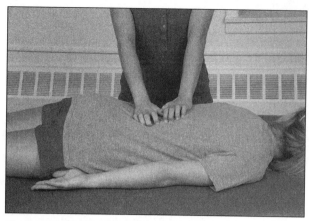

Figure 10-24 Proper positioning for thoraco-lumbar extension grades 2–0. Source: Delmar/Cengage Learning

Thoracic and Lumbar Spine Grades 2, 1, 0 (Poor, Trace, None)

POSITION OF PATIENT: Prone on treatment table (see Figure 10-24).

POSITION OF THERAPIST: At side of patient with fingers placed to palpate lumbar and thoracic extensor muscles.

TEST: Patient attempts to lift upper body off table surface.

DIRECTIONS: Say to the patient, "Try to arch your back."

GRADING:

- **Grade 2 (Poor):** Patient moves through partial range.
- **Grade 1 (Trace):** Patient shows slight motion, or contraction is palpable.
- **Grade 0 (None):** No activity noted.

Trunk Flexion

Table 10-6 presents the primary and accessory muscles responsible for trunk flexion. The rectus abdominus (see Figure 10-25), obliquus externus abdominis (see Figure 10-26), and obliquus internus abdominis (see Figure 10-27) muscles are the primary movers for trunk flexion.

TABLE 10-6	MUSCLES RESPONSIBLE FOR TRUNK FLEXION		
PRIMARY MUSCLES	**ORIGIN**	**INSERTION**	**INNERVATION**
Rectus abdominus	Pubis	Xiphoid process and costal cartilage of 5–7 ribs	7–12 intercostal nerve
Obliquus externus abdominis	Lateral lower 8 ribs	Iliac crest and linea alba	8–12 intercostal, iliohypogastric, ilioinguinal
Obliquus internus abdominis	Inguinal ligament, iliac crest, thoraco-lumbar fascia	10–12 ribs, abdominal aponeurosis	8–12 intercostal, iliohypogastric, ilioinguinal
ACCESSORY MUSCLES	**ORIGIN**	**INSERTION**	**INNERVATION**
Psoas major	Transverse processes L1–L5, T12–L5 vertebral bodies	Lesser trochanter femur	L2–L4 spinal
Psoas minor	Vertebral bodies T12–L1	Pubis, iliac fascia	L1 spinal

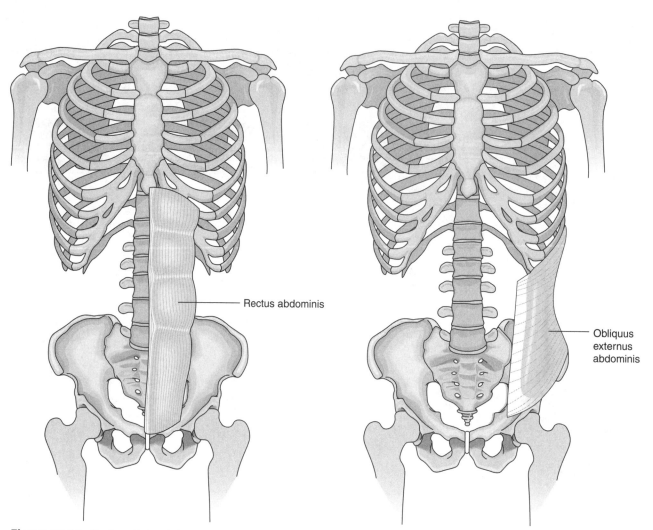

Figure 10-25 Rectus abdominis. Source: Delmar/Cengage Learning

Figure 10-26 Obliquus externus abdominis.

Source: Delmar/Cengage Learning

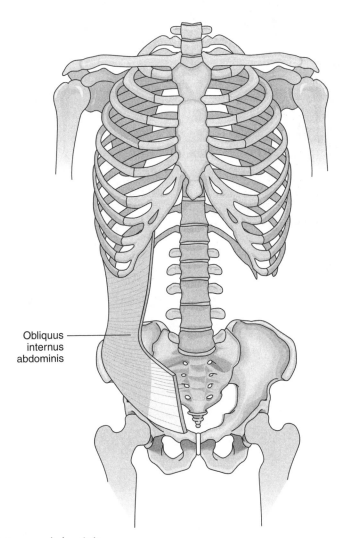

Figure 10-27 Obliquus internus abdominis. Source: Delmar/Cengage Learning

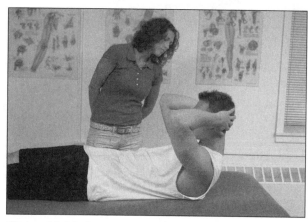

Figure 10-28 Proper positioning for trunk flexion grade 5. Source: Delmar/Cengage Learning

Testing for Trunk Flexion Grade 5 (Normal)

POSITION OF PATIENT: Supine on table with hands clasped behind head (see Figure 10-28).

POSITION OF THERAPIST: At side of patient prepared to stabilize at the pelvis if weak hip flexors are present.

TEST: Patient performs a curl-up to the point the scapulae clear the table.

DIRECTIONS: Say to the patient, "Do a partial sit-up. Lift your shoulders off the table. Hold for a count of 5."

GRADING:

- **Grade 5 (Normal):** Patient achieves position and holds.

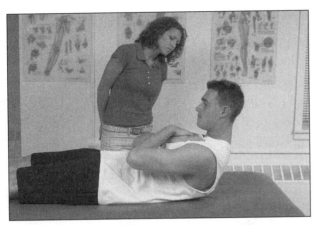

Figure 10-29 Proper positioning for trunk flexion grade 4. Source: Delmar/Cengage Learning

Testing for Trunk Flexion Grade 4 (Good)

POSITION OF PATIENT: Supine on table with arms crossed over chest (see Figure10-29).

POSITION OF THERAPIST: At side of patient prepared to stabilize at the pelvis if weak hip flexors are present.

TEST: Patient performs a curl-up to the point the scapulae clear the table.

DIRECTIONS: Say to the patient, "Do a partial sit-up. Lift your shoulders off the table. Hold for a count of 5."

GRADING:

- **Grade 4 (Good):** Patient achieves position and holds.

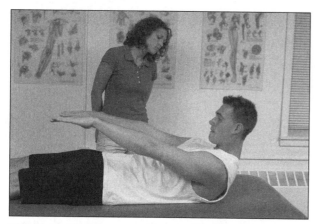

Figure 10-30 Proper positioning for trunk flexion grade 3. Source: Delmar/Cengage Learning

Testing for Trunk Flexion Grade 3 (Fair)

POSITION OF PATIENT: Supine on table with arms at sides (see Figure 10-30).

POSITION OF THERAPIST: At side of patient prepared to stabilize at the pelvis if weak hip flexors are present.

TEST: Patient performs a curl-up to the point the scapulae clear the table.

DIRECTIONS: Say to the patient, "Do a partial sit-up. Lift your shoulders off the table. Hold for a count of 5."

GRADING:

- **Grade 3 (Fair):** Patient achieves position and holds.

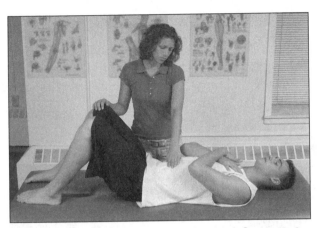

Figure 10-31 Proper positioning for trunk flexion 2–0.

Source: Delmar/Cengage Learning

Testing for Trunk Flexion
Grades 2, 1, 0 (Poor, Trace, None)

POSITION OF PATIENT: Supine on treatment table with knees flexed and feet flat on table (see Figure 10-31).

POSITION OF THERAPIST: Standing at side with fingers placed over linea alba to palpate contraction of the rectus abdominus.

TEST: Patient attempts to lift upper body off table.

DIRECTIONS: Say to the patient, "Do a partial sit-up. Lift your shoulders off the table."

ALTERNATIVE TEST: Therapist cradles the upper body in a slightly flexed position with directions to patient to lean forward from that position or cough. With either of these actions the abdominals kick in if you see any depression of the rib cage.

GRADING:

- **Grade 2 (Poor):** Patient rib cage depresses during attempt.
- **Grade 1 (Trace):** Patient shows slight motion, or contraction is palpable.
- **Grade 0 (None):** No activity noted.

Elevation of Pelvis

The primary and accessory muscles responsible for the elevation of the pelvis are presented in Table 10-7. The quadratus lumborum (refer to Figure 10-20), obliquus externus abdominis (refer to Figure 10-26), and obliquus internus abdominis (refer to Figure 10-27) muscles are the primary movers for the elevation of the pelvis.

TABLE 10-7	MUSCLES RESPONSIBLE FOR THE ELEVATION OF THE PELVIS		
PRIMARY MUSCLES	**ORIGIN**	**INSERTION**	**INNERVATION**
Quadratus lumborum	Iliac crest	Twelfth rib, transverse processes L1–L5	Twelfth thoracic and first lumbar
Obliquus externus abdominis	Lateral lower 8 ribs	Iliac crest and linea alba	8–12 intercostal, iliohypogastric, ilioinguinal
Obliquus internus abdominis	Inguinal ligament, iliac crest, thoraco-lumbar fascia	10–12 ribs, abdominal aponeurosis	8–12 intercostal, iliohypogastric, ilioinguinal
ACCESSORY MUSCLES	**ORIGIN**	**INSERTION**	**INNERVATION**
Latissimus dorsi	Spinous processes of T7–L5, posterior surface of the sacrum, iliac crest, and lower three ribs	Medial lip of the bicipital groove of the humerus	Thoracodorsal
Iliocostalis lumborum	Erector spinae tendon, thoraco-lumbar fascia, iliac crest, sacrum	Transverse processes of all lumbar vertebrae, 5–12 ribs	L1–L5 spinal

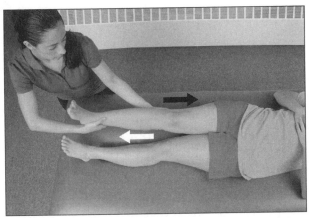

Figure 10-32 Proper positioning for elevation of pelvis grades 5, 4. Source: Delmar/Cengage Learning

Testing for Elevation of Pelvis Grades 5, 4 (Normal, Good)

POSITION OF PATIENT: Supine on treatment table (see Figure 10-32).

POSITION OF THERAPIST: Standing at foot of table holding test limb with both hands just above the ankle prepared to provide a **traction** type of resistance.

TEST: Patient decreases the distance between the pelvis and the rib cage by hiking the hip and holding against resistance.

DIRECTIONS: Say to the patient, "Hike your hip toward your rib cage and hold the position. Don't let me pull your leg down."

GRADING:

- **Grade 5 (Normal):** Patient achieves position and holds against maximum resistance.
- **Grade 4 (Good):** Patient achieves position and holds against strong (but not full) resistance.

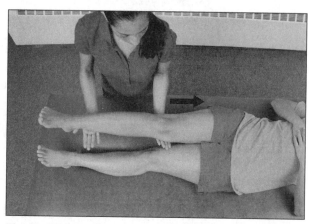

Figure 10-33 Proper positioning for elevation of pelvis grades 3, 2. Source: Delmar/Cengage Learning

Testing for Elevation of Pelvis Grades 3, 2 (Fair, Poor)

POSITION OF PATIENT: Supine on treatment table (see Figure 10-33).

POSITION OF THERAPIST: Standing at foot of table holding test limb with one hand just above the ankle and the other placed under the knee in order to lift the leg off the table slightly to decrease friction.

TEST: Patient decreases the distance between the pelvis and the rib cage by hiking the hip.

DIRECTIONS: Say to the patient, "Hike your leg toward your rib cage."

GRADING:

- **Grade 3 (Fair):** Patient achieves position.
- **Grade 2 (Poor):** Patient moves through partial range.
- **Grades 1 (Trace)** and **0 (None):** Not gradable with this test as the principle muscle lies too deeply in the lumbar region to accurately palpate.

Trunk Rotation

The primary muscles responsible for trunk rotation are presented in Table 10-8. The quadratus obliquus externus abdominis and obliquus internus abdominis muscles are the primary movers for trunk rotation (refer to Figures 10-26 and 10-27).

TABLE 10-8	MUSCLES RESPONSIBLE FOR TRUNK ROTATION		
PRIMARY MUSCLES	**ORIGIN**	**INSERTION**	**INNERVATION**
Obliquus externus abdominis	Lateral lower 8 ribs	Iliac crest and linea alba	8–12 intercostal, iliohypogastric, ilioinguinal
Obliquus internus abdominis	Inguinal ligament, iliac crest, thoraco-lumbar fascia	10–12 ribs, abdominal aponeurosis	8–12 intercostal, iliohypogastric, ilioinguinal

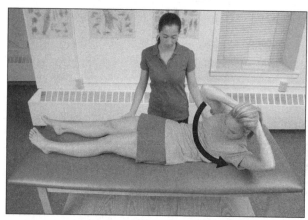

Figure 10-34 Proper positioning for trunk rotation grade 5. Source: Delmar/Cengage Learning

Testing for Trunk Rotation Grade 5 (Normal)

POSITION OF PATIENT: Supine on table with hands clasped behind head (see Figure 10-34).

POSITION OF THERAPIST: At side of patient prepared to stabilize at the pelvis if weak hip flexors are present.

TEST: Patient flexes trunk and rotates to one side. The contracting internal obliques will be on the side the patient rotates toward. The contracting external obliques will be on the opposite side.

DIRECTIONS: Say to the patient, "While performing a partial sit-up, bring your elbow toward the opposite knee and hold it for a count of 5."

GRADING:

- **Grade 5 (Normal):** Patient achieves position with the upper scapula clearing the table.

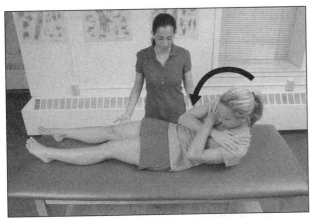

Figure 10-35 Proper positioning for trunk rotation grade 4. _{Source: Delmar/Cengage Learning}

Testing for Trunk Rotation Grade 4 (Good)

POSITION OF PATIENT: Supine on table with arms crossed over chest (see Figure 10-35).

POSITION OF THERAPIST: At side of patient prepared to stabilize at the pelvis if weak hip flexors are present.

TEST: Patient flexes trunk and rotates to one side. The contracting internal obliques will be on the side the patient rotates toward. The contracting external obliques will be on the opposite side.

DIRECTIONS: Say to the patient, "While performing a partial sit-up, bring your elbow toward the opposite knee and hold it for a count of 5."

GRADING:

- **Grade 4 (Good):** Patient achieves position with the upper scapula clearing the table.

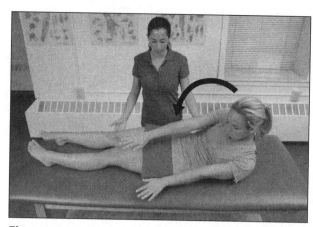

Figure 10-36 Proper positioning for trunk rotation grade 3. Source: Delmar/Cengage Learning

Testing for Trunk Rotation Grade 3 (Fair)

POSITION OF PATIENT: Supine on table with arms at sides (see Figure 10-36).

POSITION OF THERAPIST: At side of patient prepared to stabilize at the pelvis if weak hip flexors are present.

TEST: Patient flexes trunk and rotates to one side. The contracting internal obliques will be on the side the patient rotates toward. The contracting external obliques will be on the opposite side.

DIRECTIONS: Say to the patient, "Reach your hand toward the opposite knee and hold it for a count of 5."

GRADING:

- **Grade 3 (Fair):** Patient achieves position with the upper scapula clearing the table.

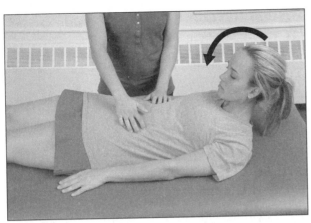

Figure 10-37 Proper positioning for trunk rotation grade 2. Source: Delmar/Cengage Learning

Testing for Trunk Rotation Grade 2 (Poor)

POSITION OF PATIENT: Supine on treatment table with arms stretched out above body (see Figure 10-37).

POSITION OF THERAPIST: Standing at side with fingers placed over obliques to palpate contraction.

TEST: Patient attempts to rotate and lift upper body off table.

DIRECTIONS: Say to the patient, "Try to lift your upper body and bring your elbow toward the opposite knee."

GRADING:

- **Grade 2 (Poor):** Patient unable to lift scapula off table.

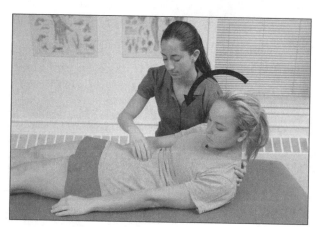

Figure 10-38 Proper positioning for trunk rotation grade 1, 0. Source: Delmar/Cengage Learning

Testing for Trunk Rotation Grades 1, 0 (Trace, None)

POSITION OF PATIENT: Supine on treatment table with hips and knees flexed, feet flat on table (see Figure 10-38).

POSITION OF THERAPIST: One arm cradles the head as patient attempts to rotate to one side. Other hand palpates the internal obliques on the side the patient is rotating toward and then the external obliques on the opposite side.

TEST: Patient attempts to lift and rotate upper body off table.

DIRECTIONS: Say to the patient, "Try to lift your upper body and bring your elbow toward the opposite knee."

GRADING:

- **Grade 1 (Trace):** Patient shows slight motion, or contraction is visible or palpable.
- **Grade 0 (None):** No activity noted.

Substitutions

Important substitutions to watch for during MMT of the trunk are as follows:

- If the sternocleidomastoid muscles are weak or inactive, the platysma may substitute. This can be observed by a downward pulling on the corner of the mouth during the activity. Superficial muscle activity in the anterior neck region may also be noted.
- During elevation of the pelvis, the patient may substitute using the abdominals or the trunk extensors. With this substitution it is very difficult to detect an inefficient quadratus lumborum because of the difficulty of palpation.

RANGE OF MOTION

Spinal ROM can be measured by several different means. The methods used in this text are the most basic and can be done in any setting without special equipment. If your facility has access to **inclinometers, double inclinometers** can be used to measure spinal ROM. Another option is a device called a **CROM,** which uses both **gravity inclinometers** and **compass inclinometers** attached to a headpiece to measure all cervical motions. Make sure to familiarize yourself with the process prior to attempting measurement with patients.

Cervical Flexion

Cervical flexion occurs in a sagittal plane around a frontal (medial/lateral) axis. Normal ROM is 45°, according to the American Academy of Orthopaedic Surgeons (1965). The normal end-feel for cervical flexion is firm due to the stretching of the posterior soft tissue structures in the cervical spine.

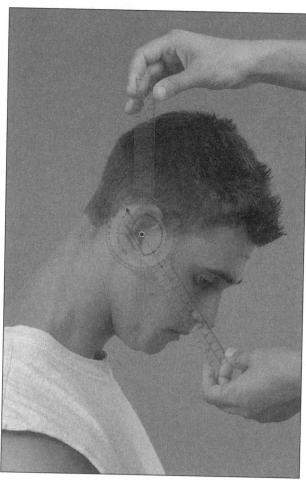

Figure 10-39 Proper positioning for cervical flexion ROM. Source: Delmar/Cengage Learning

POSITION OF PATIENT: Sitting with spine in good postural position. Patient then tilts chin toward the chest.

POSITION OF THERAPIST: To patient's side to align goniometer and stabilize the shoulder girdle, if needed, to prevent thoraco-lumbar flexion during activity.

POSITION OF GONIOMETER:

- **Fulcrum:** Over the external auditory meatus (see Figure 10-39)
- **Stationary arm:** Perpendicular to the ground, pointing up
- **Movable arm:** Aligned with the base of the nares

Cervical Extension

Cervical extension is a motion that occurs in a sagittal plane around a frontal (medial/lateral) axis. The normal ROM for cervical extension is 45°, according to the American Academy of Orthopaedic Surgeons (1965). The normal end-feel is firm due to the stretch of anterior soft tissue structures in the cervical area.

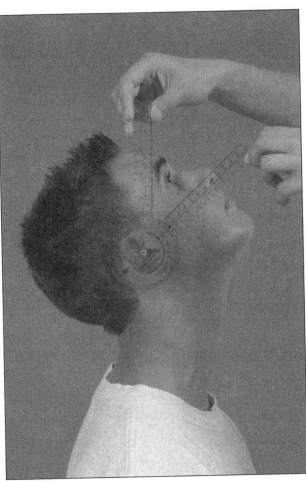

POSITION OF PATIENT: Sitting with spine in good postural position. Patient then lifts chin toward the ceiling.

POSITION OF THERAPIST: To patient's side to align goniometer and stabilize the shoulder girdle, if needed, to prevent thoraco-lumbar extension during activity.

POSITION OF GONIOMETER:

- **Fulcrum:** Over the external auditory meatus (see Figure 10-40)
- **Stationary arm:** Perpendicular to the ground, pointing up
- **Movable arm:** Aligned with the base of the nares

Figure 10-40 Proper positioning for cervical extension ROM. Source: Delmar/Cengage Learning

Cervical Lateral Flexion (Side-bend)

Lateral flexion occurs in the frontal plane around a sagittal (anterior-posterior) axis. The normal ROM is 45°, according to the American Academy of Orthopaedic Surgeons (1965). Normal end-feel for this motion is firm due to the stretch of soft tissue structures in the cervical area.

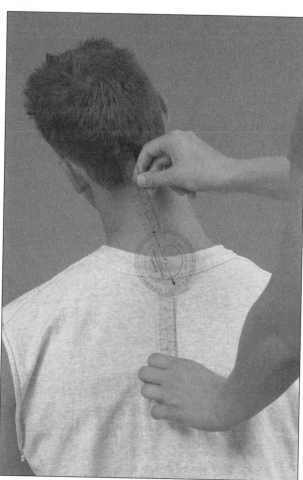

Figure 10-41 Proper positioning for cervical lateral flexion ROM. Source: Delmar/Cengage Learning

POSITION OF PATIENT: Sitting with spine in good postural position. Patient then tilts head toward one shoulder.

POSITION OF THERAPIST: Behind patient to align goniometer and stabilize the shoulder girdle, if needed, to prevent thoraco-lumbar lateral flexion during activity.

POSITION OF GONIOMETER:

- **Fulcrum:** Over the spinous process of C7 (see Figure 10-41)
- **Stationary arm:** Perpendicular to the ground, aligned with the thoracic spinous process
- **Movable arm:** Aligned with the occipital protuberance

Cervical Rotation

Cervical rotation occurs in the transverse plane around a vertical axis. The normal ROM is 60°, according to the American Academy of Orthopaedic Surgeons (1965). The end-feel for rotation is firm due to the stretch of soft tissue structures in the cervical area.

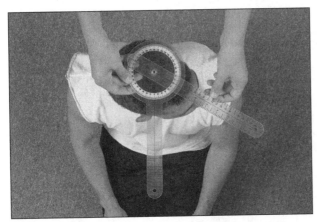

Figure 10-42 Proper positioning for cervical rotation ROM. Source: Delmar/Cengage Learning

POSITION OF PATIENT: Sitting with spine in good postural position. Patient then turns head as if to look over the shoulder. Patient may hold a tongue depressor between front teeth to extend the alignment point for easier visualization by therapist.

POSITION OF THERAPIST: Behind patient to align goniometer and stabilize the shoulder girdle, if needed, to prevent thoraco-lumbar rotation during activity.

POSITION OF GONIOMETER:

- **Fulcrum:** Center of the superior cranium (see Figure 10-42)

- **Stationary arm:** Aligned with an imaginary line that bisects the acromion processes

- **Movable arm:** Aligned with the tip of the nose (or centered on the tongue depressor)

Thoraco-Lumbar Flexion

Thoracic and lumbar flexion occurs in the sagittal plane around a frontal (medial/lateral) axis. The normal ROM is 4 cm. The end-feel is firm due to the stretch of soft tissue structures in the thoraco-lumbar area.

POSITION OF PATIENT: Standing with good posture and prepared to forward bend to a point just before the pelvis tips anteriorly.

POSITION OF THERAPIST: Behind patient to take preliminary measurement, then prepared to guide patient into position and prevent anterior pelvic tilt. As patient holds position, therapist uses tape measure to assess ROM.

POSITION OF TAPE MEASURE: Align tape measure with wax pencil markings or tape you have placed at C7 and S1. Take preliminary measurement with the patient in the upright position (see Figure 10-43). Move patient to the forward bent testing position and remeasure (see Figure 10-44). The difference between your two measurements is the thoraco-lumbar flexion.

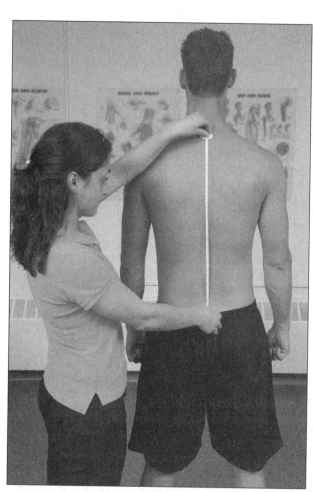

Figure 10-43 Proper starting position for thoraco-lumbar flexion ROM. Source: Delmar/Cengage Learning

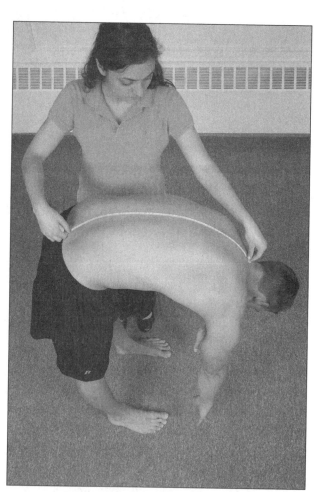

Figure 10-44 Proper ending position for thoraco-lumbar flexion ROM. Source: Delmar/Cengage Learning

Lumbar Flexion

Lumbar flexion occurs in the sagittal plane around a frontal (medial/lateral) axis. The end-feel is firm due to the stretch of soft tissue structures in the lumbar area.

POSITION OF PATIENT: Standing with good posture and prepared to forward bend to a point just before the pelvis tips anteriorly.

POSITION OF THERAPIST: Behind patient to take preliminary measurement, then prepared to guide patient into position and prevent anterior pelvic tilt. As patient holds position, therapist uses tape measure to assess ROM.

POSITION OF TAPE MEASURE: Using the MMST (Modified–Modified Schober Test), align tape measure with wax pencil markings or tape you have placed on the spine in line with the two posterior superior iliac spines and at a point 15 cm superior from the first marking (Van Adrichem & van der Korst, 1973). Take preliminary measurement with the patient in the upright position (see Figure 10-45). Move patient to the forward bent testing position and remeasure (see Figure 10-46). The difference between your two measurements is the lumbar flexion.

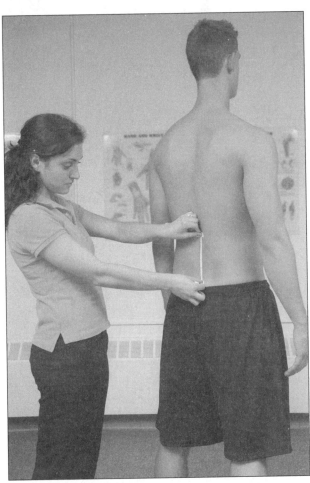

Figure 10-45 Proper starting position for lumbar flexion ROM. Source: Delmar/Cengage Learning

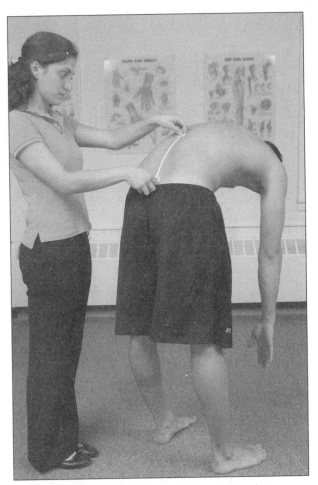

Figure 10-46 Proper ending position for lumbar flexion ROM. Source: Delmar/Cengage Learning

Thoraco-Lumbar Extension

Thoracic and lumbar extension occurs in the sagittal plane around a frontal (medial/lateral) axis. The end-feel is firm due to the stretch of soft tissue structures in the thoraco-lumbar area.

POSITION OF PATIENT: Standing with good posture and prepared to backward bend to a point just before the pelvis tips posteriorly.

POSITION OF THERAPIST: Behind patient to take preliminary measurement, then prepared to guide patient into position and prevent posterior pelvic tilt. As patient holds position, therapist uses tape measure to assess ROM.

POSITION OF TAPE MEASURE: Align tape measure with wax pencil markings or tape you have placed at C7 and S1. Take preliminary measurement with the patient in the upright position (see Figure 10-47). Move patient to the backward bent testing position and remeasure (see Figure 10-48). The difference between your two measurements is the thoraco-lumbar extension.

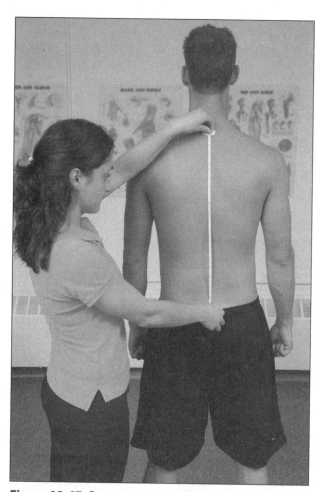

Figure 10-47 Proper starting position for thoraco-lumbar extension ROM. Source: Delmar/Cengage Learning

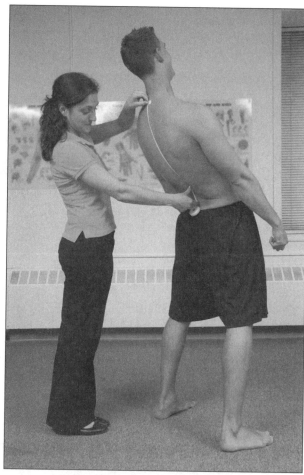

Figure 10-48 Proper ending position for thoraco-lumbar extension ROM. Source: Delmar/Cengage Learning

Lumbar Extension

Lumbar extension occurs in the sagittal plane around a frontal (medial/lateral) axis. The end-feel is firm due to the stretch of soft tissue structures in the lumbar area.

POSITION OF PATIENT: Standing with good posture and prepared to backward bend to a point just before the pelvis tips posteriorly.

POSITION OF THERAPIST: Behind patient to take preliminary measurement, then prepared to guide patient into position and prevent posterior pelvic tilt. As patient holds position, therapist uses tape measure to assess ROM.

POSITION OF TAPE MEASURE: Using the MMST (Modified–Modified Schober Test), align tape measure with wax pencil markings or tape you have placed on the spine in line with the two posterior superior iliac spines and at a point 15 cm superior from the first marking (Van Adrichem & van der Korst, 1973). Take preliminary measurement with the patient in the upright position (see Figure 10-49). Move patient to the backward bent testing position and remeasure (see Figure 10-50). The difference between your two measurements is the lumbar extension.

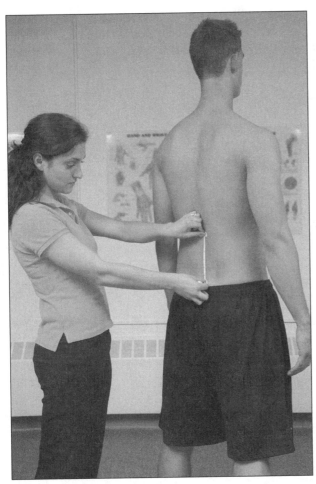

Figure 10-49 Proper starting position for lumbar extension ROM. Source: Delmar/Cengage Learning

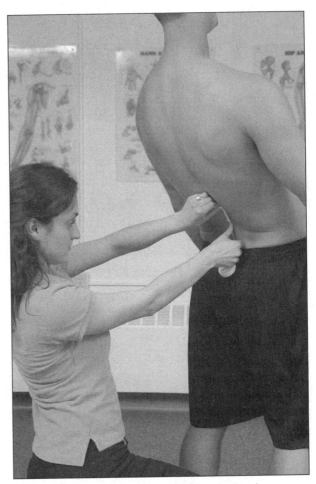

Figure 10-50 Proper ending position for lumbar extension ROM. Source: Delmar/Cengage Learning

Thoraco-Lumbar Lateral Flexion (Side-bend)

Lateral flexion of the spine occurs in a frontal plane around a sagittal axis. Normal ROM is 35°. The end-feel for this motion is firm due to the stretch of soft tissue structures in the thoraco-lumbar area.

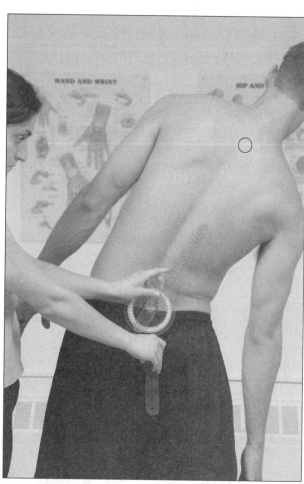

Figure 10-51 Proper positioning for thoraco-lumbar lateral flexion ROM. Source: Delmar/Cengage Learning

POSITION OF PATIENT: Standing with good posture and prepared to side-bend to a point just before the pelvis tips laterally.

POSITION OF THERAPIST: Behind patient to guide into the testing position and to align and read the goniometer.

POSITION OF GONIOMETER:

- **Fulcrum:** Over S1 (see Figure 10-51)
- **Stationary arm:** Perpendicular to the ground
- **Movable arm:** Aligned with C7

Thoraco-Lumbar Rotation

Thoraco-lumbar rotation occurs in a transverse plane around a vertical axis. Normal ROM is 45°, according to the American Academy of Orthopaedic Surgeons (1965). The end-feel is firm due to the stretch of soft tissue structures in the thoraco-lumbar area.

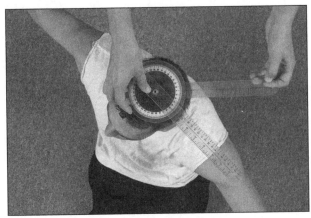

Figure 10-52 Proper positioning for thoraco-lumbar rotation ROM. Source: Delmar/Cengage Learning

POSITION OF PATIENT: Sitting with feet flat on the floor to help with stabilization. Patient prepares to rotate upper body to the side.

POSITION OF THERAPIST: Behind and above patient to align goniometer and stabilize pelvis as needed.

POSITION OF GONIOMETER:

- **Fulcrum:** Center of the superior cranium (see Figure 10-52)

- **Stationary arm:** Aligned with an imaginary line that bisects the two iliac crests

- **Movable arm:** Aligned with an imaginary line that bisects the two acromion processes

FUNCTIONAL APPLICATION

Adequate motion of the spine is necessary for most daily activities. ROM in the cervical area is necessary for activities such as answering the telephone, looking both ways before crossing a street, and drinking from a cup. ROM in the lumbar spine is necessary for ADLs of the lower body such as putting on shoes and socks or moving from the sit to stand/stand to sit positions. According to Norkin and White (1995), 40°–50° of cervical extension is required to look up at the ceiling, and 60°–70° of rotation is required to look over the shoulder for oncoming traffic while driving. Hsieh and Pringle (1994) determined that 56°–66° of lumbar flexion is required for sit-to-stand activities and that picking something up from the floor requires about 60° of flexion. After studying these chapters on individual joints, you can see that, by design, the human body functions well if normal ROM and muscle strength are present. Any deficits require the body to compensate through the use of surrounding joints or by altering its posture. Therefore, posture is the next subject to discuss in Chapter 11.

LEARNER CHALLENGE

1. Describe the bony structures of the spine and their joint motions. Then identify the plane and axis in which they occur.

2. Create a chart including the prime movers for all trunk motions as well as their innervations.

3. Palpate the following landmarks: Occipital protuberance, C7, spinous processes of the thoracic vertebrae, sacrum, SI joint.

4. On a lab partner, use a china marker to shade in the rectus abdominus and the obliques with your partner in supine. With your partner in prone, shade in the quadratus lumborum, intertransversarii, and interspinales. Instruct lab partner to perform appropriate trunk motions and observe/palpate the movement under your shaded areas.

POSTURE

OBJECTIVES

Upon completion of this chapter, the reader will be able to:

- Define posture and give examples of both static and dynamic posture.

- Identify the four normal curves of the spine.

- Define a plumb line and how it is used.

- Identify the proper positioning of the plumb line through the appropriate body segments for anterior, posterior, and lateral views.

- Recognize the common red flags for postural deviations when assessing posture in the anterior, posterior, and lateral views.

- Explain the proper alignment of body segments for ideal posture.

- Describe common abnormal standing postures.

- Describe the components of proper sitting and lying posture.

- Recognize abnormal sitting and lying postures.

ROLE OF PROPER POSTURE

The importance of good posture and the role it plays in overall function and mobility is often over-looked. The muscles in the body are continually working and making adjustments to maintain good posture against gravity. Posture is how one carries oneself. It is the relationship of body parts to one another as the body maintains itself against gravity. Proper posture helps promote back health by aligning the body segments, allowing the muscles to work properly and efficiently, reducing the stress on the ligaments of the spine, decreasing muscle fatigue by encouraging proper functioning, reducing the risk of muscle strain and overuse, and helping to minimize the abnormal wear and tear of the surface of the spinal joints.

Proper posture is maintained by the unique structure of the spine. Instead of being straight, the spine is comprised of a series of anterior and posterior curves that work together to counterbalance each other. To help decrease the risk of injury and to absorb shock, these curves should be maintained at all times. The four curves that make up the spine are the cervical, thoracic, lumbar, and sacral curves. The cervical and lumbar curves are convex anteriorly and counter the concave thoracic and sacral curves (see Figure 11-1).

Although the position of the spinal curves is the key to good posture, the pelvis also plays an important role. The position of the pelvis can greatly influence the lumbar region of the spine. For proper posture, the pelvis should be in neutral because this results in the appropriate amount of

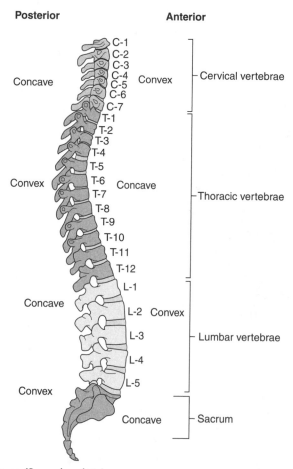

Figure 11-1 Spinal column curves *(See color plate).* Source: Delmar/Cengage Learning

curvature in the lumbar spine. The pelvis is in neutral when the anterior superior iliac spine (ASIS) and the posterior superior iliac spine (PSIS) are level with each other.

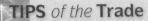

TIPS *of the* **Trade**

Place your hands on your hips with each index finger over the ASIS. Now tilt the pelvis forward in an exaggerated motion, and then tilt it backward. The index fingers will move forward during anterior tilt and back for posterior tilt. Neutral position is somewhere in between the two exaggerated motions.

Tilting the pelvis forward or anteriorly increases lumbar curvature and is called a **lordosis.** Tilting the pelvis back or posteriorly decreases the amount of lumbar curvature and is known as flat back.

The muscles responsible for contracting to stay upright in both static and dynamic postures are the hip, knee, trunk, and neck extensors. Collectively, they are known as the *antigravity muscles.* The trunk and neck flexors, lateral benders, hip abductors and adductors, and the ankle pronator and supinator muscles are also involved but do not play a major role. A person would fall to the ground if all these muscles relaxed.

The ankle plantar flexor and dorsiflexor muscles help control **postural sway.** Postural sway takes place due to the motion occurring at the ankles resulting in the forward and backward motion of the entire body when standing. The motion at the ankles is a result of the continual displacement of the body's center of gravity (COG) and the adjustments made within the base of support (BOS) to correct this displacement. The higher the COG and the smaller the BOS, the more postural sway is felt.

TIPS *of the* **Trade**

Try comparing standing up with your feet apart versus standing on your toes with the feet touching. More postural sway should be felt in the latter position due to the higher COG and smaller BOS.

Posture can be static or dynamic. Standing, sitting, and lying down are all considered **static posture** because the body stays in one place. Moving from one place to another or one position to another is considered **dynamic posture.** Assessing posture is easier to do when the patient is in a static position because the body is not moving. However, most of the guidelines for assessing static posture can be applied to dynamic posture. Postural assessment and evaluation are crucial parts of the rehab process because they help identify where stress and strain are being placed on the body, which in turn can cause poor posture. Evaluating posture can also provide information on potential problems by recognizing muscles weaknesses and imbalances that can result in pain and problems over time.

Posture is typically assessed in the standing position. The use of a **plumb line** is highly recommended when assessing standing posture. A plumb line is a string usually suspended from the ceiling with a weight attached to the end. The weight on the end makes a perfectly straight vertical line of gravity to use as a reference point. The plumb line can also be hooked to a **posture grid.** The patient stands in front of the posture grid and the therapist uses it as a point of reference. The plumb line is aligned with the feet because they provide the most stable reference point. The plumb line can be used to assess posture from an anterior, posterior, or lateral view.

Anterior View

When assessing posture from the anterior view, the plumb line should divide the body in two equal halves by passing through the middle of the body (see Figure 11-2A). The proper positioning of the body parts in relation to the plumb line should be as follows:

- **Head:** Level and in a neutral position without any flexion or hyperextension
- **Shoulders:** Even without any elevation or depression
- **Sternum:** Plumb line hangs through the center
- **Hips:** ASISs are even
- **Legs:** Regular BOS with feet shoulder width apart
- **Knees:** Even without signs of any **genu valgum** (knock knees) or **genu varum** (bow legs)
- **Ankles:** Arches are normal without a flattened or high longitudinal arch
- **Feet:** Toeing outward to some extent

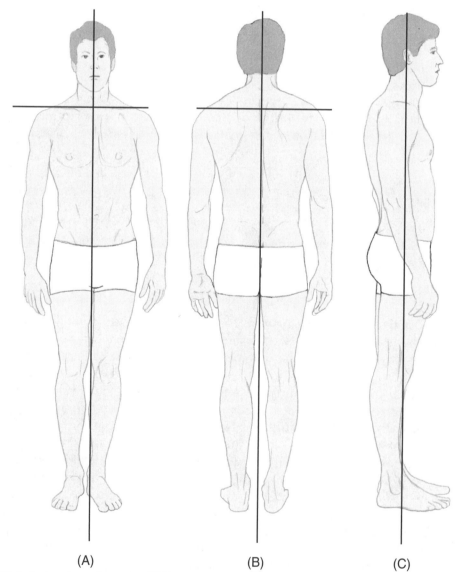

(A)   (B)   (C)

Figure 11-2 (A) Anterior view of posture (B) Posterior view of posture (C) Lateral view of posture *(See color plate).*

Source: Delmar/Cengage Learning

Once the patient is in this position, the therapist begins to systematically go through each body part to look for postural deviations. The following are common red flags to look for when observing posture from the anterior view:

- **Head**
  — Tilted/side bent
  — Rotated
  — Uneven mandibles
- **Shoulders**
  — Elevation
  — Depression

TIPS *of the* Trade

You can usually tell a person's dominant hand by observing the position of the shoulders. The shoulder on the dominant side will be slightly depressed or lower than the nondominant side.

- **Pelvis**
  — Uneven ASISs and iliac crests through palpation
- **Hips**
  — Medial rotation
  — Lateral rotation
  — Uneven greater trochanters meaning possible leg length discrepancy
- **Knees**
  — External/lateral **tibial torsion**
  — Internal/medial tibial torsion
  — Malaligned patella
- **Ankles**
  — Flattened longitudinal arch from a pronated foot with medial malleolus turning in
  — High arch from a supinated foot with lateral positioning of the lateral malleolus
- **Toes**
  — Hallux valgus: Great toe adducts toward the second toe
  — Claw toes: Extension of MTP joint with flexion of PIP and DIP joints
  — Hammer toes: Flexion of PIP joint, usually on second toe
  — Mallet toes: Flexion of DIP joint of toe

Posterior View

When assessing posture from the posterior view, the plumb line also divides the body into halves with similar positioning of the body segments (see Figure 11-2B). The body parts should be aligned with the plumb line as follows:

- **Head:** Level and in a neutral position without any flexion or hyperextension
- **Shoulders:** Even without any elevation or depression
- **Spinous processes:** Centered down the middle
- **Hips:** PSISs even
- **Legs:** Regular BOS with feet shoulder width apart
- **Knees:** Even without signs of any genu valgum or genu varum
- **Ankles:** Straight calcaneus

Again, with the patient and plumb line in position, the therapist can go through each body segment to look for postural deviations. Common red flags to be aware of in the posterior view are as follows:

- **Head**
  - Tilted/side bending
  - Rotated
- **Shoulders**
  - Elevation
  - Depression
- **Scapulae**
  - Protraction/abduction where the scapula moves away from the spine
  - Retraction/abduction where the scapula moves toward the spine
  - Winged where scapula demonstrates prominent inferior angles
- **Thoracic spine**
  - Lateral curvature/**scoliosis**
- **Lumbar spine**
  - Lateral curvature
- **Pelvis**
  - Lateral pelvic tilt discovered through PSIS palpation
  - Rotation
- **Knees**
  - Genu valgum or knock knees
  - Genu varum or bow legged
- **Ankles**
  - **Pes planus** or flat fleet due to fallen arches
  - **Pes cavus** or high arches

Lateral View

When assessing posture from the lateral view, the plumb line is set up to divide the body into front and back halves (see Figure 11-2C). The plumb line should pass through the body segments in the following way:

- **Head:** Through the middle of the ear lobe
- **Shoulders:** Through the lateral end or tip of the acromion process
- **Thoracic spine:** Slightly anterior to the vertebral bodies
- **Lumbar spine:** Bisecting the vertebral bodies
- **Pelvis:** Middle of the iliac crest
- **Hips:** Through the greater trochanter
- **Knees:** Slightly posterior to the patella of the extended knee
- **Ankles:** Slightly anterior to the lateral malleolus of the ankle in neutral position

With the patient in proper positioning, the therapist can go through each landmark and observe any postural deviations. Common red flags to look for in the lateral view are as follows:

- **Head**
  - Forward resulting in a forward head posture
- **Cervical spine**
  - Decreased or flattened curve
  - Increased or exaggerated curve
- **Shoulders**
  - Rounded
- **Thoracic spine**
  - Kyphosis or exaggerated curve
- **Lumbar spine**
  - Decreased or flattened curve
  - Increased or exaggerated curve
- **Pelvis**
  - Anterior tilt resulting in an increased lumbar curve
  - Posterior tilt resulting in a decreased lumbar curve
- **Knees**
  - Flexion of knees
  - **Genu recurvatum** or hyperextension of the knees
- **Ankles**
  - Longitudinal arch flattened
  - Longitudinal arch exaggerated

Good Standing Posture

Now that each specific view has been discussed, it is time to put the pieces together for proper posture. When all the body segments are aligned correctly, ideal posture is achieved. A person with ideal posture demonstrates the head in neutral position with no bending, tilting, or rotation, resulting in a normal cervical curve. The shoulders are level and the scapulae in neutral with the medial borders basically parallel and equal distance from the spine. The spinal curves are all normal with no exaggerations, flattening, or lateral curvatures. The pelvis is in neutral with even ASISs and PSISs. The hips and knees are neither flexed nor hyperextended with each hip joint and each knee joint level with each other respectively. There is no hip abduction or adduction or knee genu valgum, varum, or recurvatum present. The ankles are in neutral with the toes slightly pointing outward. The feet are slightly apart with no ankle supination or pronation.

As for the muscles during ideal posture, all the anterior and posterior muscles are in balance as the abdominal muscles pull up and the legs pull down, keeping the pelvis in neutral. Core stability is provided to the trunk through contraction of the abdominal and back extensor muscles. The antigravity muscles are strong and balanced to contract and keep the body upright against gravity (see Figure 11-3). It is important to remember every patient is different, and slight variations from ideal posture can be present and not result in any pain or postural problems. These slight variations can be normal for that person. Problems occur when the variations progress and begin to cause pain and discomfort. Over time, the body compensates and faulty postures can emerge.

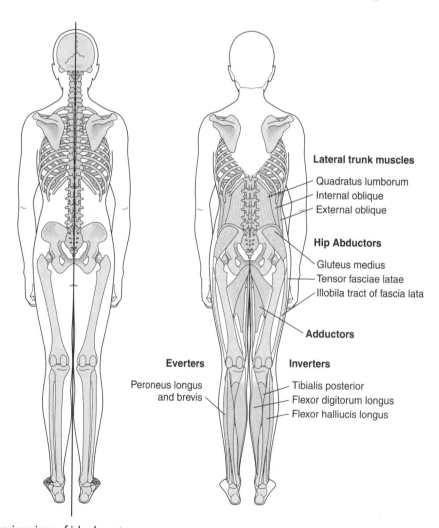

Figure 11-3 Posterior view of ideal posture. Source: Delmar/Cengage Learning

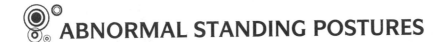

ABNORMAL STANDING POSTURES

Any pronounced deviation from ideal or good posture is considered to be faulty or abnormal posture. The causes of these deviations are many and can range from structural problems, congenital deformities, acquired deformities from a trauma, neurological conditions, muscle imbalances, or functional/nonstructural problems that stem from bad habits like repetitive slouching. As a general rule, postures with increased curves result in short and strong muscles on the concave side and longer weaker muscles on the convex side of the curve. The following section discusses a few of the more common abnormal postures. However, this is by no means a comprehensive list.

Kyphosis-Lordosis Posture

A kyphosis-lordosis posture occurs when one or more of the vertebral curves become out of balance, thus affecting all four spinal curves. A person with this abnormal posture demonstrates a forward head positioning resulting in hyperextension of the upper cervical spine, flexion of the lower cervical spine, and flexion of the upper thoracic spine. Overall, the entire thoracic spine demonstrates increased flexion or kyphosis resulting in a rounded or protruding upper back (see Figure 11-4). Because of the thoracic kyphosis, the scapulae are protracted. This hunched back appearance is typically seen in the elderly population due to compression fractures. The entire lumbar spine shows increased hyperextension or lordosis, resulting in anterior pelvis tilt. This in turn causes hip flexion and slight hyperextension of the knees, pushing the legs backward. This backward movement of the legs then causes slight plantar flexion of the ankle joints.

With the body segments all out of alignment, the muscles become unbalanced. Over time, the one-joint hip flexor muscles, the neck extensor muscles, and the low back muscles all shorten. In addition, the neck flexors, erector spinae, external oblique, and hamstring muscles all elongate and weaken. The unbalanced muscles increase risk of injury to all the joints involved.

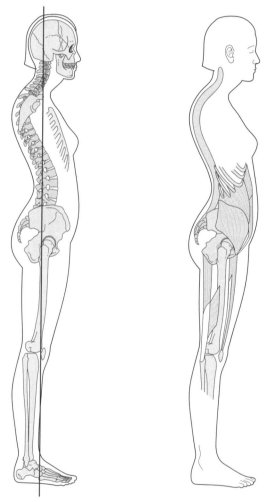

Figure 11-4 Kyphosis-lordosis posture. Source: Delmar/Cengage Learning

Sway Back

Sway back posture is often mistaken for the kyphosis-lordosis posture. As with the kyphosis posture, the curves of the back are out of balance. Like the previous posture, a person with sway back demonstrates a forward head positioning, resulting in hyperextension of the upper cervical spine and flexion of the lower cervical spine. The patient also presents with an elongated thoracic spine that is easily observed when using the plumb line (see Figure 11-5). The thoracic spine is posteriorly displaced in relation to the plumb line. The lumbar spine demonstrates a decrease in lordosis or curvature. This decrease in lordosis results in a posterior pelvic tilt, which in turn creates a hyperextension of the hip joint. The body compensates by forwardly displacing the pelvis. This helps to stabilize the body weight when the trunk is being displaced posteriorly. The knees hyperextend but the ankles can remain in neutral.

Because the curves of the body are out of alignment, the length of the muscles change over time. The cervical flexor, upper back extensor, external oblique, and the one joint hip flexor muscles all become weak and elongated. The hamstring, upper fibers of the internal oblique, and low back extensor muscles all become short and strong. Again this muscle imbalance opens the door for all sorts of injuries.

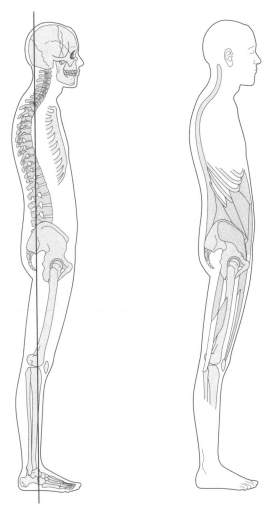

Figure 11-5 Sway back posture. Source: Delmar/Cengage Learning

Military Posture

Military posture is often thought of to be a good posture because a person stands so straight and tall. At times, it can be mistaken for normal or ideal posture. Military posture is considered a faulty posture because the curves of the spine are out of alignment (see Figure 11-6). While the head can be in neutral, it is usually thrust forward, demonstrating axial extension and a decrease in the cervical lordosis. In this posture, the chest is also pushed forward with the shoulders tightly pulled back, resulting in a straight upright thoracic spine. The lumbar spine shows an increased lordosis, causing the pelvis to anteriorly tilt and the hips to flex. The anterior tilt causes the knees to hyperextend or lock. The hamstring muscles work to resist the tendency of the hips to flex, while the calf muscles resist the tendency of the ankles to dorsiflex due to the knees being locked. As time passes and this posture remains, the muscles of the chest are elongated and weak while the upper back muscles are tight and strong.

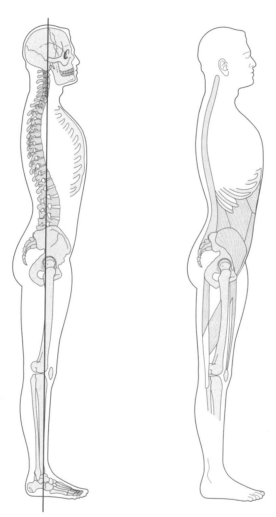

Figure 11-6 Military posture. Source: Delmar/Cengage Learning

Scoliosis

To this point, we have reviewed faulty postures with exaggerated or flattened curves of the spine. A lateral curvature of the spine is called *scoliosis*. From the posterior view, the spine may resemble the letters S or C (see Figure 11-7). Scoliosis may result from a congenital, **idiopathic,** or neuromuscular condition or be a secondary symptom from another condition. A person with scoliosis may present with uneven shoulders or waist or with the head off center. As with all other faulty postures, the curves are out of alignment, causing muscular imbalances that result in pain and dysfunction.

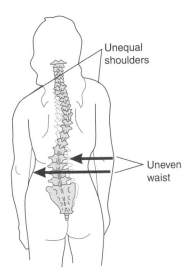

Unequal shoulders

Uneven waist

Figure 11-7 Scoliosis posture. Source: Delmar/Cengage Learning

SITTING AND SUPINE POSTURES

While standing is the most common position used to assess posture, sitting and lying down may also be assessed. Especially for people who spend a lot of time seated, this position can place a great deal of pressure on the disks in the spine. Merely sitting with good posture can result in far more pressure on the disks of the back than when standing. Sitting improperly over long periods of time can result in an increased chance of injury to these disks. Just leaning forward to shift weight will further increase the pressure on the disks. Add to that reaching or picking up an object, and the disc pressure continues to increase. Sitting without back support, or what is commonly called *slouched posture,* can also increase the pressure on the disks due to the decrease in the lumbar curve (see Figure 11-8). The lack of a back support results in the constant contraction of the core muscles to keep the body upright. These are just a few of the reasons why sitting with good posture and support are so important.

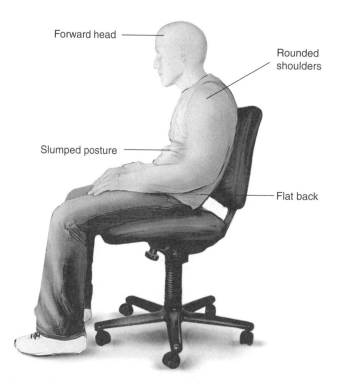

Figure 11-8 Abnormal/slouched sitting posture. Source: Delmar/Cengage Learning

What is proper sitting posture? It entails sitting with the normal curves maintained by (see Figure 11-9):

- Having the back straight
- The shoulders back
- Using a chair with back support and a towel roll for lumbar support
- Distributing weight evenly through both hips
- Knees bent
- Feet flat on the floor
- Changing positions every 30 minutes

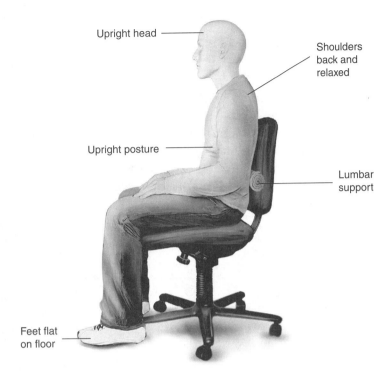

Upright head

Shoulders back and relaxed

Upright posture

Lumbar support

Feet flat on floor

Figure 11-9 Proper sitting posture. Source: Delmar/Cengage Learning

By being aware of one's posture, corrections can be made throughout the day to decrease the risk of a faulty postural habit forming, which in turn can result in pain and dysfunction.

Contrary to sitting posture, properly lying supine places the least amount of pressure on the disks in the back and is considered a resting position (see Figure 11-10). The body is basically in the same position as standing so a plumb line running horizontally would intersect the same body segments as if standing. Sidelying is also a common resting position. When in the sidelying position, the bottom leg is extended and the top leg is flexed with a pillow between the knees to keep the hips in good alignment. When lying down in any position, the surface should support the normal curves of the body. A common cause of poor lying posture is a surface that is too soft or too firm. This places the curves of the spine in an unbalanced position (see Figure 11-11).

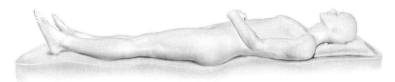

Figure 11-10 Proper supine lying posture. Source: Delmar/Cengage Learning

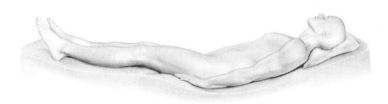

Figure 11-11 Abnormal supine lying posture. Source: Delmar/Cengage Learning

FUNCTIONAL APPLICATION

Overall, good posture should be maintained whatever the body's position. Using good body mechanics and maintaining the normal spinal curves are keys to decreasing the amount of stress and strain on the trunk and muscles of the body. This in turn helps decrease the chance of faulty postural habits forming that over time can lead to pain, injury, and dysfunction. The therapist plays a crucial role in early identification of postural deviations and muscles imbalances. Once they are identified, proper interventions can be implemented to correct the postural deviations before structural changes occur. The sooner problems are identified, the sooner and more easily they can be corrected.

LEARNER CHALLENGE

1. Using a plumb line and postural grid, if available, practice the proper positioning of the plumb line through the appropriate body segments on your lab partner in the anterior, posterior, and lateral views. Then switch roles.

2. Once the plumb line is properly positioned on your lab partner, go through each body segment and look for the common red flags for postural deviations in the anterior, posterior, and lateral views. Then switch roles and compare each other's findings.

3. Between you and your partner, list the components of good posture in sitting, standing, and lying down.

4. With a lab partner, research a condition or disease that affects posture like scoliosis, ankylosing spondylitis, or pregnancy. Analyze the information and discuss how that patient would present, how the spinal curves would be affected, what muscles would be weak and elongated, what muscles would be short and strong, and how other systems are affected.

GAIT

OBJECTIVES

Upon completion of this chapter, the reader will be able to:

- Define the gait cycle.

- Explain the difference between stride length and step length.

- Identify the five stages of the stance phase and describe the muscle actions involved.

- Identify the three stages of the swing phase and describe the muscle actions involved.

- Define periods of double support, single support, and nonsupport during the gait cycle.

- Define the determinants of gait and describe the role of the pelvis in them.

- Describe common abnormal gait patterns and how the body compensates for them.

THE GAIT CYCLE

Most people give little thought to the process of walking. It is often taken for granted as one moves through the day from place to place. Walking is the general term used to describe moving about on foot. *Human gait* refers specifically to the style or manner of walking. It is the result of various complex interactions between the joints and muscles of the lower extremities, with support from the trunk and upper extremities. While it is true that each person has a unique style of gait, the same basic components make up the normal gait cycle. This cycle consists of the activity that occurs from the time of initial contact of the heel of one foot until that same heel comes back into contact with the ground.

Definitions

The distance of one gait cycle is known as **stride length.** It is measured using the distance from the heel strike of one foot to the distance of the next heel strike of the same foot (see Figure 12-1).

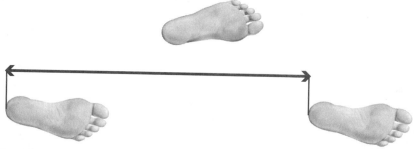

Figure 12-1 Stride length. Source: Delmar/Cengage Learning

Step length is different from stride length. Step length is the distance between heel strikes of the right and left foot (see Figure 12-2). By taking a step, one experiences a period of double support, single support, and a stance and swing phase.

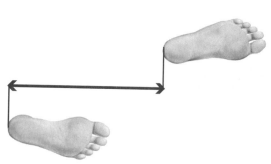

Figure 12-2 Step length. Source: Delmar/Cengage Learning

The **gait cycle** can be broken down into the stance phase and the swing phase. The **stance phase** pertains to the activity that occurs when the foot is in contact with the ground. This phase begins when one foot touches the ground and goes on until that foot leaves the ground. The stance phase provides stability as the lower extremity supports the body so it can move over the supporting limb; this phase accounts for 60% of the gait cycle. The stance phase is divided into the following five stages: heel strike, foot flat, midstance, heel off, and toe off (see Figure 12-3). The **swing phase** begins when the toe of the extremity leaves the ground and ends when the heel of the same extremity hits the ground.

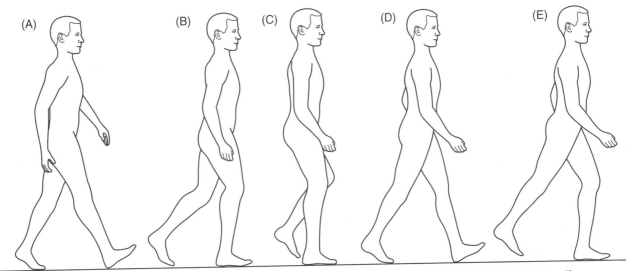

(A) (B) (C) (D) (E)

Figure 12-3 Five stages of the stance phase (A) Heel strike (B) Foot flat (C) Midstance (D) Heel off (E) Toe off.

Source: Delmar/Cengage Learning

Heel strike is the moment the heel makes initial contact with the ground and signals the start of the stance phase. The ankle of the foot is in neutral while the hip and knee begin to flex, resulting in some shock absorption. The trunk remains erect and is rotated to the opposite side. The opposite arm is forward and the same side arm is back in hyperextension of the shoulder. Heel strike is the weight-loading portion of the stance phase as the body weight begins to shift to the stance leg.

During heel strike, one foot is initially contacting the ground while the other foot is supporting the body weight. It is here that the first period of double support is observed. Double support is when both feet are touching the ground at the same time and occurs twice during each gait cycle (see Figure 12-4). One period occurs when the left leg is ending its stance phase and the other occurs when the right leg is ending its stance phase.

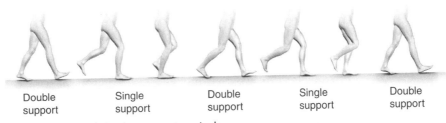

Double support Single support Double support Single support Double support

Figure 12-4 Double support and single support periods. Source: Delmar/Cengage Learning

The amount of time spent with double support can vary according to one's **cadence,** or walking speed. Cadence is measured by counting the number of steps per minute. Walking slower increases the time both feet are on the ground or in double support, while walking faster decreases it. While walking includes periods of double support and single support, which will be discussed later, it does not entail a period of nonsupport. Nonsupport is a period of time in which neither foot is in contact with the ground. This is seen only in running and represents the biggest difference between the gait cycles of these two movements.

Stance Phase

Although it does not look complex, a lot of muscle activity occurs during heel strike. At the beginning, the dorsiflexors are actively keeping the ankle in neutral. Next, the quadriceps muscles begin to contract eccentrically to minimize knee flexion, while the hip extensors contract to minimize any further hip flexion. Finally, the trunk is kept upright by the erector spinae muscles actively contracting, and the pelvis is anteriorly rotated.

The second stage of the stance phase is called *foot flat*. This occurs just after heel strike and is when the foot is flat on the ground. Here the ankle plantar flexes slightly. The foot is kept from slapping flat on the ground by the eccentric contraction of the dorsiflexor muscles. The pelvis continues to rotate anteriorly, and the upper body begins to catch up with the leg as the hip moves into extension and the knee slightly flexes. The weight of the body continues to move onto the stance limb.

The third stage is called *midstance,* which occurs as the weight of the body passes over the stance limb and the body reaches its highest point in the gait cycle. During midstance, a person can balance on one leg, thus supporting the entire weight of the body. This is known as *single support* (see Figure 12-4). Two periods of single support occur during a gait cycle, first when the left foot is the only limb on the ground supporting the body weight and second when the right foot is the only limb on the ground. Here the plantar flexors contract to control the rate the limb progresses over the ankle, putting it into slight dorsiflexion. The pelvis is now rotating posteriorly, and the trunk continues to be in neutral with both arms parallel to it in shoulder extension. The knee and hip continue to extend.

The fourth stage occurs when the heel rises off the ground and is appropriately known as *heel off.* In this stage, the weight of the body starts to transfer onto the other leg as the stance foot is preparing to leave the ground. Ankle dorsiflexion and plantar flexion occur as the heel comes off the ground, signaling the start of the *push-off* phase. During the push-off phase, the ankle plantar flexor muscles contract, propelling the body forward. The knee joint is almost fully extended with the hip in hyperextension, abduction, and external rotation. The trunk starts to rotate to the same side, as the shoulders move into flexion, swinging the arms forward.

The fifth and final stage of the stance phase is *toe off.* Toe off includes the time before and during which the toes leave the ground. The ankle slightly plantar flexes while the hip and knee flex. This signals the end of the stance phase and the beginning of the second phase of the gait cycle known as the *swing phase.*

Swing Phase

The swing phase pertains to all non-weight-bearing activities during gait when the foot is not in contact with the ground. There are three stages of the swing phase: acceleration, midswing, and deceleration (see Figure 12-5). During acceleration, the hip and knee rapidly flex as the ankle dorsiflexes to help the limb behind the body move forward to catch up. The pelvis is in posterior rotation. With the ankle now in neutral, the knee at full flexion and the hip slightly flexed, the swing leg is brought up to the stance leg, allowing the foot to clear the ground as it swings through. This is known as *midswing*. Finally, deceleration occurs as the ankle remains in neutral through active contraction of the dorsiflexor muscles, while the hamstring muscles eccentrically contract to slowly extend the knee. This allows the swing leg to slow down to prepare for heel strike. The pelvis begins to move into anterior rotation from posterior rotation.

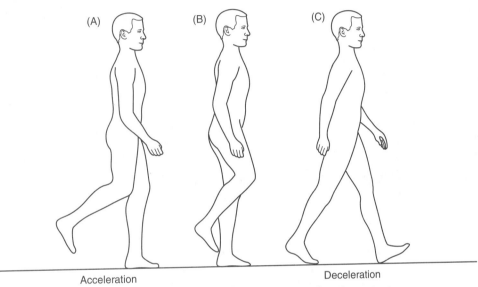

Figure 12-5 Swing phases of gait (A) Acceleration (B) Midswing (C) Deceleration. Source: Delmar/Cengage Learning

It is important to note the terms used to describe the phases of gait in this text are traditional terms. However, another set of terminology developed by the Gait Laboratory at Rancho Los Amigos Medical Center has become quite common. Both sets of terminology divide the gait cycle into the stance and swing phases, with five components in the stance phase and three in the swing phase. As noted previously, traditional terminology refers to the five components of the stance phase as heel strike, foot flat, midstance, heel off, and toe off. Rancho Los Amigos terminology refers to these components as initial contact, loading response, midstance, terminal stance, and preswing. Traditional terms for the components of swing phase are acceleration, midswing, and deceleration, while Rancho Los Amigos labels these as initial swing, midswing, and terminal swing. The main distinction between the two sets of terms is that the traditional terms refer to *points in time* during the gait cycle, and the Rancho Los Amigos terms refer to *periods of time* during the gait cycle (Lippert, 2000).

Other Factors

The previous discussion of the phases of gait has focused mainly on the actions of the lower extremities with brief mention of the trunk and upper extremities. Other determinants of gait are the adjustments made by the body to keep its center of gravity in place. During ambulation, the center of gravity is both vertically and horizontally displaced equally.

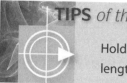

TIPS *of the* Trade

Hold a piece of chalk in your hand with your arm stretched out to the side and walk the length of the chalkboard. The line moving up and down like a wave represents the vertical displacement of your center of gravity.

The adjustments or determinants of gait help to minimize the horizontal and vertical displacement of the center of gravity. The pelvis plays a big role in minimizing displacement. When walking, the pelvis laterally tilts up and down in the frontal plane.

TIPS *of the* Trade

Place your hands on your hips and walk across the room. It is easy to feel how the hips move up and down as your pelvis drops slightly on each side.

Lateral pelvic tilt occurs at toe off as the weight of the body is taken off the lower extremity (see Figure 12-6). This lateral tilt or dip is very small secondary to the actions of the hip abductor muscles on the opposite side and the erector spinae muscles on the same side. The two muscles contract together to keep the pelvis fairly level. For example, when the pelvis on the non-weight-bearing side, or right, tilts down during toe off, the left or weight-bearing hip has no choice but to adduct.

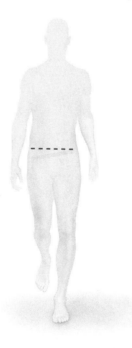

Figure 12-6 Lateral pelvic tilt. Source: Delmar/Cengage Learning

To off set this left hip adduction and keep the pelvis level, the left hip abductors contract. The erector spinae muscles on the right side also play a role. They attach to the pelvis and contract to pull up on the side of the pelvis, which would otherwise tilt excessively to drop (see Figure 12-7).

The pelvis also shifts side to side and rotates during gait. Shifting side to side helps center the upper body and trunk over the stance leg. This results in decreased lateral movement of the body's center of gravity and helps to maintain balance. Pelvis rotation also helps maintain balance, decrease the body's center of gravity, and regulate the speed of walking. The pelvis rotates one way, and the trunk rotates in the opposite direction.

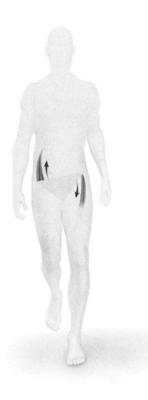

Figure 12-7 Abductor and erector spinae muscles working together to minimize pelvic tilt. Source: Delmar/Cengage Learning

ABNORMAL GAIT

Now that we have examined normal gait cycle, we can move on to abnormal gait. Many patients present with problems resulting in abnormal gait. These problems can range from muscle weakness to decreased joint ROM to pain to neurological involvement. When working with patients with gait problems, it is best to observe them from the side, front, and back to get the entire picture. Side observations give the best view of step length, lower extremity activity, arm swing, and trunk and head position. The anterior and posterior views offer the best look at the head and shoulder position, lateral pelvic tilt, and **step width.** Step width is the distance between the two feet. It is found by drawing lines through the midpoints of each heel and measuring the distance between them (see Figure 12-8).

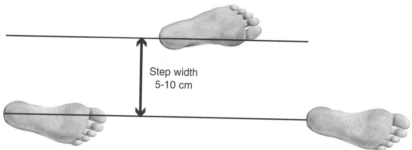

Step width
5-10 cm

Figure 12-8 Step width. Source: Delmar/Cengage Learning

Common Abnormal Gait Patterns

A review of some common abnormal gait patterns provides a brief introduction to the causes and results of these abnormalities.

- **Trendelenberg Gait:** Also known as *gluteus medius gait,* this pattern occurs when the gluteus medius muscle on one side is weak. For example, a weak right gluteus medius or hip abductor muscle results in the left side of the pelvis significantly dropping when the left lower extremity leaves the ground to begin the swing phase. The person shifts the trunk to the affected side during stance phase to compensate.

- **Rocking Horse Gait:** Also known as *gluteus maximus gait,* this occurs when the gluteus maximus muscle is weak, resulting in continual hip extension during the stance phase. The trunk quickly shifts posterior to compensate. The excessive forward and backward shifting of the trunk during gait resembles that of a rocking horse.

- **Quadriceps Gait:** This occurs when the quadriceps muscles are weak, resulting in the inability to extend the knee during the stance phase. The body compensates with forward flexion of the trunk and strong plantar flexion of the ankle, resulting in hyperextension of the knee.

- **Hamstring Weakness:** When the hamstrings are weak, both the stance and the swing phase are affected. During the stance phase, the knee demonstrates genu recurvatum or excessive knee hyperextension. During deceleration of the swing phase, the knee slaps into extension because the hamstring muscles are not strong enough to slow down the forward swing of the lower extremity.

- **Foot Slap:** The foot slaps onto the ground during heel strike due to weak dorsiflexor muscles. The ankle is not able to support the weight of the body at heel strike.

- **Foot Drop:** Also known as *steppage gait,* this occurs when the dorsiflexor muscles are weak or paralyzed. This weakness results in the inability of the toes to clear during the swing phase. The body compensates by lifting the knee higher to allow the foot drop or plantar-flexed ankle to clear the floor. Instead of heel strike, there is toe strike because the dorsiflexor muscles are not strong enough to dorsiflex the ankle.

- **Sore Foot Limp:** Most noticeable when walking up hills, this occurs when the gastrocnemius and soleus, or triceps surae group, are weak. The ankle demonstrates decreased ability to plantar flex or heel rise at push off. The body compensates by displaying a shortened step length on the affected side.

- **Waddling Gait:** This pattern presents with shoulders behind the hips when standing with little or no reciprocal pelvis or trunk rotation. To compensate, the entire side of the body must swing forward to progress the leg forward in a waddling motion. This waddling is often accompanied by a lumbar lordosis and steppage gait. This gait pattern is commonly seen in people with muscular dystrophy.

- **Antalgic Gait:** This gait pattern typically occurs when a person has pain in any of the joints in the lower extremity. The result is a shortened stance phase because it hurts to stand on it. The painful side usually demonstrates a short abducted stance phase resulting in a fast and short step length on the uninvolved side. The reciprocal arm swing also compensates by shortening.

- **Hemiplegic Gait:** This pattern is seen in patients who suffered from a cerebrovascular accident (CVA), and the severity of the gait depends on the severity of the CVA, as well as the degree of **spasticity** or **flaccidity** present. Typically, the person shifts the body to the uninvolved side to be able to circumduct the involved leg during the swing phase. Circumduction is necessary to compensate for the weak or paralyzed dorsiflexor muscles. The involved foot lands flat footed or toe first instead of the normal heel strike usually seen during the stance phase. The involved side demonstrates a longer step length and little or no reciprocal arm swing due to the flexed pattern of the involved upper extremity.

- **Ataxic Gait:** A person with this pattern ambulates with a wide base of support with jerky and unsteady movements of both upper and lower extremities. They demonstrate difficulty ambulating in a straight line and tend to stagger.

- **Scissors Gait:** Spasticity in the hip adductor muscles result in the swing phase limb crossing midline to hit the stance limb during ambulation.

- **Parkinsonian Gait:** This pattern presents with a shuffling gait, flexed trunk and lower extremities, as well as decreased reciprocal arm swing and stride length. Overall, the person demonstrates diminished movement and difficulty initiating movements. The flexed trunk results in a forward center of gravity. A **festinating gait** is observed in advanced cases secondary to the forward center of gravity. To regain balance and refrain from falling, a person ambulates with many short and rapid steps.

- **Crouch Gait:** This is common when there is injury or disease to both lower extremities. An exaggerated reciprocal arm swing is present to compensate for excessive lumbar lordosis, anterior pelvic tilt, hip and knee flexion, and ankle plantar flexion.

- **Equinus Gait:** This results from a leg length discrepancy and varies in severity. A minimal discrepancy results in the dropping of the pelvis on the affected side, placing increased stress on the lower back. A person with a moderate discrepancy will walk on the ball of the foot of the shorter leg because merely dropping the pelvis is no longer effective. Severe discrepancies result in dropping of the pelvis and walking on the ball of the foot on the shorter side, as well as flexing the knee of the longer limb.

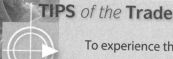

TIPS *of the* **Trade**

To experience the equinnus gait, walk with one leg on a curb and the other on the road.

FUNCTIONAL APPLICATION

The previous section lists only a few of the gait abnormalities you may encounter in your work. The human gait is a complex combination of muscle and joint movements that work together to allow ambulation. Having some basic knowledge of the events that occur during a normal gait cycle and familiarity with some abnormal gait patterns can help identify and treat patients with gait problems. It is important to observe the entire person to develop a complete picture of the extent of the problem. Pain in one area can be the result of a problem in a different area altogether. The body is efficient at compensating when problems arise. However, these compensations can lead to more problems and abnormalities down the road. Therefore, it is crucial to identify and correct the issue as soon as possible to avoid further complications and functional limitations.

LEARNER CHALLENGE

1. Sprinkle baby powder on the floor and have your lab partner step in it with both feet and take a few steps. Take a tape measure and measure step width and stride length using the foot prints made with the baby powder. Then switch roles.

2. Pick three different abnormal gait patterns from the chapter and demonstrate them one at a time to your lab partner while he or she determines which one it is and explains the deficits. Then switch roles.

3. With your lab partner, visit a busy spot on campus. Pick one person and observe him or her ambulating. Each person is to record observations on the person's gait pattern and note any abnormalities. Then compare your observations and discuss the findings.

·NOTES

APPENDIX A: MUSCLE AND NERVE CHARTS

Courtesy of Lisa Kihl. Reprinted with permission.

Ankle and Foot Muscles

POSTERIOR (SUPERFICIAL)

MUSCLE	MUSCLE ACTION	INNERVATION	SPINAL SEGMENT	ORIGIN	INSERTION
Gastrocnemius: medial head*	Knee flexion Ankle plantar flexion	Tibial	S1,S2	Medial condyle of femur	Posterior calcaneus
Gastrocnemius: lateral head	Knee flexion Ankle plantar flexion	Tibial	S1,S2	Lateral condyle of femur	Posterior calcaneus
Soleus	Ankle plantar flexion	Tibial	S1,S2	Posterior tibia and fibula	Posterior calcaneus
Plantaris*	Weak knee flexion Plantar flexion	Tibial	L4,L5,S1	Posterior lateral condyle of femur	Posterior calcaneus

*Indicates a two-joint muscle.

POSTERIOR DEEP TO THE GASTROCNEMIUS

MUSCLE	MUSCLE ACTION	INNERVATION	SPINAL SEGMENT	ORIGIN	INSERTION
Tibialis posterior	Ankle inversion Assists plantar flexion	Tibial	L5,S1	Interosseous membrane Adjacent tibia and fibula	Navicular Most tarsals and metatarsals
Flexor digitorum longus*	Flexes 4 lesser toes Ankle inversion Plantar flexion	Tibial	L5,S1	Posterior tibia	Distal phalanx of 4 lesser toes

*Indicates a two-joint muscle.

continues

POSTERIOR DEEP TO THE GASTROCNEMIUS (continued)

MUSCLE	MUSCLE ACTION	INNERVATION	SPINAL SEGMENT	ORIGIN	INSERTION
Flexor digitorum brevis	Flexion 4 lesser toes	Medial plantar	S2,S3	Calcaneus	MP joint 2–5 toes
Flexor hallucis longus*	Flexes great toe Assists inversion Plantar flexion	Tibial	L5,S1,S2	Posterior fibula Interosseous membrane	Distal phalanx of great toe
Flexor hallucis brevis*	Flexion of great toe Flexion of MP joints and toes	Medial plantar	S2,S3	Cuboid bone plantar surface	Proximal phalanx great toe both sides of base

*Indicates a two-joint muscle.

ANTERIOR (FROM KNEE TO ANKLE)

MUSCLE	MUSCLE ACTION	INNERVATION	SPINAL SEGMENT	ORIGIN	INSERTION
Tibialis anterior	Ankle inversion Dorsiflexion	Deep peroneal	L4,L5,S1	Lateral tibia Interosseous membrane	1st cuneform Metatarsal
Extensor hallucis longus*	Extends 1st toe Ankle inversion Dorsiflexion	Deep peroneal	L4,L5,S1	Fibula interosseous membrane	Distal phalanx of great toe
Extensor digitorum longus*	Extends 4 lesser toes Ankle dorsiflexion	Deep peroneal	L4,L5,S1	Fibula interosseous membrane and tibia	Distal phalanx of 4 lesser toes
Extensor digitorum brevis*	Extend toes MP joint	Fibular nerve	S1,S2	Anterior part calcaneus bone	Base of great toe

*Indicates a two-joint muscle.

LATERAL GROUP (FROM KNEE TO ANKLE)

MUSCLE	MUSCLE ACTION	INNERVATION	SPINAL SEGMENT	ORIGIN	INSERTION
Peroneus longus	Eversion	Superficial peroneal	L4,L5,S1	Lateral proximal fibula Interosseus membrane	Plantar surface of 1st cuniform and metatarsal
Peroneus brevis	Eversion	Superficial peroneal	L4,L5,S1	Lateral distal fibula	Base of 5th metatarsal
Peroneus tertius	Dorsiflexion Eversion	Deep peroneal	L4,L5,S1	Distal medial fibula	Base of 5th metatarsal

Brachial Plexus

AXILLARY NERVE SPINAL CORD SEGMENT C5,C6

	MUSCLE INNERVATION
Brachial plexus C5–T1	Deltoid
Brachial plexus C5–T1	Teres minor

MUSCULOCUTANEOUS NERVE SPINAL CORD SEGMENT C5,C6

	MUSCLE INNERVATION
Brachial plexus C5–T1	Coracobrachialis
Brachial plexus C5–T1	Biceps
Brachial plexus C5–T1	Brachialis

RADIAL NERVE SPINAL CORD SEGMENT C6–T1

	MUSCLE INNERVATION
Brachial plexus C5–T1	Triceps
Brachial plexus C5–T1	Anconeus
Brachial plexus C5–T1	Brachioradialis
Brachial plexus C5–T1	Supinator
Brachial plexus C5–T1	Extensor carpi radialis longus and brevis
Brachial plexus C5–T1	Extensor digitorum
Brachial plexus C5–T1	Extensor digiti minimi
Brachial plexus C5–T1	Extensor carpi ulnaris
Brachial plexus C5–T1	Extensor pollicis longus and brevis
Brachial plexus C5–T1	Extensor indicis
Brachial plexus C5–T1	Abductor pollicis longus

MEDIAN NERVE SPINAL CORD SEGMENT C6–T1

	MUSCLE INNERVATION
Brachial plexus C5–T1	Pronator teres
Brachial plexus C5–T1	Flexor carpi radialis
Brachial plexus C5–T1	Palmaris longus
Brachial plexus C5–T1	Flexor digitorum superficialis
Brachial plexus C5–T1	Flexor digitorum profundus
Brachial plexus C5–T1	Flexor pollicis longus
Brachial plexus C5–T1	Pronator quadratus
Brachial plexus C5–T1	Abductor pollicis brevis
Brachial plexus C5–T1	Opponens pollicis

ULNAR NERVE SPINAL CORD SEGMENT C8,T1

	MUSCLE INNERVATION
Brachial plexus C5–T1	Flexor carpi ulnaris
Brachial plexus C5–T1	Flexor digitorum profundus
Brachial plexus C5–T1	Adductor pollicis
Brachial plexus C5–T1	Palmaris brevis
Brachial plexus C5–T1	Abductor digiti minimi
Brachial plexus C5–T1	Opponens digiti minimi
Brachial plexus C5–T1	Flexor digiti minimi
Brachial plexus C5–T1	3rd and 4th lumbricals
Brachial plexus C5–T1	Dorsal and palmar interossei

Hip Muscles

HIP FLEXORS (ANTERIOR)

MUSCLE	MUSCLE ACTION	INNERVATION	SPINAL SEGMENT	ORIGIN	INSERTION
Iliopsoas: psoas major	Hip flexion	Ventral rami	L1,L2,L3	Surfaces of T12-L5	Lesser trochanter
Iliopsoas: iliacus	Hip flexion	Femoral	L2,L3	Iliac fossa	Lesser trochanter
Rectus femoris*	Hip flexion Knee extension	Femoral	L2,L3,L4	AIIS	Tibial tuberosity
Sartorius*	Hip flexion Knee flexion Lateral rotation Hip abduction	Femoral	L2,L3	ASIS	†Proximal medial aspect of tibia

*Indicates a two-joint muscle.
†Pes Anserine- Common distal attachment for 3 muscles Sartorius, Gracilis, Semitendinosis on the anterior medial proximal tibia.

ADDUCTORS (MEDIAL)

MUSCLE	MUSCLE ACTION	INNERVATION	SPINAL SEGMENT	ORIGIN	INSERTION
Pectineus	Hip flexion Hip adduction	Femoral	L2,L3,L4	Superior ramus of pubis	Pectineal line of femur
Adductor longus	Hip adduction	Obturator	L3, L4	Pubis	Middle 3rd of the linea aspera
Adductor brevis	Hip adduction	Obturator	L3, L4	Pubis	Pectineal line proximal linea aspera
Adductor magnus	Hip adduction	Obturator sciatic	L3, L4	Ischium and pubis	Entire linea aspera and adductor tubercle
Gracilis*	Hip adduction	Obturator	L2,L3	Pubis	†Anterior medial surface of proximal end of tibia

*Indicates a two-joint muscle.
†Pes Anserine- Common distal attachment for 3 muscles Sartorius, Gracilis, Semitendinosis on the anterior medial proximal tibia.

HIP EXTENSORS (POSTERIOR)

MUSCLE	MUSCLE ACTION	INNERVATION	SPINAL SEGMENT	ORIGIN	INSERTION
Gluteus maximus	Hip extension Hyperextension Lateral rotation	Inferior gluteal	L5,S1,S2	Posterior sacrum and ilium	Posterior femur distal to greater trochanter and iliotibial band

continues

HIP EXTENSORS (POSTERIOR) *(continued)*

MUSCLE	MUSCLE ACTION	INNERVATION	SPINAL SEGMENT	ORIGIN	INSERTION
HAMSTRINGS					
Semimembranosus*	Extends hip Flexes knee	Sciatic	L5,S1,S2	Ischial tuberosity	Posterior of medial condyle of tibia
Semitendinosus*	Extends hip Flexes knee	Sciatic	L5,S1,S2	Ischial tuberosity	†Anterior medial surface of proximal tibia
Biceps femoris: short head*	Flexes knee	Common peroneal	L5,S1,S2	Linea aspera	Fibular head
Bicep femoris: long head*	Extends hip Flexes knee	Sciatic	S1,S2,S3	Ischial tuberosity	Fibular head

*Indicates a two-joint muscle.
†Pes Anserine- Common distal attachment for 3 muscles Sartorius, Gracilis, Semitendinosis on the anterior medial proximal tibia.

ABDUCTORS (LATERAL)

MUSCLE	MUSCLE ACTION	INNERVATION	SPINAL SEGMENT	ORIGIN	INSERTION
Gluteus medius	Hip abduction	Superior gluteal	L4,L5,S1	Lateral ilium	Greater trochanter
Gluteus minimus	Hip abduction Medial rotation	Superior gluteal	L4,L5,S1	Lateral ilium	Greater trochanter
Tensor fascia latae*	Abduction Hip flexion	Superior gluteal	L4,L5	ASIS	Lateral condyle of tibia

*Indicates a two-joint muscle.

DEEP ROTATORS (POSTERIOR)

MUSCLE	MUSCLE ACTION	INNERVATION	SPINAL SEGMENT	ORIGIN	INSERTION
Obturator externus	Hip lateral rotation	Obturator	L5,S1	Ramus of pubis	Greater trochanter
Obturator internus	Hip lateral rotation	Nerve to obturator interus	L5,S1	Ramus of pubis	Trochanteric fossa
Quadratus femoris	Hip lateral rotation	Nerve to quadratus femoris	L5,S1	Ischial tuberosity	Greater trochanter
Piriformis	Hip lateral rotation	Anterior rami	S1,S2	Ischium	Greater trochanter
Gemellus superior	Hip lateral rotation	Nerve to obturator interus	L5,S1	Ischium	Greater trochanter
Gemellus inferior	Hip lateral rotation	Nerve to quadratus femoris	L5,S1	Ischium	Greater trochanter

Extrinsic Muscles of Hand

EXTRINSIC FLEXOR MUSCLES OF FINGER (ANTERIOR)

MUSCLE	MUSCLE ACTION	INNERVATION	SPINAL SEGMENT	ORIGIN	INSERTION
Flexor digitorum superficialis*	Flexes MCP and PIP joints	Median nerve	C7,C8,T1	Common flexor tendon Coronoid process and radius	Sides of middle phalanx of the 4 fingers
Flexor digitorum profundus*	Flexes all 3 joints of the finger	Median Ulnar	C8,T1	3/4 of ulnar shaft	Distal phalanx of 4 fingers

*Indicates a two-joint muscle.

EXTRINSIC EXTENSOR MUSCLES OF FINGER (POSTERIOR)

MUSCLE	MUSCLE ACTION	INNERVATION	SPINAL SEGMENT	ORIGIN	INSERTION
Extensor digitorum*	Extends all 3 joints of the finger	Radial nerve	C6,C7,C8	Lateral epicondyle of humerus	Base of distal phalanx of 2nd-5th fingers
Extensor digiti minimi*	Extends all 3 joints of 5th finger	Radial nerve	C6,C7,C8	Distal ulna	Base of distal phalanx of 5th fingers
Extensor indicis*	Extends all 3 joints of 2nd finger	Radial nerve	C6,C7,C8	Distal ulna	Base of distal phalanx of 2nd fingers

*Indicates a two-joint muscle.

DEEP POSTERIOR FOREARM

MUSCLE	MUSCLE ACTION	INNERVATION	SPINAL SEGMENT	ORIGIN	INSERTION
Flexor pollicis longus	Flexes all 3 joints of the thumb	Median nerve	C8,T1	Radius anterior surface	Distal phalanx of thumb
Abductor pollicis longus*	Abducts thumb	Radial nerve	C7,C8,T1	Posterior radius interosseous membrane	Base of 1st metacarpal

continues

DEEP POSTERIOR FOREARM *(continued)*

MUSCLE	MUSCLE ACTION	INNERVATION	SPINAL SEGMENT	ORIGIN	INSERTION
Extensor pollicis brevis*	Extends CMC and MCP joint of thumb	Radial nerve	C6,C7	Posterior distal radius	Base of proximal phalanx of thumb
Extensor pollicis longus*	Extends all 3 joints of the thumb	Radial nerve	C6,C7,C8	Middle posterior ulna and interosseous membrane	Base of distal phalanx of thumb

*Indicates a two-joint muscle.

Knee Muscles

KNEE EXTENSORS (ANTERIOR)

MUSCLE	MUSCLE ACTION	INNERVATION	SPINAL SEGMENT	ORIGIN	INSERTION
QUADS					
Rectus femoris*	Knee extension Hip flexion	Femoral nerve	L2,L3,L4	AIIS	Tibial tuberosity
Vastus lateralis	Knee extension	Femoral nerve	L2,L3,L4	Greater trochanter	Tibial tuberosity via patellar tendon
Vastus medialis	Knee extension	Femoral nerve	L2,L3,L4	Greater trochanter	Tibial tuberosity via patellar tendon
Vastus intermedialis	Knee extension	Femoral nerve	L2,L3,L4	Anterior femur	Tibial tuberosity via patellar tendon

*Indicates a two-joint muscle.

KNEE FLEXORS (POSTERIOR)

MUSCLE	MUSCLE ACTION	INNERVATION	SPINAL SEGMENT	ORIGIN	INSERTION
Popliteus	Knee flexion	Tibial	L4,L5,S1	Lateral condyle of femur	Posterior medial condyle of tibia
Gastrocnemius*	Knee flexion Ankle plantar flexion	Tibial	S1,S2	Medial and lateral condyles	Posterior calcaneus
HAMSTRINGS					
Semimembranosus*	Extends hip Flexes knee	Sciatic	L5,S1,S2	Ischial tuberosity	Posterior of medial condyle of tibia
Semitendinosus*	Extends hip Flexes knee	Sciatic	L5,S1,S2	Ischial tuberosity	Anteromedial surface of proximal tibia
Biceps femoris: short head	Flexes knee	Common peroneal	L5,S1,S2	Lateral lip if linea aspera	Fibular head
Biceps femoris: long head*	Extends hip Flexes knee	Sciatic	S1,S2,S3	Ischial tuberosity	Fibular head

*Indicates a two-joint muscle.

Head, Neck, and Trunk Muscles

HEAD AND NECK MUSCLES

MUSCLES	ACTION	INNERVATION	ORIGIN	INSERTION
Masseter	Closes lower jaw	Mandibular division of trigeminal nerve	Zygomatic process of maxilla and zygomatic arch	Lateral mandible
Temporalis	Closes lower jaw	Mandibular division of trigeminal nerve	Temporal fossa	Coronoid process
Scm	**Bilaterally:** Flexes neck and hyperextends **Unilaterally:** Bends the neck; rotates head to the opposite side	Accessory	Sternum and medial clavicle	Mastoid process
Semispinalis capitis	Extends Rotates the head	Spinal nerve	Transverse process C4–C7 and T1–T2	Occipital bone
Semispinalis cervicis	Extends Rotates the head	Spinal nerve	Transverse process T1–T5	Spinous processes C2–C7
Splenius capitis	**Bilateral:** Extends the head **Unilateral:** Rotates the head to same side	Spinal nerve	Lower half of nuchal ligament Spinous process C7–T3	Mastoid process and occipital bone
Splenius cervicis	Extends cervical vertebrae	Spinal nerve	Nuchal Ligamentum Spinous process C7	Spinous process of axis C2
Longissismus capitis	Extends Rotates the head	Cervical nerves	Transverse processes of T1–T5 Articular processes of C5–C7	Posterior mastoid process
Anterior scalene	**Bilateral:** Assists in neck flexion	Lower cervical nerve	Transverse process C3–C6	Inserts first rib
Middle scalene	Unilateral neck flexion	Lower cervical nerve	Transverse process C2–C7	Inserts first rib
Posterior scalene	Neck lateral bending	Lower cervical nerve	Transverse process C5–C7	Inserts second rib

TRUNK MUSCLES

MUSCLES	ACTION	INNERVATION	ORIGIN	INSERTION
Rectus abdominis	Trunk flexion Abdominal compression	7–12 intercostal nerves	Pubis	Cartilage of 5–7 ribs
External oblique	**Bilaterally:** Trunk flexion; compression of abdomen **Unilaterally:** Lateral bending; rotation to opposite side	8–12 intercostal nerves	Ribs 4–12	Iliac crest and abdominal aponeurosis to linea alba
Internal oblique	**Bilaterally:** Trunk flexion; compression of abdomen **Unilaterally:** Lateral bending; rotation to same side	8–12 intercostal nerves	Inguinal ligament; iliac crest	Ribs 9–12; abdominal aponeurosis
Transverse abdominis	Compression of abdomen	7–12 intercostal nerves	Inguinal ligament; iliac crest Thoracolumbar fascia; lower 6 Ribs	Abdominal aponeurosis to linea alba
Quadratus lumborum	Trunk lateral bending	L12–L1	Iliac crest	Twelfth rib; transverse process of all 5 lumbar vertebrae
Erector spinae	Extends bilaterally	Spinal nerves	Spinous and transverse processes Ribs from the occiput to sacrum and ilium	Spinous and transverse processes Ribs from the occiput to sacrum and ilium

Shoulder Girdle

POSTERIOR SHOULDER GIRDLE

MUSCLE	MUSCLE ACTION	INNERVATION	SPINAL SEGMENT	ORIGIN	INSERTION
Upper trapezius	Scapular elevation Upward rotation	Spinal accessory (cranial nerve XI)	C3,C4	Occipital bone, Nuchal ligament	Outer 3rd of clavicle acromion process
Middle trapezius	Scapular retraction	Spinal accessory (cranial nerve XI)	C3,C4	Spinous process of C7–T3	Scapular spine
Lower trapezius	Scapular depression Upward rotation	Spinal accessory (cranial nerve XI)	C3,C4	Spinous process of middle and lower thoracic vertebrae	Base of scapular spine
Levator scapula	Scapular elevation Downward rotation	3rd and 4th cervical nerves Dorsal scapular nerve	C5	Transverse process of 1st 4 cervical vertebrae	Vertebral border of scapula between superior angle and spine
Rhomboid	Scapular retraction Elevation Downward rotation	Dorsal scapular nerve	C5	Spinous process C7–T5	Vertebral border of scapula between spine inferior angle

ANTERIOR LATERAL SHOULDER GIRDLE

MUSCLE	MUSCLE ACTION	INNERVATION	SPINAL SEGMENT	ORIGIN	INSERTION
Serratus anterior	Scapular protraction Upward rotation	Long thoracic nerve	C5,C6,C7	Lateral surface of the 8 ribs	Vertebral border of scapula anterior surface

ANTERIOR SHOULDER GIRDLE

MUSCLE	MUSCLE ACTION	INNERVATION	SPINAL SEGMENT	ORIGIN	INSERTION
Pectoralis minor (lies deep to the pectoralis major; only shoulder girdle muscle located on the anterior surface)	Scapular depression Protraction downward rotation and tilt	Medial pectoral nerve	C8, T1	Anterior surface 3rd–5th ribs	Coracoid process of the scapula

LATERAL SHOULDER JOINT

MUSCLE	MUSCLE ACTION	INNERVATION	SPINAL SEGMENT	ORIGIN	INSERTION
Anterior deltoid (line of pull horizontal)	Shoulder abduction Flexion Internal rotation Horizontal adduction	Axillary nerve	C5, C6	Lateral 3rd of the clavicle	Deltloid tuberosity
Middle deltoid (line of pull vertical)	Shoulder abduction	Axillary nerve	C5, C6	Acromion process	Deltloid tuberosity
Posterior deltoid (line of pull horizontal)	Shoulder abduction Extension Hyperextension External rotation Horizontal abduction	Axillary nerve	C5, C6	Spine of scapula	Deltloid tuberosity

POSTERIOR SHOULDER JOINT

MUSCLE	MUSCLE ACTION	INNERVATION	SPINAL SEGMENT	ORIGIN	INSERTION
Supraspinous	Shoulder abduction	Lateral medial pectoral nerve	C5–C8, T1	Supraspinous fossa of the scapula	Greater tubercle of the humerus
Infraspinatus	Shoulder external rotation Horizontal abduction	Lateral medial pectoral nerve	C5–C8, T1	Infraspinous fossa of scapula	Greater tubercle of the humerus

continues

POSTERIOR SHOULDER JOINT *(continued)*

MUSCLE	MUSCLE ACTION	INNERVATION	SPINAL SEGMENT	ORIGIN	INSERTION
Pectoralis major (clavicular vertical line of pull)	Shoulder adduction Internal rotation Horizontal adduction Shoulder flexion first 60 degrees (from 180–120)	Lateral medial pectoral nerve	C5–C8, T1	Medial 3rd clavicle	Lateral lip of bicipital groove of humerus
Pectoralis major sternal	Shoulder extension (1st 60 degrees from 180–120)	Lateral medial pectoral nerve	C5–C8, T1	Sternocostal cartilage of 1st 6 ribs	Lateral lip of bicipital groove of humerus
Latissismus dorsi	Shoulder extension Adduction Internal rotation Hyper-extension	Thoracodorsal nerve	C6,C7,C8	Spinous processes of T7–L5 posterior surface of sacrum, iliac crest, and lower three ribs	Medial lip of bicipital groove of humerus
Teres major	Shoulder extension Adduction Internal rotation	Subscapular nerve	C5,C6	Axillary border of scapula near inferior angle	Crest below lesser tubercle next to latissimus dorsi attachment
Teres minor	Shoulder external rotation Horizontal abduction	Axillary nerve	C5,C6	Axillary border of scapula near inferior angle	Greater tubercle of the humerus
Subscapularis (deep to the scapula horizontal line of pull)	Shoulder internal rotation	Subscapular nerve	C5,C6	Subscapular fossa of scapula	Lesser tubercle of humerus
Coracobrachialis	Stablizes shoulder joint	Musculocutaeous nerve	C6,C7	Coracoid process of scapula	Medial surface of the humerus near midpoint

Lumbo-Sacral Plexus

FEMORAL NERVE SPINAL CORD SEGMENT L2–L4

Lumbar plexus L1–L5	MUSCLE INNERVATION
	Hip flexors: Iliopsoas: iliacus
	Sartorius
	Pectineus
	Quads: Rectus femoris
	Vastus lateralis
	Vastus medialis
	Vastus intermedialis

OBTURATOR EXTERNUS SPINAL CORD SEGMENT L2–L4

Lumbar plexus L1–L5	MUSCLE INNERVATION
	Adductors: Adductor externus
	Adductor longus
	Adductor brevis
	Adductor magnus
	Gracilis

SCIATIC NERVE SPINAL CORD SEGMENT L4–S3

Sacral plexus L4–S4	MUSCLE INNERVATION
	Hamstrings: Semimembranous
	Semitendinosus
	Bicep femoris: longhead

TIBIAL NERVE SPINAL CORD SEGMENT L4–S3

Sacral plexus L4–S4	MUSCLE INNERVATION
	Knee Flexor: Popliteus
	Plantar Flexors: Soleus
	Plantaris
	Gastroc: medial/lateral heads
	Tibialis posterior
	Flexor digitorum longus
	Flexor hallucis longus

Elbow and Wrist Muscles

ELBOW JOINT

MUSCLE	MUSCLE ACTION	INNERVATION	SPINAL SEGMENT	ORIGIN	INSERTION
Brachialis (deep to biceps)	Elbow flexion	Musculocutaneous nerve	C5,C6	Distal half of humerus anterior surface	Coronoid process of the ulna
Biceps brachii*	Elbow flexion Forearm supination	Musculocutaneous nerve	C5,C6	**Long head:** Supraglenoid tubercle of scapula **Short Head:** Coracoid process of scapula	Radial tuberosity, bicipital aponeurosis
Brachioradialis	Elbow flexion	Radial nerve	C7,C8	Lateral supracondylar ridge on the humerus	Lateral shaft of radius just proximal to the styloid process
Triceps*	Elbow extension	Radial nerve	C7,C8	**Long Head:** Infraglenoid tubercle of scapula **Medial Head:** Posterior surface of humerus **Lateral Head:** inferior to greater tubercle on posterior humerus	Proximal posterior surface of the olecranon process, capsule of the elbow
Anconeus	Assists in elbow extension	Radial nerve	C7,C8	Lateral epicondyle of humerus	Lateral aspect of the olecranon, posterior surface of the upper ¼ shaft of the ulna
Pronator teres	Forearm pronation assistive in elbow flexion	Median nerve	C6,C7	Medial epicondyle of humerus coronoid process of ulna	Middle portion of the lateral shaft of the radius
Pronator quadratus	Forearm pronation	Median nerve	C8, T1	Distal one fourth of radius	Distal ¼ of the anterior surface of the radius
Supinator	Forearm supination	Radial nerve	C6	Lateral epicondyle of humerus and adjacent ulna	Radial tuberosity, proximal ⅓ of lateral shaft of the radius

*Indicates a two-joint muscle.

WRIST JOINT

MUSCLE	MUSCLE ACTION	INNERVATION	SPINAL SEGMENT	ORIGIN	INSERTION
Flexor carpi ulnaris	Wrist flexion Ulnar deviation	Ulnar nerve	C8, T1	Medial epicondyle of humerus	Pisiform, Hamate, 5th metacarpal, flexor retinaculum
Flexor carpi radialis	Wrist flexion Radial deviation	Median nerve	C6, C7	Medial epicondyle of humerus	Base of 2nd and 3rd metacarpals, palmar surface
Palmaris longus	Assists wrist flexion	Median nerve	C6, C7	Medial epicondyle of humerus	Flexor retinaculum, palmar aponeurosis
Extensor carpi radialis longus	Wrist extension Radial deviation	Radial nerve	C6, C7	Supracondylar ridge of humerus	Base of 2nd metacarpal, dorsal surface
Extensor carpi radialis brevis	Wrist extension	Radial nerve	C6, C7	Lateral epicondyle of humerus	Base of 3rd metacarpal dorsal surface
Extensor carpi ulnaris	Wrist extension Ulnar deviation	Radial nerve	C6, C7, C8	Lateral epicondyle of humerus	Base of 5th metacarpal, tubercle on ulnar side

APPENDIX B:
JOINT MOVEMENTS

JOINT MOVEMENTS

JOINT	MOTION	PLANE	AXIS
Hip	Flexion	Sagittal	Frontal
	Extension	Sagittal	Frontal
	Abduction	Frontal	Sagittal
	Adduction	Frontal	Sagittal
	Lateral/external rotation	Transverse	Vertical
	Medial/internal rotation	Transverse	Vertical
Knee	Flexion	Sagittal	Frontal
	Extension	Sagittal	Frontal
Ankle	Dorsiflexion	Sagittal	Frontal
	Plantarflexion	Sagittal	Frontal
	Inversion	Frontal	Sagittal
	Eversion	Frontal	Sagittal
Toes	Flexion	Sagittal	Frontal
	Extension	Sagittal	Frontal
Shoulder	Flexion	Sagittal	Frontal
	Extension	Sagittal	Frontal
	Abduction	Frontal	Sagittal
	Adduction	Frontal	Sagittal
	Horizontal abduction	Transverse	Vertical
	Horizontal adduction	Transverse	Vertical
	Lateral/external rotation	Transverse	Vertical
	Medial/internal rotation	Transverse	Vertical
Elbow	Flexion	Sagittal	Frontal
	Extension	Sagittal	Frontal
Forearm	Supination	Transverse	Vertical
	Pronation	Transverse	Vertical

continues

JOINT MOVEMENTS *(continued)*

JOINT	MOTION	PLANE	AXIS
Wrist	Flexion	Sagittal	Frontal
	Extension	Sagittal	Frontal
	Ulnar deviation	Frontal	Sagittal
	Radial deviation	Frontal	Sagittal
Hand	Finger flexion	Sagittal	Frontal
	Finger extension	Sagittal	Frontal
	Finger abduction	Frontal	Sagittal
	Finger adduction	Frontal	Sagittal
	Thumb flexion	Frontal	Sagittal
	Thumb extension	Frontal	Sagittal
	Thumb abduction	Sagittal	Frontal
	Thumb adduction	Sagittal	Frontal
Neck	Flexion	Sagittal	Frontal
	Extension	Sagittal	Frontal
	Lateral flexion	Frontal	Sagittal
	Rotation	Transverse	Vertical
Trunk	Flexion	Sagittal	Frontal
	Extension	Sagittal	Frontal
	Lateral flexion	Frontal	Sagittal
	Rotation	Transverse	Vertical

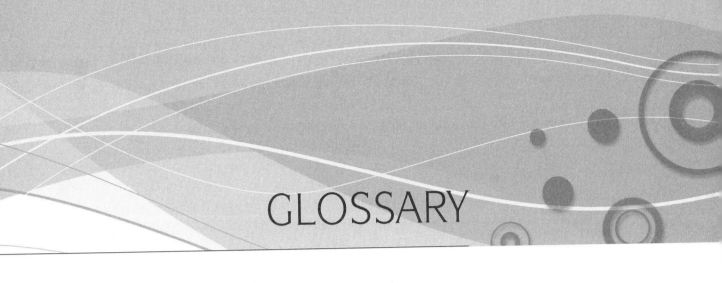

GLOSSARY

abduction: any movement away from the midline of the body.

active insufficiency: the point at which a two-joint muscle can no longer actively contract.

active range of motion (AROM): the unassisted and voluntary motion of a joint.

activities of daily living (ADLs): activities done in the context of a normal day such as dressing, personal hygiene, locomotion.

adduction: any movement toward the midline of the body.

against gravity: positioning patients so they are lifting the body part using gravity as part of the resistance; gravity must be overcome to move the body part.

ambulation: walking or going from one place to the other.

anatomical position: the position of standing erect, feet flat, and palms facing forward.

anterior: referring to the front side of the body, the abdominal or ventral side.

appendicular skeleton: the part of the skeleton that moves around a fixed axial base and pertains to the structures of the arms and legs.

axial skeleton: the base of support around which appendicular muscles pull for movement; includes the skull, vertebral column, and rib cage.

axis of motion: the point around which a movement occurs.

break test: procedure used to test muscle strength in which the clinician applies pressure in the opposite direction of the body part's movement, thereby trying to force the body part back in the direction it came.

cadence: walking speed, measured by counting the number of steps per minute.

capsular: specific and expected pattern of restriction in joints.

caudal: pertaining to the tail.

cephalad: refers to the head.

circumduction: the action of moving a limb in a cone-shaped figure.

compass inclinometers: measuring tools that use a compass face to indicate changes in position.

concave: a hollow indentation forming a bowl-like structure.

connective tissue: tissue that binds and supports other structures or tissues in the body.

contractile tissue: structures that can contract or shorten like muscles and their tendonous attachments to the bone.

contractures: when a joint is in a permanent flexed position from the shortening of muscles.

contralateral: opposite side of the point of reference.

convex: curved evenly or arched.

CROM: a specific device that measures cervical range of motion using a headpiece containing two gravity inclinometers and a compass inclinometer.

deep: under another structure or away from the surface.

depression: the downward motion of a structure.

distal: a position away from the trunk of the body.

dorsal: toward the back.

dorsiflexion: motion at the ankle bringing the toes up toward the shin.

double inclinometers: the use of two inclinometers to assess range of motion.

downward rotation: an angular motion describing the movement of the scapula going down and toward the vertebral column.

dynamic posture: moving from one place to another or one position to another.

elevation: upward motion of a structure.

end-feel: characteristic feeling of resistance to motion experienced by the examiner as he or she passively takes a joint to its end range.

eversion: movement that brings the sole of the foot outward.

extension: straightening motion that increases the angle of a joint.

external/lateral rotation: rotation of a joint away from the center or midline of the body.

fascia: fibrous tissue that covers muscles.

festinating gait: gait pattern in which the person's speed gets increasingly faster to compensate for the displaced center of gravity from the forward flexed posture.

fine motor movements: coordinated and precise movements from the use of small muscle groups.

flaccidity: weakness due to the lack of normal muscle tone.

flexion: bending movement that decreases the angle of a joint.

frontal axis: pivot point allowing motion only in the sagittal plane.

frontal plane: plane that divides the body into front and back sections.

fundamental position: essentially the same as anatomical position except the palms face the sides of the body.

gait: style or manner of walking.

gait cycle: activity that occurs from the time of initial contact of the heel of one foot until that same heel comes back into contact with the ground.

genu recurvatum: hyperextension of the knee joints.

genu valgum: condition in which the knees are positioned toward midline, forming an L; also known as knock knees.

genu varum: condition in which the knees are positioned laterally, also known as bow legged.

goniometer: a device used to measure joint angle, specifically angles created by the movement of human joints.

goniometry: medical term that refers to the measuring of joint movements.

gravity decreased: positioning the patient to allow for the motion to be done with as little gravitational interference as possible; gravity plays less of a role in the added resistance.

gravity inclinometers: devices used to measure range of motion based on gravitational pull.

gravity minimal: positioning the patient to allow for the motion to be done with as little gravitational interference as possible; gravity plays less of a role in the added resistance.

gravity resisted: positioning patients so they are lifting the body part using gravity as part of the resistance, gravity must be overcome to move the body part.

gross motor movements: bigger, more general movements using the large muscle groups in the body.

hinge joint: joint that allows movement only in the sagittal plane around a frontal axis.

horizontal abduction: movement bringing the arm across the chest toward midline with the shoulder at 90° of flexion.

horizontal adduction: movement bringing the arm away from midline with the shoulder at 90° of flexion.

hyperextension: straightening motion that increases the angle of a joint beyond its normal limits or beyond 0°.

idiopathic: no known cause.

impingement: a pinching of soft tissue, often a tendon between two hard surfaces, often bones or cartilage.

inclinometers: devices used to measure range of motion based on measuring the angles of movement through gravity or compass readings.

inferior: below or underneath.

internal/medial rotation: rotation of a joint toward the center or midline of the body.

inversion: movement that brings the sole of the foot in toward the ankle.

kyphosis: an increased or exaggerated curve of the thoracic spine, rounding of upper back or hunchback.

kyphotic curve: spinal curve that curves outward away from the center of the body.

lateral: away from midline or to the side.

lateral flexion: bending of a structure like the trunk to the right or left, also known as side-bending.

lordosis: increase in the lumbar curvature, an exaggerated lumbar curve.

lordotic curve: spinal curve that curves inward toward the center of the body.

medial: toward midline.

noncapsular patterns: when other conditions involving structures other than the joint capsule cause limitation in range of motion.

noncontractile tissue: refers to structures that cannot contract like ligaments, joint capsules, bursae, and fascia.

one-joint muscle: muscle that crosses only one joint.

passive range of motion (PROM): movement without any assistance from the patient.

pes cavus: high arches.

pes planus: flat fleet due to fallen arches.

planes of motion: how the body is divided.

plantar flexion: motion at the ankle resulting in the toes pointing down.

plumb line: tool used to assess posture, consisting of a string suspended from the ceiling with a weight attached to the end.

posterior: refers to a structure located on the backside of the body.

postural sway: the forward and backward motion of the entire body when standing due to the motion occurring at the ankles.

posture: the relationship of body parts to one another as the body maintains itself against gravity.

posture grid: a grid that goes behind a patient and is used as an assessment tool to correct and evaluate posture.

pronation: movement of the forearm inward resulting in the palm facing back or posteriorly.

prone: position described as lying horizontal with the face down.

protraction: any movement away from the midline in a plane parallel to the ground.

proximal: refers to an anatomical structure that is closer to the trunk of the body or closer to another structure.

radial deviation: lateral movement of the hand from anatomical position toward the radial side.

repeatability: able to reproduce the same results over and over.

retraction: movement in a parallel plane to the ground going away from midline.

rotation: the movement of a structure around its longitudinal axis.

sagittal axis: a pivot point allowing motion only in the frontal plane.

sagittal plane: the plane through the body that divides it into right and left sections.

scaption: midway between flexion and abduction.

scoliosis: a lateral curvature of the spine.

sesamoid bone: short bone that is usually found within the tendon of a muscle.

side-bending: bending of a structure like the trunk to the right or left, also known as lateral flexion.

spasticity: increased muscle tone.

stance phase of gait: activity that occurs when the foot is in contact with the ground and begins when one foot touches the ground and goes on until that foot leaves the ground.

static posture: when the body stays in one place.

step length: distance between heel strikes of the right and left foot.

step width: distance between the two feet found using the midpoints of each heel.

stride length: distance of one gait cycle measured using the distance from the heel strike of one foot to the distance of heel strike of the same foot again.

superficial: referring to the surface.

superior: higher than or above another structure.

supination: movement of the forearm outward, resulting in the palm facing upward.

supine: lying horizontal on the back with the face toward the ceiling.

swing phase: the part of the gait cycle in which the toe of the extremity leaves the ground and does not end until the heel of the same extremity hits the ground.

syndemosis joint: structure that supports the nonmovable joints between the bones.

synovial joint: freely movable joint consisting of a joint cavity filled with synovial fluid.

tibial torsion: a twisting of the tibia.

traction: putting a structure under tension with gentle pulling.

transverse plane: plane that divides the body into top and bottom parts.

two-joint muscle: muscle that crosses two joints.

ulnar deviation: medial movement of the hand from anatomical position toward the ulnar side.

uniaxial joint: joint with movement around one axis in one plane.

upward rotation: angular motion describing the movement of the scapula going up and away from the vertebral column.

valgus: positioned outward away from the midline.

varus: positioned inward toward the midline.

ventral: toward the belly and opposite of dorsal.

vertical axis: perpendicualr to the horizontal axis.

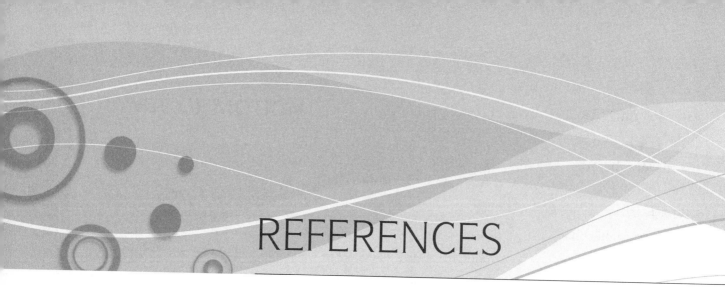

REFERENCES

American Academy of Orthopaedic Surgeons. (1965). *Joint motion: Methods of measuring and recording.* Chicago: Author.

Cyriax, J., & Coldham, M. (1984). *Treatment by manipulation, massage and injection. Textbook of orthopedic medicine, Vol. 2* (11th ed.). London: Bailliere-Tindall.

Hislop, H. J., & Montgomery, J. (2002). *Muscle testing: Techniques of manual examination* (7th ed.). Philadelphia: W. B. Saunders.

Hsieh, C. Y., & Pringle, R. K. (1994). Range of motion of the lumbar spine required for four activities of daily living. *Journal of Manipulative & Physiological Therapeutics, 17*(6), 353–358.

Jevsevar, D. S., Riley, P. O., Hodge, W. A., & Krebs, D. E. (1993, April). Knee kinematics and kinetics during locomotor activities of daily living in subjects with knee arthroplasty and in healthy control subjects. *Physical Therapy, 73*(4), 229–239.

Lippert, L. S. (2000). *Clinical kinesiology for physical therapist assistants* (3rd ed.). Philadelphia: F. A. Davis.

Livingston, L. A., Stevenson, J. M., & Olney, S. J. (1991, May). Stairclimbing kinematics on stairs of different dimensions. *Archives of Physical Medicine and Rehabilitation, 72*(6), 398–402.

Matsen, F. A., Sidles, J. A., & Harryman, D. T. (1994). *Practical evaluation and management of the shoulder.* Philadelphia: W. B. Saunders.

Norkin, C., & White, J. D. (1995). *Measurement of joint motion: A guide to goniometery.* Philadelphia: F. A. Davis.

Professional Staff Association, Rancho Los Amigos Medical Center. (1989). *Observational gait analysis handbook.* Downey, CA: Author.

Ryu, J. Y., Cooney, W. P., Askew, L. J., An, K. N., & Chao, E. Y. (1991, May). Functional ranges of motion of the wrist joint. *Journal of Hand Surgery, 16A*(3), 409–419.

Saunders, D. H. (1994). *Evaluation, treatment and prevention of musculoskeletal disorders: Vol. 2 Extremities* (3rd ed.). Chaksa, MN: Saunders.

Van Adrichem, J. A. M., & van der Korst, J. K. (1973). Assessment of the flexibility of the lumbar spine: A pilot study in children and adolescents. *Scandinavian Journal of Rheumatology, 2*(2), 87–91.

INDEX

Student CD-ROM to Accompany Therapeutic Measurement and Testing: The Basics of ROM, MMT,
Posture, and Gait Analysis
By Lisa Jennings Weaver, PTA, CMT and Amanda L. Ferg, B.S., PTA
ISBN-10: 1-4180-8080-2
ISBN-13: 978-1-4180-8080-8

Set Up Instructions:
PC:

1. Insert disc into CD-ROM drive. The installation program should start automatically. If it does not, go to step 2.
2. From My Computer, double-click the icon for the CD drive.
3. Double-click the *start.exe* file to start the program.

System Requirements:
PC:

Operating System: Windows 2000 w/ SP4, XP w/ SP2, Vista
8x CD-ROM drive or faster
Hard Drive: 200MB
Memory: 512 MB
Monitor: Minimum 800 x 600, 16-bit color
An Internet connection, Firefox 2, Internet Explorer 6 & 7
Microsoft® Word 95 (or newer) is required to edit the
Instructor's Manual and Microsoft PowerPoint® 97 (or
newer) is required to edit the presentations.

Microsoft® and PowerPoint® are registered trademarks
and Windows® and Windows XP® and Windows Vista® are
trademarks of Microsoft Corporation. Microsoft Word®
and Microsoft PowerPoint® are trademarks of the Microsoft
Corporation.

TECH SUPPORT:
1-800-648-7450
8:30 AM to 6:30 PM Eastern Time
Email: **Delmar.help@cengage.com**

IMPORTANT! READ CAREFULLY: This End User License Agreement ("Agreement") sets forth the conditions by which Cengage Learning will make electronic access to the Cengage Learning-owned licensed content and associated media, software, documentation, printed materials, and electronic documentation contained in this package and/or made available to you via this product (the "Licensed Content"), available to you (the "End User"). BY CLICKING THE "I ACCEPT" BUTTON AND/ OR OPENING THIS PACKAGE, YOU ACKNOWLEDGE THAT YOU HAVE READ ALL OF THE TERMS AND CONDITIONS, AND THAT YOU AGREE TO BE BOUND BY ITS TERMS, CONDITIONS, AND ALL APPLICABLE LAWS AND REGULATIONS GOVERNING THE USE OF THE LICENSED CONTENT.

1.0 SCOPE OF LICENSE
1.1 <u>Licensed Content</u>. The Licensed Content may contain portions of modifiable content ("Modifiable Content") and content which may not be modified or otherwise altered by the End User ("Non-Modifiable Content"). For purposes of this Agreement, Modifiable Content and Non-Modifiable Content may be collectively referred to herein as the "Licensed Content." All Licensed Content shall be considered Non-Modifiable Content, unless such Licensed Content is presented to the End User in a modifiable format and it is clearly indicated that modification of the Licensed Content is permitted.

1.2 Subject to the End User's compliance with the terms and conditions of this Agreement, Cengage Learning hereby grants the End User, a nontransferable, nonexclusive, limited right to access and view a single copy of the Licensed Content on a single personal computer system for noncommercial, internal, personal use only. The End User shall not (i) reproduce, copy, modify (except in the case of Modifiable Content), distribute, display, transfer, sublicense, prepare derivative work(s) based on, sell, exchange, barter or transfer, rent, lease, loan, resell, or in any other manner exploit the Licensed Content; (ii) remove, obscure, or alter any notice of Cengage Learning's intellectual property rights present on or in the Licensed Content, including, but not limited to, copyright, trademark, and/or patent notices; or (iii) disassemble, decompile, translate, reverse engineer, or otherwise reduce the Licensed Content.

2.0 TERMINATION
2.1 Cengage Learning may at any time (without prejudice to its other rights or remedies) immediately terminate this Agreement and/or suspend access to some or all of the Licensed Content, in the event that the End User does not comply with any of the terms and conditions of this Agreement. In the event of such termination by Cengage Learning, the End User shall immediately return any and all copies of the Licensed Content to Cengage Learning.

3.0 PROPRIETARY RIGHTS
3.1 The End User acknowledges that Cengage Learning owns all rights, title and interest, including, but not limited to all copyright rights therein, in and to the Licensed Content, and that the End User shall not take any action inconsistent with such ownership. The Licensed Content is protected by U.S., Canadian and other applicable copyright laws and by international treaties, including the Berne Convention and the Universal Copyright Convention. Nothing contained in this Agreement shall be construed as granting the End User any ownership rights in or to the Licensed Content.

3.2 Cengage Learning reserves the right at any time to withdraw from the Licensed Content any item or part of an item for which it no longer retains the right to publish, or which it has reasonable grounds to believe infringes copyright or is defamatory, unlawful, or otherwise objectionable.

4.0 PROTECTION AND SECURITY

4.1 The End User shall use its best efforts and take all reasonable steps to safeguard its copy of the Licensed Content to ensure that no unauthorized reproduction, publication, disclosure, modification, or distribution of the Licensed Content, in whole or in part, is made. To the extent that the End User becomes aware of any such unauthorized use of the Licensed Content, the End User shall immediately notify Cengage Learning. Notification of such violations may be made by sending an e-mail to infringement@cengage.com.

5.0 MISUSE OF THE LICENSED PRODUCT

5.1 In the event that the End User uses the Licensed Content in violation of this Agreement, Cengage Learning shall have the option of electing liquidated damages, which shall include all profits generated by the End User's use of the Licensed Content plus interest computed at the maximum rate permitted by law and all legal fees and other expenses incurred by Cengage Learning in enforcing its rights, plus penalties.

6.0 FEDERAL GOVERNMENT CLIENTS

6.1 Except as expressly authorized by Cengage Learning, Federal Government clients obtain only the rights specified in this Agreement and no other rights. The Government acknowledges that (i) all software and related documentation incorporated in the Licensed Content is existing commercial computer software within the meaning of FAR 27.405(b)(2); and (2) all other data delivered in whatever form, is limited rights data within the meaning of FAR 27.401. The restrictions in this section are acceptable as consistent with the Government's need for software and other data under this Agreement.

7.0 DISCLAIMER OF WARRANTIES AND LIABILITIES

7.1 Although Cengage Learning believes the Licensed Content to be reliable, Cengage Learning does not guarantee or warrant (i) any information or materials contained in or produced by the Licensed Content, (ii) the accuracy, completeness or reliability of the Licensed Content, or (iii) that the Licensed Content is free from errors or other material defects. THE LICENSED PRODUCT IS PROVIDED "AS IS," WITHOUT ANY WARRANTY OF ANY KIND AND CENGAGE LEARNING DISCLAIMS ANY AND ALL WARRANTIES, EXPRESSED OR IMPLIED, INCLUDING, WITHOUT LIMITATION, WARRANTIES OF MERCHANTABILITY OR FITNESS FOR A PARTICULAR PURPOSE. IN NO EVENT SHALL CENGAGE LEARNING BE LIABLE FOR: INDIRECT, SPECIAL, PUNITIVE OR CONSEQUENTIAL DAMAGES INCLUDING FOR LOST PROFITS, LOST DATA, OR OTHERWISE. IN NO EVENT SHALL CENGAGE LEARNING'S AGGREGATE LIABILITY HEREUNDER, WHETHER ARISING IN CONTRACT, TORT, STRICT LIABILITY OR OTHERWISE, EXCEED THE AMOUNT OF FEES PAID BY THE END USER HEREUNDER FOR THE LICENSE OF THE LICENSED CONTENT.

8.0 GENERAL

8.1 <u>Entire Agreement</u>. This Agreement shall constitute the entire Agreement between the Parties and supercedes all prior Agreements and understandings oral or written relating to the subject matter hereof.

8.2 <u>Enhancements/Modifications of Licensed Content</u>. From time to time, and in Cengage Learning's sole discretion, Cengage Learning may advise the End User of updates, upgrades, enhancements and/or improvements to the Licensed Content, and may permit the End User to access and use, subject to the terms and conditions of this Agreement, such modifications, upon payment of prices as may be established by Cengage Learning.

8.3 <u>No Export</u>. The End User shall use the Licensed Content solely in the United States and shall not transfer or export, directly or indirectly, the Licensed Content outside the United States.

8.4 <u>Severability</u>. If any provision of this Agreement is invalid, illegal, or unenforceable under any applicable statute or rule of law, the provision shall be deemed omitted to the extent that it is invalid, illegal, or unenforceable. In such a case, the remainder of the Agreement shall be construed in a manner as to give greatest effect to the original intention of the parties hereto.

8.5 <u>Waiver</u>. The waiver of any right or failure of either party to exercise in any respect any right provided in this Agreement in any instance shall not be deemed to be a waiver of such right in the future or a waiver of any other right under this Agreement.

8.6 <u>Choice of Law/Venue</u>. This Agreement shall be interpreted, construed, and governed by and in accordance with the laws of the State of New York, applicable to contracts executed and to be wholly preformed therein, without regard to its principles governing conflicts of law. Each party agrees that any proceeding arising out of or relating to this Agreement or the breach or threatened breach of this Agreement may be commenced and prosecuted in a court in the State and County of New York. Each party consents and submits to the nonexclusive personal jurisdiction of any court in the State and County of New York in respect of any such proceeding.

8.7 <u>Acknowledgment</u>. By opening this package and/or by accessing the Licensed Content on this Web site, THE END USER ACKNOWLEDGES THAT IT HAS READ THIS AGREEMENT, UNDERSTANDS IT, AND AGREES TO BE BOUND BY ITS TERMS AND CONDITIONS. IF YOU DO NOT ACCEPT THESE TERMS AND CONDITIONS, YOU MUST NOT ACCESS THE LICENSED CONTENT AND RETURN THE LICENSED PRODUCT TO CENGAGE LEARNING (WITHIN 30 CALENDAR DAYS OF THE END USER'S PURCHASE) WITH PROOF OF PAYMENT ACCEPTABLE TO CENGAGE LEARNING, FOR A CREDIT OR A REFUND. Should the End User have any questions/comments regarding this Agreement, please contact Cengage Learning at Delmar.help@cengage.com.